W9-BVJ-252

Medical Management of Lipid Disorders:

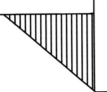

Focus on Prevention of Coronary Artery Disease

Edited and Co-Authored by

WILLIAM H. FRISHMAN M.D.
Professor and Associate Chairman, Department of Medicine
Professor, Department of Epidemiology & Social Medicine
The Albert Einstein College of Medicine

Director of the Clinical Pharmacology and Therapeutic Trials Unit
Weiler Hospital of the Albert Einstein College of Medicine/
Montefiore Medical Center
Bronx, New York

with a Foreword by
Howard A. Eder M.D.

**Futura Publishing
Company, Inc.**
Mount Kisco, NY

Library of Congress Cataloging-in-Publication Data

Medical management of hyperlipidemia : focus on prevention of coronary
  artery diseases / edited and co-authored by William H. Frishman with
  a foreword by Howard Eder.
      p.   cm.
    Includes bibliographical references and index.
    ISBN 0-87993-523-5
    1. Hyperlipidemia—Treatment.   2. Coronary heart disease—
Prevention.   I. Frishman, William H., 1946– .
    [DNLM: 1. Coronary Disease—prevention & control.
2. Hyperlipidemia—complications.   3. Hyperlipidemia—therapy.   WD
200.5.H8 M489]
RC632.H87M43   1992
616.3'99706—dc20
DNLM/DLC
for Library of Congress   92-970
                                                                        CIP

This book has been printed on acid-free paper.

Copyright 1992
Futura Publishing Company, Inc
2 Bedford Ridge Road
Mount Kisco, New York 10549

L.C. No.:'92-970
ISBN No.:0-87993-5235

Every effort has been made to ensure that the information in this book is
as up to date and accurate as possible at the time of publication. However,
due to the constant developments in medicine, neither the author, nor the
editor, nor the publisher can accept any legal or any other responsibility
for any errors or omissions that may occur.

All rights reserved.
No part of this book may be translated or reproduced in any form without
written permission of the publisher.

Printed in the United States of America

To Esther ▪ ▪ ▪
Without Her There Would Be Nothing

Contributors

Miriam Aronson, Ed.D.   Departments of Neurology & Epidemiology, The Albert Einstein College of Medicine, Bronx, New York

Martin Ast, M.D.   Department of Medicine, Long Island Jewish Medical Center/ The Albert Einstein College of Medicine, Bronx, New York

Marcia Brown, M.D.   Department of Medicine, Booth Memorial Hospital, Flushing, New York

Marjorie F. Dannis, M.D.   Department of Medicine, University of Miami School of Medicine/Jackson Memorial Hospital, Miami, Florida

Margaret A. Danylchuk, Pharm.D.   Drug Information Service, University of Massachusetts Medical Center, Worcester, Massachusetts

Melanie P. Derman, M.D.   Department of Medicine, Harvard Medical School/Beth Israel Hospital, Boston, Massachusetts

Jeffrey M. Drood, M.D.   Department of Medicine, Georgetown University School of Medicine, Washington, D.C.

Lynn Edlen-Nezin, M.A.   Department of Epidemiology & Social Medicine, The Albert Einstein College of Medicine, Bronx, New York

William H. Frishman, M.D.   Departments of Medicine and Epidemiology, The Albert Einstein College of Medicine/Montefiore Medical Center, Bronx, New York

Mark Gloger, M.D.   Department of Medicine, New York University Medical Center, New York, New York

Brian F. Johnson, M.D.   Department of Medicine, University of Massachusetts School of Medicine and Medical Center, Worcester, Massachusetts

Shoshonah Kahn, M.D.   Department of Medicine, Columbia University College of Physicians and Surgeons/Presbyterian Hospital, New York, New York

Eliot J. Lazar, M.D.   Departments of Medicine & Anesthesiology, The Albert Einstein College of Medicine/Montefiore Medical Center, Bronx, New York

Jason Lazar, M.D.   Department of Medicine, University of Pittsburgh School of Medicine, Pittsburgh, Pennsylvania

Harold Lipsky, M.D.   Department of Medicine, University of Miami School of Medicine, Miami, Florida

Yale B. Mitchel, M.D.   Department of Medicine, The Albert Einstein College of Medicine, Bronx, New York

Judith Mitchell, M.D.   Department of Medicine, The Albert Einstein College of Medicine, Bronx, New York

Wee Lock Ooi Dr. PH.   HRCA, Research and Training Institute, Boston, Massachusetts

George Pulos, M.D.   Department of Medicine, Booth Memorial Hospital Center, Flushing, New York

Judith Wylie-Rosett Ed.D., R.D.   Departments of Medicine & Social Medicine, The Albert Einstein College of Medicine, Bronx, New York

Peter Zimetbaum, M.D.   Department of Medicine, Harvard Medical School/Beth Israel Hospital, Boston, Massachusetts

Foreword

Although the relationship between cholesterol and atherosclerosis was noted 150 years ago, the acceptance of the lipid hypothesis by the medical community has only occurred within the past several years. The lipid hypothesis is based on the premise that the elevated levels of serum or plasma lipids (and of certain lipoproteins) increase the risk of developing coronary heart disease (CHD). An enormous body of research has contributed to the validation of the lipid hypothesis. This has involved pathology, animal studies, molecular and cell biology, and epidemiology. For example the interest in cholesterol has led to the elucidation of its structure, synthesis, transport, and cellular metabolism (for which five Nobel Prizes have been awarded). Studies of the molecular biology of the lipoproteins and their receptors and of the role of growth factors and cytokines in atherogenesis have resulted in important contributions to fundamental biology. Of clinical significance is the corollary to the lipid hypothesis: that decrease in serum lipid levels will decrease risk for CHD. Numerous clinical trials performed in recent years have validated this hypothesis. This has resulted in the consensus that abnormalities in serum lipids and lipoproteins should be treated.

Because this consensus has been achieved only within the last few years, many physicians have had little experience in this area. It is difficult to obtain an understanding of the field from textbooks or from highly technical peer-reviewed publications. Perhaps the best teacher in a new area of expertise is someone whose background is that of a clinical cardiologist who has been confronted with these problems and who has put in the time and energy necessary to understand the fundamentals of lipid and lipoprotein disorders. Dr. Frishman is an experienced cardiologist who has made important contributions to the clinical pharmacology of beta blockers and calcium channel blockers and who has now made the effort to apply his expertise to lipid and lipoprotein disorders at a level that will be comprehensible to practicing cardiologists, internists, and family practitioners. Dr. Frishman and his colleagues are to be commended for this effort.

Howard A. Eder, M.D.
Professor of Medicine, Emeritus
Albert Einstein College of Medicine
January 9, 1992

Preface

"The prevention of disease today is one of the most important factors in the line of human endeavor." CHARLES H. MAYO, 1913
"Prevention is better than cure." PROVERB

Coronary artery disease remains the leading cause of death in Western society. In recent years, the medical profession has directed a great deal of effort toward the management of life-threatening cardiovascular illness. At the same time it has been recognized that relatively simple preventive interventions could reduce the incidence of these cardiovascular crises, and important inroads have been made in this area.

There is now indisputable evidence that the long-term treatment of systolic and diastolic hypertension can reduce the incidence of cardiovascular morbidity and mortality in both middle-aged and elderly men and women. β-Adrenergic blockers and some calcium-entry blockers can reduce the risk of death and nonfatal reinfarction in survivors of an acute myocardial infarction. Aspirin and warfarin can reduce the incidence of reinfarction and death in patients with myocardial infarction, and can prevent strokes in high-risk patients. Estrogen replacement may reduce the incidence of coronary heart disease in high-risk postmenopausal women. Angiotensin-converting enzyme inhibitors can reduce the risk of death in patients with congestive heart failure and prevent the development of clinical symptoms in patients with asymptomatic left ventricular dysfunction. Changes in the American lifestyle in recent years (cessation of cigarette smoking, modification of diet, and exercise) have contributed to a marked reduction in coronary heart events. Clearly, the cardiovascular disease prevention era is upon us.

There is also strong evidence that disorders in plasma lipids and lipoproteins can have an unfavorable influence on the incidence of coronary artery disease. The results of clinical studies have demonstrated that treatment of these disorders with lifestyle interventions and/or drugs can favorably impact on the risk of coronary heart disease. Recent data also suggest that the coronary atherosclerotic process not only can be prevented, but when present, can be arrested and even reversed by specific treatments.

The purpose of this book is twofold: to discuss current knowledge and thoughts about lipid and lipoprotein disorders as risk factors for coronary artery disease, and to bring together current information regarding the prevention of coronary artery disease through lifestyle modification and drug treatment.

The book is divided into four major sections. The first section reviews lipid and lipoprotein metabolism, the epidemiology of coronary artery disease and the importance of lipid disorders as risk factors, and finally, general treatment strategies for adults and children. The second section discusses nonpharmacological treatment approaches and includes dietary interventions and exercise. The third and largest section of the book deals with specific drug treatments and innovative medical approaches in the management of lipid disorders. In the final section, there is a special chapter that reviews the effects of cardiovascular drugs, specifically antihypertensive and antianginal agents, on plasma lipids and lipoproteins. The final chapter addresses the growing concerns about lipid disorders in the elderly and whether treatment interventions will be necessary.

This text was inspired by the ongoing interest at our institution in the areas of preventive cardiology and was not designed to cover every detail of the subjects on lipids and coronary artery disease prevention. However, over 1000 recently published references are cited for the reader who wishes to research an area in more detail.

The book is largely the result of many individual efforts. It is impossible to acknowledge the names of the many medical students, house officers, fellows, and colleagues from the Albert Einstein College of Medicine and Montefiore Medical Center from whom I absorbed many ideas and who have been indispensable as research collaborators, co-authors, critics, and constant sources of stimulation. I would like to express my sincere gratitude to Dr. Howard Eder who has taught thousands of us about the importance of lipid and lipoprotein disorders as risk factors for coronary artery disease. I acknowledge the outstanding effort of my secretary, Joanne Cioffi, in preparing this manuscript. I will always be indebted to the National Heart, Lung, and Blood Institute for supporting my early work in cardiac disease prevention through the Preventive Cardiology Academic Award and for their support of our epidemiologic studies and clinical trials in cardiac disease prevention. I wish to acknowledge Steven Korn and Helen Powers of Futura Publishing for their help and guidance in seeing the book through to completion. Finally, my most important collaborators have always been my wife, Esther Rose, and our children, Sheryl, Amy, and Michael Aaron, on whose constant love, patience, devotion, and forbearance I have always relied.

As we enter the next century, I am convinced the major breakthroughs in medical inquiry and practice will occur in the areas of disease prevention where future research will bear the greatest fruit.

William H. Frishman, M.D.
Bronx, New York
February 1992

Contents

Foreword   Howard Eder, M.D. vii

Preface   William H. Frishman, M.D. ix

Part I.   The Problem

Chapter 1.   Lipids and Lipoproteins: Atherosclerotic Risk and
Management
*William H. Frishman, M.D., Melanie P. Derman, M.D.,
Yale B. Mitchel, M.D., Lynn Edlen-Nezin, M.A.*   3

Part II.   Nonpharmacological Approaches

Chapter 2.   Dietary Therapy for Hyperlipidemia
*Lynn Edlen-Nezin, M.A., Judith Wylie-Rosett, Ed.D., R.D.,
William H. Frishman, M.D.*   45

Chapter 3.   Effects of Exercise on Lipid and Lipoprotein Levels
*Marjorie F. Dannis, M.D., William H. Frishman, M.D.,
Eliot J. Lazar, M.D.*   89

Part III.   Pharmacological Approaches

Chapter 4.   Bile-Acid Sequestrants
William H. Frishman, M.D., Martin Ast, M.D. 103

Chapter 5.   Effects of Gemfibrozil and Other Fibric Acid
Derivatives on Blood Lipids and Lipoproteins
*Peter Zimetbaum, M.D., William H. Frishman, M.D.,
Shoshonah Kahn, M.D.* 125

Chapter 6.   HMG-CoA Reductase Inhibitors
*William H. Frishman, M.D., Peter Zimetbaum, M.D.,
Melanie Derman, M.D.* 153

Chapter 7.   Nicotinic Acid
*William H. Frishman, M.D., Jeffrey M. Drood, M.D.,
Peter Zimetbaum, M.D.* 181

Chapter 8.   Probucol
              Peter Zimetbaum, M.D., William H. Frishman, M.D. 205

Chapter 9.   Dietary Fiber for Reducing Blood Cholesterol:
              Psyllium
              William H. Frishman, M.D., Harold Lipsky, M.D.,
              Mark Gloger, M.D. 217

Chapter 10.   Other Medical Approaches for Managing
              Hyperlipidemia: Past, Present, and Future
              William H. Frishman, M.D., Melanie P. Derman, M.D.,
              Judith Mitchell, M.D., Jason Lazar, M.D. 227

Part IV.   Special Articles

Chapter 11.   The Effects of Cardiovascular Drugs on Plasma
              Lipids and Lipoproteins
              William H. Frishman, M.D., Brian F. Johnson, M.D.,
              George Pulos, M.D., Margaret A. Danylchuk, Pharm.D.,
              Marcia Brown, M.D., Eliot J. Lazar, M.D. 253

Chapter 12.   Lipids, Vascular Disease, and Dementia with
              Advancing Age: Epidemiologic Considerations
              William H. Frishman, M.D., Peter Zimetbaum, M.D.,
              Wee Lock Ooi, Dr.PH., Miriam Aronson, Ed.D. 301

Index 319

Part I

The Problem

Chapter 1

Lipids and Lipoproteins: Atherosclerotic Risk and Management

William H. Frishman M.D., Melanie P. Derman M.D., Yale B. Mitchel M.D., Lynn Edlen-Nezin M.A.

A direct relationship between elevated serum cholesterol levels, especially elevated low-density lipoprotein (LDL) cholesterol levels, and the incidence of coronary artery disease (CAD) is well established.[1-3] Lowering LDL levels by means of diet and/or drug therapy has been shown to reduce the progression of coronary artery lesions and the incidence of coronary artery events.[4-13] As predicted from the Framingham Study, a 10% decrease in cholesterol levels is associated with a 20% decrease in the incidence of combined morbidity and mortality related to CAD.[14,15] Elevations in triglycerides and reductions in high-density lipoprotein (HDL) levels may also be contributing to an increased CAD risk.[3,15-20]

Advances in our understanding of lipid metabolism and the development of new drugs and dietary strategies for the treatment of lipid and lipoprotein disorders have made effective therapy of hyperlipidemia, and thus coronary heart disease risk intervention, an understandable and attainable goal.[20,21]

In this introductory chapter, a framework for understanding the treatment of lipid disorders is provided by introducing the concepts of lipoproteins and lipoprotein metabolism. The chapter will also discuss how abnormalities in this metabolism can result in various acquired and genetic forms of hyperlipidemia. Finally, recommendations are provided, based on the recent expert panel report of the National Choles-

From *Medical Management of Lipid Disorders: Focus on Prevention of Coronary Artery Disease,* edited by William H. Frishman, M.D. © 1992, Futura Publishing Inc., Mount Kisco, NY.

terol Education Program,[14] regarding screening and dietary and drug interventions in human populations with hyperlipidemia at risk for premature CAD.

Lipoproteins

The major circulatory form of cholesterol, cholesterol ester, and triglyceride are both insoluble in water. To circulate in an aqueous environment, they are complexed with phospholipid and protein in complexes known as lipoproteins. The protein components of these complexes are referred to as apoproteins and serve important functions in the normal processing of the lipoproteins.[22]

Cell surface lipases and lipoprotein receptors, necessary for lipid catabolism, recognize specific apoprotein moieties of the different lipoproteins rather than the lipid components. Apoproteins, therefore, serve at least two major functions. They are necessary, together with phospholipids, for the solubility of fats in blood, an aqueous medium, and, as discussed below, they also regulate cellular lipid uptake and catabolism.[22]

The six major lipoprotein classes can be distinguished by their size, density, and composition (Table 1). The particles as a group range from 50 Å to 10,000 Å in diameter. They also vary appreciably in density from <0.95 to >1.2 g/mL. The variation in density reflects their constituents, in particular the ratio of lipid to protein. The smaller the particle, the lower the lipid to protein ratio and the greater the density. The largest and least dense of the lipoproteins, the chylomicrons, contain primarily triglyceride and about 2% protein, while the smallest and most dense, the HDL, contains about 50% protein.

Lipoprotein Metabolism

Lipoprotein metabolism can be divided into an exogenous and an endogenous pathway (Fig. 1).[23] The exogenous pathway allows for the absorption of dietary fat in the postprandial state, and its subsequent distribution to the tissues. The endogenous pathway is responsible for the delivery of cholesterol and triglyceride to tissues in the fasting state.

Table 1.
Lipoprotein Classes and Composition

| Lipoprotein | Density (water = 1.000) | Composition (Weight %) | | | Major Apoprotein |
		C	TG	Protein	
Chylomicron	0.940	5	85–90	1–2	B-48, E, C-II
VLDL	0.940–1.006	20	60–70	5–10	B-100, E, C-II
Chylomicron remnant	1.006–1.019	30	30	15–20	B-48, E
VLDL remnant (IDL)	1.006–1.019	30	30	15–20	B-100, E
LDL	1.019–1.063	50–60	4–8	20	B-100
HDL	1.063–1.210	15–20	2–7	45–55	A-I, A-II

C = cholesterol; TG = triglyceride; VLDL = very low-density lipoprotein; IDL = intermediate-density lipoprotein; LDL = low-density lipoprotein; HDL = high-density lipoprotein.

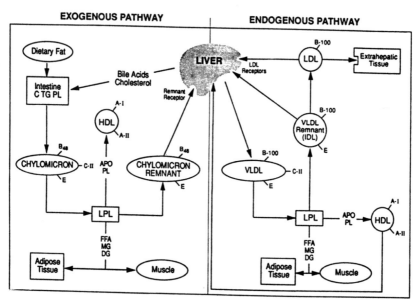

Figure 1: *Exogenous and endogenous pathways of lipoprotein metabolism. C = cholesterol; TG = triglyceride; MG = monoglyceride; DG = diglyceride; FFA = free fatty acid; LPL = lipoprotein lipase; APO = apoprotein; PL = phospholipids. (From Ref. 23 with permission.)*

Exogenous Pathway

The exogenous pathway begins with the absorption of dietary cholesterol and free fatty acids into intestinal microvilli, where they are esterified to cholesterol esters and triglycerides, respectively, and packaged into chylomicrons. These are very large particles composed primarily of a hydrophobic core of triglycerides and a hydrophilic surface of phospholipids and apoproteins. Chylomicrons contain apoproteins B-48, E, and C-II, and are not atherogenic. Once formed, they are secreted into the lymphatic system and enter the systemic circulation. In the capillaries of adipose tissue and muscle, they interact with an enzyme, lipoprotein lipase. This interaction is dependent on the presence of apoprotein C-II on the chylomicron. Lipoprotein lipase cleaves the core triglycerides into monoglycerides, diglycerides, and free fatty acids that are taken up by the surrounding tissue. The reduction in the core size of the chylomicron due to triglyceride hydrolysis results in an excess of surface components that are transferred to HDL. Thus, during the metabolism of chylomicrons, HDL components are generated. The remaining particle, now referred to as a chylomicron remnant, is greatly reduced in size, contains approximately equal amounts of cholesterol and triglyceride, and acquires atherogenic potential. The chylomicron remnants are rapidly removed from the circulation by the liver through a receptor-mediated process. The putative receptor is known as the chylomicron remnant receptor and recognizes apoprotein E on the chylomicron remnant. Cholesterol and triglyceride thus delivered can be stored in the liver, broken down to simpler molecules, or packaged into lipoproteins of the endogenous pathway. The cholesterol can also be disposed of by secretion into the bile in the form of bile acids. The exogenous pathway is predominantly functional in the postprandial state, and virtually no chylomicrons or chylomicron remnants are present in the blood after a 10-hour fast.

Endogenous Pathway

The endogenous pathway begins with the synthesis and secretion of very low-density lipoprotein (VLDL) by the liver. VLDL is also a triglyceride-rich lipoprotein, although not as large as the chylomicron, and contains the apoproteins B-100 (distinct from B-48 of chylomicrons), E, and C-II. VLDL also interacts with lipoprotein lipase located in the capillaries of adipose tissue and muscle, and triglycerides within the core of the particle are cleaved and taken up by the surrounding fat and muscle.

Again, the redundant surface components are transferred to the HDL fractions, and the remaining particle is referred to as a VLDL remnant or intermediate-density lipoprotein (IDL). This is a smaller lipoprotein, similar to the chylomicron remnant in its lipid composition and atherogenic potential. About 50% of VLDL remnants are removed by the liver by another receptor known as the LDL receptor. This receptor, first described by Brown and Goldstein,[24] recognizes apoprotein E on the VLDL remnant. The other half of VLDL remnants are transformed into LDL in the blood by further triglyceride and apoprotein removal. LDL, a highly atherogenic particle, contains mostly cholesteryl ester and only one apoprotein, B-100. LDL functions to deliver cholesterol to cholesterol-requiring tissues such as the gonads, adrenals, and rapidly dividing cells. The liver also plays a major role in the removal of LDL from the blood. These tissues remove LDL from the blood via the LDL receptor (which also recognizes apoprotein B-100). Approximately two thirds of LDL is removed from the blood in this fashion. The remaining LDL is removed by a non-LDL-receptor-mediated pathway which exists in Kupfer cells, smooth muscle cells, and macrophages. Some of this uptake occurs through receptors known as scavenger receptors.[25] The scavenger receptor recognizes a modified form of LDL, oxidized LDL. The LDL modification probably occurs in the extravascular space and is believed to transform LDL into a more atherogenic form. It is believed that this non-LDL-receptor-mediated uptake of LDL, which occurs in blood vessel walls, is a major factor in the development of foam cells and atherosclerosis.[26,27]

HDL, which seems to exert a protective effect on the development of atherosclerosis,[28,29] is synthesized both in the liver and the intestine and receives components during the lipoprotein lipase reaction. HDL is composed of approximately 50% protein, primarily apoprotein A-I and A-II, and 20% cholesterol. HDL exists in two major subfractions in the blood, HDL_2 and HDL_3; HDL_3 is a smaller, denser particle, which is believed to be the precursor of the larger, cholesterol-enriched HDL_2. The transfer of surface components during the lipoprotein lipase reaction is felt to be important in the formation of HDL_2 from HDL_3. The HDL_2 subfraction is thought to be associated with the protective effects of HDL against the development of atherosclerosis, although this is still controversial.[16] One mechanism suggested for the protective effect of HDL is believed to occur through its participation in reverse cholesterol transport, the picking up of cholesterol from cells involved in atherosclerotic process, and delivery to the liver for excretion.[29] HDL levels are higher in women than in men, possibly contributing to the lower prevalence of CAD among women.

There has been recent interest in cholesteryl ester transfer protein (CETP), which is involved with the enzyme lecithin cholesterol acyl transferase (LCAT) in driving the reverse cholesterol transport process—the net movement of cholesterol from peripheral tissues into the plasma and then from plasma back to the liver.[30,33] CETP facilitates the transfer of cholesteryl esters from HDL to VLDL and VLDL remnants. The latter are then removed from the blood through the previously described hepatic LDL receptor pathway. CETP may also regulate the in vivo catabolism of HDL-cholesteryl esters. Metabolic studies in individuals with congenital CETP deficiency and normal LCAT activity have demonstrated increased levels of apoprotein E- enriched HDL-cholesterol, a particle that may promote tissue cholesterol removal and delivery to the liver.[34] There is no history of CAD in families with congenital CETP deficiency.[34,35] This is in line with animal models, such as the rat and dog, which have absent CETP activity, a predominance of HDL lipoprotein, and resistance to the development of atherosclerosis.[36] These findings have immense implications for understanding the mechanism for the protective effects of HDL. They also provide a future pharmacological approach for possibly reducing the risk of CAD through the development of agents that interfere with the actions of CETP. In addition, subjects with CETP deficiency have reduced LDL, which may be related to decreased transfer of cholesteryl esters into LDL.

Hyperlipoproteinemia

In the fasting state, the predominant circulatory lipoproteins are LDL and HDL (accounting for most of the blood cholesterol), and VLDL (which carries most of the triglyceride and a small amount of cholesterol). Hyperlipoproteinemia results from the accumulation of lipoproteins in the blood. This may occur from either increased production or decreased removal of lipoproteins. If chylomicrons and VLDL accumulate, the patient will present with hypertriglyceridemia. If remnant particles accumulate, then the cholesterol and the triglycerides will be elevated, while the accumulation of LDL will result in hypercholesterolemia. Since LDL is a product of VLDL metabolism, overproduction of VLDL can result in hypertriglyceridemia as well as hypercholesterolemia.

The causes of hyperlipoproteinemia can be divided into acquired and genetic etiologies. In many cases, however, an acquired defect can coexist with a genetic one.

Acquired Causes of Hyperlipoproteinemia (Table 2)

Among the acquired disorders, diabetes mellitus, both insulin-dependent (IDDM) and noninsulin-dependent (NIDDM) may result in hyperlipidemia. The mechanism of hyperlipidemia in IDDM involves increased production and decreased removal of the triglyceride-rich lipoproteins.[37] Lipoprotein lipase is an insulin-dependent enzyme; reduced activity has been demonstrated in patients with IDDM. Reduced lipase activity results in accumulation of VLDL and chylomicrons and

Table 2.
Some Acquired Causes of Hyperlipidemia

Condition	Lipoprotein Accumulating	Lipid Phenotype	HDL Level
Diabetes			
IDDM	Chylomicron, VLDL	↑ TG	↓
NIDDM	VLDL	↑ TG	↓
Obesity	VLDL	↑ TG	— or ↓
Alcohol	VLDL	↑ TG	— or ↑
Oral contraceptives	VLDL	↑ TG	— or ↑
Hypothyroidism	LDL	↑ C	—
Nephrotic syndrome	VLDL, LDL	↑ TG, ↑ C	— or ↑
Renal failure	VLDL, LDL	↑ TG, ↑ C	— or ↑
Primary biliary cirrhosis	LDL	↑ C	
Acute hepatitis	VLDL	↑ TG	— or ↓

IDDM = insulin-dependent diabetes mellitus; NIDDM = noninsulin-dependent diabetes mellitus; HDL = high-density lipoprotein; VLDL = very low-density lipoprotein; LDL = low-density lipoprotein; TG = triglyceride; C = cholesterol; ↑ = increase; ↓ = decrease; — = no change.

hypertriglyceridemia. The increased free fatty acids noted in poorly controlled diabetes stimulate the synthesis and secretion of VLDL by the liver, also contributing to the hypertriglyceridemia of IDDM. Patients with poorly controlled IDDM have low HDL levels, perhaps because of decreased lipoprotein lipase activity with decreased generation of lipoprotein surface components. Insulin therapy and improvement in glycemic control usually causes a reversal of the hyperlipidemia and the low HDL levels.

The situation in NIDDM is somewhat more complicated. First, many patients with NIDDM are obese and have pre-existing abnormalities in lipoprotein metabolism.[38] Patients with NIDDM are a more heterogeneous group with varying degrees of insulin deficiency and other risk factors for hyperlipidemia. These patients frequently present with hypertriglyceridemia due to increased synthesis of VLDL and decreased removal of triglyceride-rich lipoproteins. In contrast to IDDM, improvement in glycemic control with oral agents or insulin is not always associated with a reversal of the lipid abnormalities.

Although some investigators have reported both an increase in HDL cholesterol and a decrease in the incidence of CAD in men who consume light to moderate amounts of alcohol, ingestion of alcohol in large quantities may induce secondary hypertriglyceridemia.[39]

Genetic Causes of Hyperlipoproteinemia (Table 3)

Individuals with hyperlipidemia frequently are classified according to Frederickson phenotypes I-V or in terms of familial versus polygenic disease. Frederickson phenotypes are determined by electrophoretic or lipid analysis. Phenotype I represents those patients with severe chylomicronemia. Type II patients have elevated LDL concentrations. Type IIa represents those patients with increased LDL, while type IIb patients have elevated LDL and VLDL. Type III patients have increased pre-beta or intermediate density lipoproteins manifested as elevated cholesterol and triglyceride. Type IV patients have elevated VLDL with normal LDL, and type V patients have elevated VLDL and chylomicrons. Type IIa, IIb and IV are the most common phenotypes. Type I is the most rare. Types II and III are particularly associated with increased cardiovascular disease risk. Types I and V are associated with triglyceride-related complications such as pancreatitis.

Table 3.
Genetic Causes of Hyperlipoproteinemia

Disorder	Lipoprotein Accumulating	Lipid Phenotype	HDL Level
LPL deficiency (Type I)	Chylomicron	↑ TG (massive)	↓
Apo C-II deficiency (Type I)	Chylomicron	↑ TG (massive)	↓
Familial hypertriglyceridemia (Type IV or V)	VLDL	↑ TG (moderate)	↓
Familial combined hyperlipoproteinemia (Type IIa, IIb, IV, and rarely V)	VLDL, LDL	↑ TG and/or ↑ C	—
Dysbetalipoproteinemia (Type III)	Chylomicron remnant VLDL remnant	↑ TG, ↑ C	—
Familial hypercholesterolemia (Type IIa)	LDL	↑ C	↓
Polygenic hypercholesterolemia	LDL	↑ C	—

HDL = high-density lipoprotein; LPL = lipoprotein lipase; TG = triglyceride; VLDL = very low-density lipoprotein; LDL = low-density lipoprotein; C = cholesterol; ↑ = increase; ↓ = decrease; — = no change.

Another way to classify hyperlipoproteinemia is by genotype (Table 3).[22] A deficiency in lipoprotein lipase corresponds to type I. Patients with lipoprotein lipase deficiency cannot metabolize chylomicrons or VLDL.[40] These lipoproteins accumulate and result in massive triglyceride elevations in the 22.58-112.9 mm/L (2000-10,000 mg/dl) range. Patients present early in life with pancreatitis but they do not have accelerated CAD, attesting to the nonatherogenic nature of the chylomicrons. Since apoprotein C-II is required for normal lipoprotein lipase activity, patients with a deficiency of apoprotein C-II, an extremely rare condition, present in the same fashion as the lipoprotein lipase deficient patient.

A more common form of hypertriglyceridemia is familial hypertriglyceridemia, which corresponds to the type IV lipoprotein pattern. This disorder is due to decreased removal of triglyceride-rich lipoproteins, primarily VLDL. Patients have moderate elevations of triglycerides (4.51-9.03 mm/L [400-800 mg/dl]) and probably are not at increased risk of CAD. This is in contrast to another common cause of hypertriglyceridemia, familial combined hyperlipoproteinemia, in which patients have increased production of VLDL and may present with moderate hypertriglyceridemia, hypercholesterolemia, or both, and are predisposed to CAD. The defect is thought to be an overproduction of apolipoprotein B-containing lipoproteins. The patients can be identified by a strong family history of both premature CAD and mixed hyperlipidemia.

An interesting and not uncommon genetic form of hyperlipidemia is dysbetalipoproteinemia or broad beta disease, which corresponds to the type III pattern. These patients are homozygous for the allele E2, which encodes apoprotein E.[41] Apoprotein E is the ligand for hepatic receptors for chylomicron remnants and VLDL remnants.[42] The abnormal apoprotein E is poorly recognized by the receptor and results in the accumulation of chylomicron and VLDL remnant particles in the blood. Since remnants contain equal amounts of cholesterol and triglycerides, patients present with moderate elevations in cholesterol and triglycerides. The homozygous state occurs with a frequency of $\frac{1}{100}$ in the population but symptomatic type III occurs in only $\frac{1}{10,000}$. Most individuals, therefore, can compensate for this defect, and an inability to do so may be caused by another inherited lipid defect or by an acquired one. Since this lipoprotein pattern is associated with an increased risk of CAD, acquired and reversible causes should be vigorously addressed.

The chylomicronemia syndrome corresponds to type V disease with extremely elevated triglycerides due to chylomicron accumulation and low LDL. Patients have increased risk of pancreatitis. There is also a strong interaction between genetic and acquired lipid disorders in this syndrome.

Perhaps the best understood genetic form of hypercholesterolemia is familial hypercholesterolemia, which corresponds to the type IIa phenotype.[41] The defect in these patients results from varying degrees of LDL receptor defectiveness or deficiency causing an accumulation of LDL in the blood. The disease is transmitted in an autosomal dominant pattern with incomplete penetrance. The heterozygous form is estimated to occur in $\frac{1}{500}$ of the general population and represents only 4% of patients with hypercholesterolemia. This disorder is believed to be responsible for 5% of myocardial infarction survivors < 60 years of age. These patients express about one half of the usual number of functional LDL receptors and can present with tendinous xanthomas (nodules over extensor tendons) and CAD in their forties. Cholesterol levels are in the 7.76-12.93 mm/L (300-500 mg/dl) range, and are usually responsive to conventional pharmacological therapies. The homozygous form of the disease occurs rarely and there are no functional LDL receptors. Homozygous patients present with tendinous xanthomas and CAD early in life. They have enormous cholesterol elevations, in the 15.52-25.86 mm/L (600-1000 mg/dl) range, and are unresponsive to conventional pharmacological agents.

There are various mutations at the LDL receptor locus that can cause familial hypercholesterolemia. Four types of defects have been described that lead to defective or absent LDL receptors.[41] The largest class fails to produce detectable LDL receptor protein. A second class includes mutations that prevent normal transport of receptors to the cell surface. The third class results in receptors that are expressed normally on the cell surface but are defective in binding apoprotein B- or apoprotein E-containing lipoproteins or both. The fourth class involves mutations that prevent the LDL receptors from clustering and being endocytosed within coated pits. Lipoproteins are bound normally but cannot be internalized within the cytoplasm.[41]

Recently, a new genetic abnormality, familial defective apoprotein B-100, has been described. This condition is characterized by moderate hypercholesterolemia and elevated plasma LDL.[41] The accumulation is due to defective binding of LDL to the LDL receptor. A specific mutation in the LDL receptor-binding domain of apoprotein B-100, a ligand for the LDL receptor, has been identified. Estimates of the frequency of the mutation are about 1:500.

The most common, yet least understood, form of hypercholesterolemia is referred to as polygenic hypercholesterolemia, corresponding to a type IIa lipoprotein pattern. These patients have elevated cholesterol without an identified LDL receptor deficiency. Some of these patients have increased production of LDL while others have decreased removal. The interaction between a high-fat, high-cholesterol diet and, as of yet, undefined genetic lipoprotein abnormalities is felt to be an important etiologic factor.

Lipoprotein(a)

Patients with heterozygous familial hypercholesterolemia with serum cholesterol levels ranging from 300-500 mg% (7.76 to 12.9 mm) are markedly predisposed to premature CAD.[22] However, since not all patients with familial hypercholesterolemia will develop CAD, other factors must affect the atherogenicity process.

In 1963, Berg described a genetic variation of LDL, which he called lipoprotein(a).[43] This variant was carefully characterized in the 1970s.[44] Lipoprotein(a) is formed by two components: an LDL-like particle with apoprotein B-100 and a hydrophobic protein moiety known as apoprotein (a).[44]

Lipoprotein(a) has attracted considerable attention with the recent discovery that its apoprotein (a) has a close structural homology with plasminogen. It may cause perturbations of the thrombolytic system, suggesting a link between lipoprotein metabolism and thrombosis.[45] In vitro studies of apoprotein (a) reveal that this protein binds and displaces plasminogen from binding sites on fibrin, fibrinogen, and cell surfaces.[44] It inhibits activation by bacterial-activated streptokinase and has also been found to competitively inhibit plasminogen activation by tPA through steric hindrance of tPA binding sites.[44]

Accumulation of lipoprotein(a) has been demonstrated in atherosclerotic lesions[46] and is now felt to be an atherogenic lipoprotein.[44-50] Elevated plasma levels in human beings (> 30 mg/dl appear to be associated with an increased risk for the development of CAD,[51-54] with a rate of occurrence estimated to be 2 to 5 times greater than that seen in normal controls.[53,55] The mode of inheritance of hyperlipoproteinemia(a) is felt to be by autosomal codominance. Some studies restrict the identification of lipoproteinemia(a) as a risk factor for CAD only in the setting of an elevated plasma LDL level.[53,55] Others have found the condition to be an independent risk factor.[46] Diet, age, sex, smoking, body mass index, and apoprotein E polymorphism have not been found to correlate with plasma levels of lipoprotein (a). However, increased lipoprotein(a) levels have been noted in patients with diabetes mellitus, nephrotic syndrome, and in the immediate post-myocardial infarction period.[56] Other investigators have not observed changes in lipoprotein(a) levels in acute myocardial infarction or unstable angina.[57]

Of the hypolipidemic interventions, only niacin, neomycin, and extracorporeal removal of cholesterol have been shown to affect elevated lipoprotein(a) levels.[53] The results of a preliminary study reveal that lipoprotein(a) levels may also be reduced by treatment with N-acetylcysteine.[58]

Rationale for Treatment of Hyperlipidemia in Prevention of Coronary Artery Disease

The premise for the treatment of hyperlipidemia is based on the hypothesis that abnormalities in lipid and lipoprotein levels are risk factors for CAD, and that changes in blood lipids can result in decreased risk of disease and complications.[4,5,20,59] Levels of plasma cholesterol and LDL consistently have been shown to be directly correlated with the risk of CAD.[1,2,15]

There is strong evidence to suggest this association from epidemiologic, genetic and physiological, and animal studies (see Chapter 2).[1,2,22,59-62] In addition, data from the Lipid Research Clinics Coronary Prevention Trial and Helsinki Heart Study have provided conclusive evidence that a reduction in LDL-cholesterol levels in hypercholesterolemic men can result in a decreased incidence of coronary events, including fatal and nonfatal myocardial infarctions and angina.[4-6] An aggregate analysis of other randomized trials has shown that reduction of LDL-cholesterol will reduce the risk of coronary heart disease.[14] The Coronary Drug Project demonstrated a significant decrease in overall mortality in a long-term follow-up of men with myocardial infarction treated with nicotinic acid.[5] Finally, secondary prevention trials using diet and/or drug therapies have shown that reduction of cholesterol can retard and even produce regression of coronary atherosclerosis.[7-12]

Epidemiologic studies and clinical trials are consistent in supporting the observation that for individuals with serum cholesterol levels in the 6.47-7.76 mm/L (250-300 mg/dl) range, each 1% reduction in serum cholesterol would yield approximately a 2% reduction in the rate of combined morbidity and mortality from coronary heart disease.[5] The absolute magnitude of these benefits would be greater in those individuals having other risk factors for CAD, such as cigarette smoking and hypertension.[14,63] These risk relationships are the basis for recommending lower cholesterol cutpoints and goals for those who are at high risk for developing coronary heart disease.[14]

The evidence for elevated triglycerides as a risk factor for CAD is less clear.[20,64] Several prospective studies have shown a correlation between levels of plasma triglycerides and CAD.[64] Data from the Framingham study, however, have indicated that when other risk factors, such as obesity, elevated serum cholesterol (or hypercholesterolemia), hypertension, and diabetes, were accounted for, triglycerides are not an independent risk factor for CAD.[19] However, there is a select group of patients with hypertriglyceridemia that is at increased risk of coronary heart disease, and that can be identified by a strong family history of premature CAD.[14] Another important factor is that serum triglyceride levels are inversely related to HDL levels, and reductions in triglyceride levels are associated with a rise in HDL.[65] Since HDL might be protective against CAD, this provides an additional rationale for the treatment of hypertriglyceridemia.[14] However, currently, there is no evidence that lowering triglyceride levels or raising the HDL level will result in diminished risk of CAD.[20]

Risk Assessment

For many years clinicians depended upon total cholesterol and triglyceride measurements for patient management. More sophisticated lipoprotein measurements were only available in research facilities. Recent methodological advances have made lipoprotein subclass and apoprotein determinations available from many clinical laboratories.

LDL-cholesterol has been shown to be a more accurate predictor of CAD risk than total cholesterol.[20] Likewise, low levels of HDL-cholesterol and the subfractions HDL_2 and HDL_3 have been demonstrated to be more powerful predictors of CAD than total cholesterol.[15,16] Levels of plasma apoproteins are also accurate predictors of CAD risk.

It is controversial whether increases in plasma apoprotein B levels, the major apoprotein of LDL, and decreases in levels of apoproteins A-I and A-II, the major apoproteins of HDL, are better predictors of increased coronary risk than either total cholesterol, HDL-, LDL-cholesterol or the ratio of total cholesterol to HDL-cholesterol.[16,66]

Despite the availability of these more sophisticated determinations, an individual's risk of CAD can be adequately estimated by an accurate measurement of total cholesterol and a calculated LDL-cholesterol determination. For various population groups, mean serum cholesterol and calculated LDL-cholesterol values have been reported on by the National Center for Health Statistics.[14,67]

Laboratory Methods

Serum total cholesterol levels can be measured at any time of day in the nonfasting state since total cholesterol concentrations do not vary appreciably after eating.[14] Patients who are acutely ill, losing weight, pregnant, or recently had a myocardial infarction or stroke should be studied at a later time.[14,68] Venipuncture should be carried out in patients in the sitting position for at least 5 minutes, and the tourniquet applied for the briefest time possible.[14,68-70] The blood may be collected either as serum or plasma. Details of the laboratory methods and quality control procedures have been published elsewhere.[68,71-73]

Physicians would like to think that the cholesterol values from laboratories are reliable. Unfortunately, this is not always the case.[74] The Center for Disease Control, which has monitored the performance of clinical laboratories, in the past has reported great variations in accuracy between different laboratories.[75] The National Cholesterol Education Program recently has established guidelines for standardization of lipid and lipoprotein measurements.[68] It recommends that intralaboratory precision and accuracy for cholesterol determinations be ≤3% by 1992.[68] Rapid capillary blood (fingerstick) methodology for cholesterol measurement currently is under development and evaluation.[68] In a recent study assessing compact chemical analyzers for routine office determinations, some of the machines tested were shown to have accuracy and precision above the 1988 target of 5% variance.[76,77] To be useful, the new rapid desk-top methods must be capable of providing analytical measurements that can be referred directly to the National Reference System for cholesterol established by the National Committee for Clinical Laboratory Standards. If the results are biased, the magnitude and direction of the bias should be known when interpreting the results.[68]

It is now recommended that patients with cholesterol values of 5.17 mm/L (> 200 mg/dl) should have the value confirmed by repeating the test at least 1 week later; the average of the two tests is then used to guide subsequent clinical decisions.[14,68,78] Duplicate values within 0.78 mm/L (30 mg/dl) should be averaged. If the measurements are not within 0.78 mm/L (30 mg/dl), a third measurement should be taken within 2 months.

LDL-cholesterol measurements usually are derived indirectly from the following formula: LDL-cholesterol (mg/dl) = total cholesterol (mg/dl) − HDL-cholesterol (mg/dl) − (triglyceride [mg/dl]/5).[14,79] When using this formula with mm/L units, triglyceride is divided by 2.3. There is a need for a reliable direct method for measurement of LDL-cholesterol, since the analytical precision for indirect estimates of LDL-cholesterol reflects measurements of total cholesterol, HDL-cholesterol and triglycerides, each of which contributes some degree of imprecision. Since triglyceride values are influenced by food, there should be a minimum 12-hour fast before blood is obtained for an LDL-cholesterol determination. If the triglyceride values are > 4.52 mm/L (> 400 mg/dl), the LDL-cholesterol value will be less accurate. Direct measurement of LDL in a specialized laboratory using ultracentrifugation might then be useful.[14]

The newest development in laboratory evaluation is the availability of tests for specific apolipoproteins. Some laboratories can perform apoprotein A-I and A-II measurements to reflect HDL levels, apoprotein B measurements to reflect LDL levels, and measurements of lipoprotein(a).[80] These tests have proven to be accurate predictors of cardiovascular risk in various research studies.[16] Unfortunately, until more is known about their utility in clinical practice, they should not be obtained in routine clinical management.[81,82] In situations where triglycerides are high and LDL-cholesterol would be underestimated, however, an apoprotein B level might be useful. The availability of these specialized tests indicate that in the future there may be more sensitive and specific laboratory evaluations for estimating cardiovascular risk.

Who Should Be Screened For Hyperlipidemia?

The Expert Panel Report of the National Cholesterol Education Program on Detection, Evaluation and Treatment of High Blood Cholesterol in Adults (NCEP) suggests that total cholesterol be measured in all adults 20 years of age and over at least once every 5 years.[14] A recent NCEP panel recommended that cholesterol screening should not be done routinely in children unless a history of familial hyperlipidemia exists or a family history of premature CAD is present. Cholesterol values in the general pediatric population may not always predict the future development of hypercholesterolemia in adults.[83,84]

Who Should Be Treated For Hypercholesterolemia?

The NCEP has classified all adult patients into the following categories: those with desirable cholesterol values (5.17 mm/L [< 200 mg/dl]), borderline high blood cholesterol values (5.17-6.18 mm/L [200-239 mg/dl]), and high blood cholesterol values (6.21 mm/L [≥ 240 mg/dl], Fig. 2)..[14] LDL-cholesterol values 3.36 mm/L (< 130 mg/dl) are considered desirable, 3.36-4.11 mm/L (130-159 mg/dl) are borderline high risk, and 4.14 mm/L (≥ 160 mg/dl) are high risk.[14] Coronary heart disease is associated with other risk factors that should also be considered in preventive medicine (Table 4).[14]

Once the screening cholesterol values are obtained (Figs. 2 and 3), the NCEP recommends the following approach to clinical management in adults.[14] The presence of a high cholesterol should always be confirmed with a second test, and the fasting LDL-cholesterol measured in a lipoprotein analysis in order to make a more precise estimate of CAD risk.[14,78] The standard deviation of repeated measurements in an individual over time has been reported as 0.39 mm/L (15 mg/dl) for total cholesterol and 0.39 mm/L (15 mg/dl) for LDL-cholesterol. Patients should be maintained on the same diet during these initial determinations before therapy is instituted. Secondary causes of hypercholesterolemia (hypothyroidism, nephrotic syndrome, diabetes mellitus) should also be considered.[14]

The NCEP recommends an approach in adults based on LDL-cholesterol, which is shown in Figure 3. Management should always begin with dietary intervention, as outlined in Figure 4. Additional dietary strategies are discussed in Chapter 2. When response to diet is inadequate, the NCEP recommends the addition of pharmacological therapy (Fig. 5). Specific drug therapies are discussed in Chapters 4 to 10.

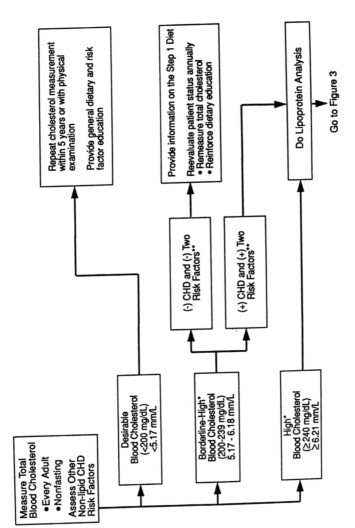

Figure 2: *Initial classification based on total cholesterol (adults). CHD = coronary heart disease; * = must be confirmed by obtaining repeated measurements and then using the average value; ** = one of which can be male sex. (From Ref. 14 with permission.)*

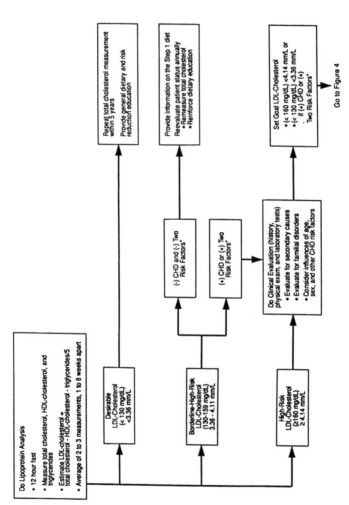

Figure 3: *Classification based on low-density lipoprotein (LDL)-cholesterol (adults). * = one of which can be male sex; CHD = coronary heart disease; HDL = high-density lipoprotein. (From Ref. 14 with permission.)*

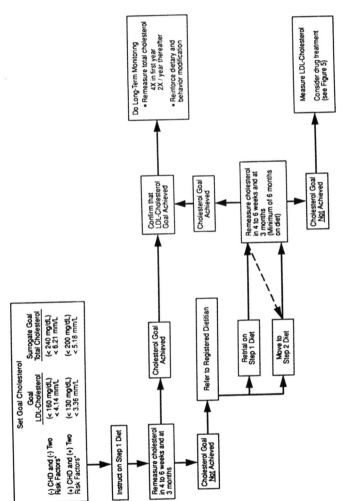

Figure 4: *Dietary treatment (adults).* * *= one of which can be male sex; LDL = low-density lipoprotein; CHD = coronary heart disease. (From Ref. 14 with permission.)*

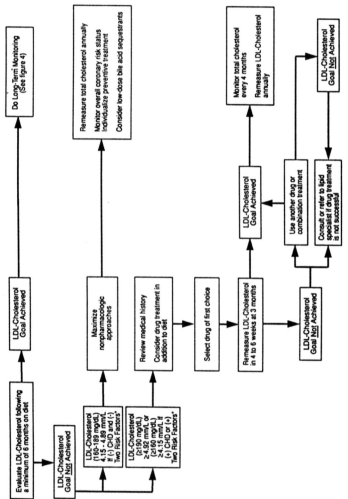

Figure 5: *Drug treatment (adults).* * = one of which can be male sex; LDL = low-density lipoprotein; CHD = coronary heart disease. (From Ref. 14 with permission.)

Table 4.
Risk Status Based on Presence of Coronary Heart Disease Risk Factors Other Than LDL Cholesterol

The patient is considered to have a high-risk status if he or she has one of the following:

–Definite CHD: the characteristic clinical picture and objective laboratory findings of either:
>Definite prior myocardial infarction, or
>Definite myocardial ischemia, such as angina pectoris

–Two Other CHD Risk Factors:
>Male sex*
>Family history of premature CHD (definite myocadial infarction or sudden death before 55 years of age in a parent or sibling)
>Cigarette smoking (currently smokes > 10 cigarettes daily)
>Hypertension
>Low HDL-cholesterol concentration (0.91 mm/L [< 35 mg/dl] confirmed by repeated measurement)
>Diabetes mellitus
>History of definite cerebrovascular or occlusive peripheral vascular disease
>Severe obesity (≥ 30% overweight)

*Male sex is considered a risk factor in this scheme because the rates of CHD are 3–4 times higher in men than in women in the middle decades of life and roughly 2 times higher in the elderly. Hence, a male with one other CHD risk factor is cnsidered to have a high-risk status, whereas a female is not so considered unless she has two other CHD risk factors. (From Ref. 14, with permission.)

Who Should Be Treated For Hypertriglyceridemia?

Interest in the link between serum triglyceride levels and coronary heart disease has grown in recent years. Triglyceride levels correlate positively with levels of LDL-cholesterol[85] and inversely with HDL.[64] Clinical trials with triglyceride-lowering drugs, nicotinic acid[5] and gemfibrozil,[6] have shown a benefit on coronary artery event frequency compared to placebo therapy. However, therapy in these trials was not targeted to patients with primary hypertriglyceridemia. The currently recommended approach to the problem of hypertriglyceridemia is presented in the report of the National Institutes of Health Consensus Development Conference on Treatment of Hypertriglyceridemia.[64]

A link between plasma triglycerides and disease is most apparent in patients with severe hypertriglyceridemia with chylomicronemia.[22]

These patients are prone to abdominal pain and/or pancreatitis. Changes in lifestyle (control of weight, increased physical activity, restriction of alcohol, restriction of dietary fat to 10% to 20% of total caloric intake), as well as drug therapy are often required.[14,64]

Much of borderline hypertriglyceridemia (2.82-5.65 mm/L [250-500 mg/dl]) is due to various exogenous or secondary factors (Table 2)[14] that include alcohol, diabetes mellitus, hypothyroidism, obesity, chronic renal disease, and drugs (Chapter 11). Changes in lifestyle and/or treatment of the primary disease process may be sufficient to reduce triglycerides.

Patients with borderline hypertriglyceridemia due to familial hypertriglyceridemia (type IV) are not at risk of having premature CAD.[22,64] Caloric restriction and increased exercise can be recommended for obese patients but drug therapy is inappropriate.[64]

Patients with familial combined hyperlipoproteinemia often will have mild hypertriglyceridemia. Patients with this condition are at risk for premature coronary heart disease. These patients should have dietary treatment first and, if necessary, drugs.[14,64] Any patient with borderline hypertriglyceridemia with clinical manifestations of CAD can be treated as if they have familial combined hyperlipoproteinemia.[14,64]

Approach to Low Serum HDL-Cholesterol

A low serum HDL-cholesterol level has emerged as the strongest single lipoprotein predictor of coronary heart disease.[15-17] In one prospective study, after adjustment for other risk factors in predicting the risk of myocardial infarction, a change in one unit in the ratio of total- to HDL-cholesterol was associated with a 53% change in risk.[16] However, it is still not known how low HDL levels are linked to CAD and whether raising HDL levels can lower coronary disease risk.[20] The major causes of reduced serum HDL-cholesterol are listed in Table 5. Clearly, attempts should be made to raise low HDL-cholesterol by hygienic means[14] (see Chapter 3). When a low HDL is associated with an increase in VLDL, the latter deserves consideration for therapeutic modification.[14] However, when the HDL is reduced without associated risk factors, attempts to raise HDL levels by drugs cannot be justified because of a lack of clinical trial evidence showing benefit.[14,20]

Table 5.
Major Causes of Reduced Serum HDL-Cholesterol

Cigarette Smoking

Obesity

Lack of exercise

Androgenic and related steroids
    Androgens
    Progestational agents
    Anabolic steroids

β-adrenergic blocking agents

Hypertriglyceridemia

Genetic factors
Primary hypoalphalipoproteinemia

Special Problems

Diabetes Mellitus

Despite the frequency of lipid abnormalities and the increased risk of CAD in diabetics, there are no prospective intervention studies in diabetes patients to show that improvement of lipid abnormalities is associated with reduced risk of morbidity and mortality from atherosclerosis or that treatment will prevent progression of disease.[86,87] Nevertheless, the NCEP recommends that LDL-cholesterol be reduced to 3.36 mm/L (<130 mg/dl) in diabetic men.[14] In diabetic women, the minimal LDL-cholesterol goal is 4.14 mm/L (<160 mg/dl) in the absence of coronary heart disease or 3.36 mm/L (<130 mg/dl) when CAD or another risk factor is present.[14] Often, careful control of plasma glucose will reduce LDL levels and raise HDL-cholesterol concentrations.

In NIDDM, hypertriglyceridemia is commonly seen. Severe hypertriglyceridemia can occur with acute pancreatitis.[14] In these patients, weight reduction must be encouraged, intake of fat must be restricted, and insulin may be required to restore normal activity of lipoprotein lipase.[14] If triglycerides remain elevated despite good diabetic control, a familial form of hyperlipidemia may also be present.

Gender

Most of the clinical trials examining the effect of lipid-lowering therapy on the incidence of CAD have examined middle-aged males. However, there is enough epidemiologic evidence to conclude that women with higher total cholesterol and LDL-cholesterol values are also at risk and, therefore, would benefit from dietary and/or drug intervention. The rates of coronary heart disease are four times higher in middle-aged men than women, and two times higher in elderly men.[88,89]

Age

Children and Adolescents

Most of the clinical trials evaluating the effects of lipid-lowering therapy for reducing the risk of CAD examined middle-aged men. Recently, the NCEP reported on the recommendations of the Expert Panel on Blood Cholesterol Levels in Children and Adolescents.[90] The panel recommended the selective screening, in the context of regular health care, of children and adolescents who have a family history of premature cardiovascular disease or at least one parent with high cholesterol.[90] In children and adolescents from families with hypercholesterolemia or premature CAD, the NCEP has established the following classifications for total cholesterol and LDL-cholesterol values. For total cholesterol, the desirable levels are < 4.40 mm/L (< 170 mg/dl), borderline levels 4.40-5.09 mm/L (170-199 mg/dl), and high levels ≥ 5.17 mm/L (≥ 200 mg/dl) (Fig. 6).[90] For LDL-cholesterol, the desirable levels are < 2.84 mm/L (< 110 mg/dl), borderline levels 2.84-3.34 mm/L (110-129 mg/dl), and high levels ≥ 3.36 mm/L (≥ 130 mg/dl).[90]

For young individuals being screened because they have one parent with high cholesterol, the initial test should be a measurement of total cholesterol. If the child's or adolescent's total cholesterol is high, a lipoprotein analysis should be done.[90] If the total cholesterol levels are borderline, a second measurement of total cholesterol should be taken, and if the average is borderline or high, a lipoprotein analysis should be obtained (Fig. 6). For young individuals being tested due to a documented history of premature cardiovascular disease, the initial test rec-

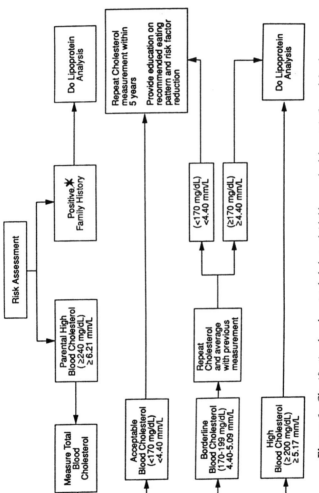

Figure 6: *Classification based on total cholesterol (children and adolescents).* * = *defined as a history of premature (before age 55 years) cardiovascular disease in a parent or grandparent. (From Ref. 89 with permission.)*

ommended is a lipoprotein analysis because a high percentage of these children will have a lipoprotein abnormality.[90]

Once the lipoprotein analysis has been obtained, it should be repeated to determine the average LDL-cholesterol levels (Fig. 7). The NCEP recommends a management approach to children and adolescents based on LDL-cholesterol (Fig. 7).

Diet therapy is the primary approach to treating children and adolescents with elevated blood cholesterol (Fig. 8).[90] Drug therapy is recommended in children aged 10 or older if the LDL-cholesterol remains above 4.91 mm/L (190 mg/dl) or the LDL-cholesterol remains >4.14 mm/L (>160 mg/dl) and there are other cardiovascular risk factors present in the child or adolescent that cannot be controlled.[90] The NCEP was only comfortable recommending bile acid sequestrants as drug therapy, until long-term safety data with other lipid-lowering drugs become available.[90]

The Elderly

There is little clinical evidence from trials that elderly patients will benefit from dietary or drug interventions. However, hyperlipidemia clearly remains a risk factor.[91,92] The subject of hyperlipidemia in the elderly is discussed in Chapter 12.

Systemic Hypertension

A recent report from the Working Group on Management of Patients with Hypertension and High Blood Cholesterol emphasized the synergistic effects of hypertension and hypercholesterolemia on the risks of cardiovascular disease.[93] There are biological interrelations between blood pressure and blood lipids that may influence the mechanisms by which blood pressure is associated with the risk of CAD.[94] Nonpharmacological therapy in the form of proper diet, exercise, and smoking cessation is the foundation for management of both hypertension and high cholesterol. Clinicians should use these nondrug measures as definitive or adjunctive therapy. Pharmacological agents also can be very beneficial in managing the risks. In selecting medications, it is important to consider benefits, costs, and potential untoward effects.[93]

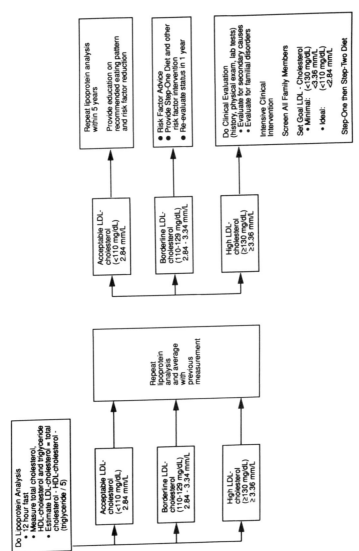

Figure 7: *Classification based on low-density lipoprotein (LDL)-cholesterol (children and adolescents). (From Ref. 89 with permission.)*

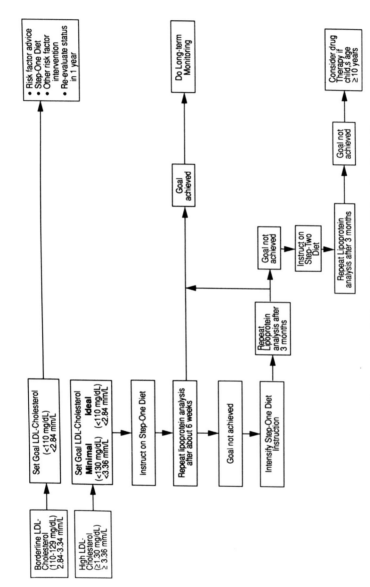

Figure 8: *Dietary and drug treatment (children and adolescents. LDL = low-density lipoprotein. (From Ref. 89 with permission.)*

Myocardial Infarction

Most of the recommendations regarding cholesterol lowering have been directed towards primary prevention and less focused on cholesterol reduction in patients with existing CAD.[95] However, elevated cholesterol and LDL levels have been shown to pose an even greater risk for men with established CAD.[96] In a recent review of observational and clinical trials, it has been concluded from the existing data on morbidity and mortality that cholesterol lowering should be a therapeutic goal of post-infarction therapy.[97] The authors recommend that all patients with known CAD have a fasting lipoprotein analysis rather than a screening test of the serum cholesterol level. Patients should have their LDL-cholesterol reduced to 3.36 mm/L (<130 mg/dl) and their total cholesterol to 5.17 mm/L (<200 mg/dl).[97]

Coronary Artery Bypass Grafts

Investigators at the Montreal Heart Institute performed angiography 1 and 10 years post-surgery to determine the patency of vein grafts in 82 patients who had undergone saphenous vein bypass surgery.[98] The 10-year examination confirmed that atherosclerotic changes are common in saphenous vein bypass grafts at that time: of 132 grafts that were patent at the 1-year examination, only 50 (37.5%) showed no change at the 10-year examination, while evidence of atherosclerosis was found in 43 (33%) and complete occlusion in 30 (29.5%). Progressive atherosclerosis was identified as the single most important cause of occlusion in these grafts. When the investigators analyzed the relationship between cardiovascular risk factors and the development of atherosclerosis, they found no significant difference for smoking, hypertension, or diabetes between the group that developed disease and the group that did not develop disease.

However, in a multivariate analysis, it was revealed that low HDL-cholesterol, high LDL-cholesterol, and high apolipoprotein B were the most significant predictors of atherosclerotic disease in grafts.[98] Almost 80% of those who did not develop disease had normal lipid levels and normal LDL and apolipoprotein B levels in contrast to 8% of patients who developed disease.

Investigators from the Montreal Heart Institute have recommended internal mammary bypass grafting as the coronary bypass procedure of choice, since atherosclerosis progresses less rapidly with these grafts than with saphenous veins. However, there is also now growing evidence that aggressive dietary and lipid-lowering drug therapy can slow down, arrest, and even reverse atherosclerotic disease in patients with saphenous vein coronary bypass grafts.[7] Additional large scale clinical trials addressing this issue are now in progress.

Coronary Angioplasty

Restenosis after successful coronary angioplasty has been observed in 25% to 40% of patients undergoing this procedure.[99,100] Attempts have been made to decrease the incidence of restenosis using a wide array of pharmacological interventions. Some studies have suggested that fish oil might reduce the incidence of restenosis.[101] Restenosis after angioplasty appears to result from intimal smooth muscle cell proliferation.[102] Results of experiments in cholesterol-fed animals after balloon injury of the arterial wall have suggested that restenosis occurs primarily from the migration and proliferation of smooth muscle cells in response to platelet-derived growth factor released from platelets adherent to the site of de-endothelialization.[103] Antiplatelet drugs and calcium channel-blocking drugs have had little or no benefit in reducing the rate of post-angioplasty restenosis.[104,105]

Recently, Gellman and associates demonstrated a benefit from using high-dose lovastatin therapy in reducing intimal hyperplasia in hypercholesterolemic-atherosclerotic rabbits undergoing femoral balloon angioplasty.[106] In a recent preliminary experience, cholesterol reduction with drug therapy was shown to reduce the incidence of restenosis after successful balloon coronary angioplasty in human beings.[107]

Heart Transplantation

Elevated plasma lipids are commonly found in recipients of cardiac transplants,[108,109] as well as an increased risk of accelerated CAD.[109,110] Although many of the drugs used to treat and/or prevent rejection (high-dose steroids, cyclosporine) can raise LDL-cholesterol,[111] hypercholesterolemia has not been found to be a primary risk factor for developing graft atherosclerosis.[112,113] Pathologically, the CAD is often different from that seen in nontransplanted patients, and is characterized as a diffuse, necrotizing vasculitis or atherosclerosis of the entire coronary arterial system.[109,114] It has been proposed that the development of CAD is a manifestation of chronic tissue rejection.[109]

Monitoring of lipids after cardiac transplantation may be worthwhile in these patients, and intake of dietary fats and cholesterol probably should be modified while on high-dose immunosuppressive therapy.[109] Use of lipid-lowering drug therapy does carry with it an increased risk of potential complications[109] and should be considered for those patients for whom there is reasonable hope of benefit, with an appreciation that this is not well defined. It is not known what plasma level of cholesterol requires therapy, and there is no cholesterol target level that has been identified. Controlled prospective studies need to be done to assess the benefits and risks of lipid-lowering drug therapy in this population.

Conclusions

Hyperlipidemia, specifically elevations in plasma cholesterol and LDL-cholesterol, is associated with an increased risk of morbidity and mortality from CAD. Elevations in plasma triglycerides and lower HDL-cholesterol values may also contribute to increased risk. It is clear now that dietary and/or drug therapy of hypercholesterolemia can favorably modify this risk.[115] Guidelines for selecting subjects for treatment have been established. In the subsequent 9 chapters, the nonpharmacological and pharmacological interventions designed to treat hyperlipidemia and disorders of lipoprotein metabolism will be presented and discussed.

References

1. Stamler J, Wentworth D, Neaton J: Is the relationship between serum cholesterol and risk of death from coronary heart disease continuous and graded? JAMA 1986; 256: 2823-2828.
2. Martin MJ, Hulley SB, Browner WS, et al: Serum cholesterol, blood pressure, and mortality: Implications from a cohort of 361,662 men. Lancet 1986; 2: 933-936.
3. McGill HC: Relationship of atherosclerosis in young men to serum lipoprotein cholesterol concentrations and smoking: a preliminary report from the Pathobiological Determinants of Atherosclerosis in Youth (PDAY) Research Group. JAMA 1990; 264: 3018-3024.

4. Lipid Research Clinics Program: The Lipid Research Clinics Coronary Primary Prevention Trial Results: I. Reduction in the incidence of coronary heart disease. JAMA 1984; 251: 351-364.
5. Canner PL, Berge KG, Wenger NK, et al: Fifteen year mortality in Coronary Drug Project patients: Long-term benefit with niacin. J Am Coll Cardiol 1986; 8: 1245-1255.
6. Frick MH, Elo MO, Haapa K, et al: Helsinki Heart Study: primary prevention trial with gemfibrozil in middle-aged men with dyslipidemia. N Engl J Med 1987; 317: 1237-1245.
7. Blankenhorn DH, Johnson RL, Nessim SA, et al: The cholesterol lowering atherosclerosis study (CLAS): design, methods and baseline results. Controlled Clin Trials 1987; 8: 356-387.
8. Ornish D, Brown SE, Scherwitz W, et al: Can lifestyle reverse coronary heart disease? Lancet 1990; 1: 129-133.
9. Kane JP, Malloy MJ, Ports TA, et al: Regression of coronary atherosclerosis during treatment of familial hypercholesterolemia with combined drug regimens. JAMA 1990; 264: 3007-3012.
10. Cashin-Hemphill L, Mack WJ, Pogoda JM, et al: Beneficial effects of colestipol-niacin on coronary atherosclerosis. JAMA 1990; 264: 3013-3017.
11. Brown G, Albers JJ, Fisher LD, et al: Regression of coronary artery disease as a result of intensive lipid-lowering therapy in men with high levels of apolipoprotein B. N Engl J Med 1990; 323: 1289-1298.
12. Buchwald H, Varco RL, Matts JP, et al: Effect of partial ileal bypass surgery on mortality and morbidity from coronary heart disease in patients with hypercholesterolemia. N Engl J Med 1990; 323: 946-955.
13. Holme I: An analysis of randomized trials evaluating the effect of cholesterol reduction on total mortality and coronary heart disease incidence. Circulation 1990; 82: 1916-1924.
14. The Expert Panel: Report of the National Cholesterol Education Program Expert Panel on detection, evaluation, and treatment of high blood cholesterol in adults. Arch Intern Med 1988; 148: 36-69.
15. Kannel WB, Castelli WP, Gordon T: Cholesterol in the prediction of atherosclerotic disease: new perspectives in the Framingham Study. Ann Intern Med 1979; 90: 85-91.
16. Stampfer MJ, Sacks FN, Salvini S, et al: A prospective study of cholesterol, apolipoproteins, and the risk of myocardial infarction. N Engl J Med 1991; 325: 373-381.
17. Gordon DJ, Probstfeld JL, Garrison RJ, et al: High-density lipoprotein cholesterol and cardiovascular disease: four prospective American series. Circulation 1989; 79: 8-15.
18. Guianturco SH, Bradley WA: Lipoprotein mediated cellular mechanisms for atherogenesis in hypertriglyceridemia. Semin Thromb Hemost 1988; 14: 165-169.
19. Castelli WP: The triglyceride issue: a view from Framingham. Am Heart J 1986; 112: 432-437.
20. Grundy SM: Cholesterol and coronary heart disease. Future directions. JAMA 1990; 264: 3053-3059.

21. Schucker B, Wittes JT, Santanello NC, et al: Changes in cholesterol awareness and action: results from national physician and public surveys. Arch Intern Med 1991; 151: 666-673.
22. Schaefer EJ, Levy RI: Pathogenesis and management of lipoprotein disorders. N Engl J Med 1985; 312: 1300-1310.
23. Mitchel Y: Hyperlipidemia, Part 1. Background. Pract Diabet 1987; 6: 6-13.
24. Brown MS, Goldstein JL: A receptor-mediated pathway for cholesterol homeostasis. Science 1986; 232: 34-47.
25. Kodama T, Freeman M, Rohrer L, et al: Type I macrophage scavenger receptor contains a-helical and collagen-like coiled coils. Nature 1990; 343: 531-535.
26. Steinberg D, Parthasarathy S, Carew TE, et al: Beyond cholesterol: modifications of low-density lipoproteins that increase its atherogenicity. N Engl J Med 1989; 320: 915-923.
27. Steinberg D, Witztum JL: Lipoproteins and atherogenesis. Current concepts. JAMA 1990; 264: 3047-3052.
28. van Tol A: Reverse cholesterol transport. In Steinmetz A, Kaffarnik H, Schneider J (eds): Cholesterol Transport Systems and Their Relation to Atherosclerosis. New York, Springer-Verlag, 1989; 85-91.
29. Khoo JC, Miller E, McLoughlin P, et al: Prevention of low-density lipoprotein aggregation by high-density lipoprotein or apolipoprotein A-I. Lipid Res 1990; 3l: 645-658.
30. Brown ML, Hesler C, Tall AR: Plasma enzymes and transfer proteins in cholesterol metabolism. Curr Opin Lipid 1990; 1: 122-127.
31. Hesler CB, Swenson TL, Tall AR: Purification and characterization of a human plasma cholesteryl ester transfer protein 1987; J Biol Chem 1987; 262: 2275-2282.
32. Tall A: Plasma lipid transfer proteins. J Lipid Res 1986; 27: 361-367.
33. Schmitz G, Williamson E: High-density lipoprotein metabolism reverse cholesterol transport and membrane protection. Curr Opin Lipid 1991; 2: 177-179.
34. Yamashita S, Sprecher DL, Sakai N, et al: Accumulation of apoprotein E-rich high-density lipoproteins in hyperalphalipoproteinemic human subjects with plasma cholesteryl ester transfer protein deficiency. J Clin Invest 1990; 86: 688-695.
35. Brown ML, Inazu A, Hesler CB, et al: Molecular basis of lipid transfer protein deficiency in a family with increased high-density lipoproteins. Nature 1989; 342: 448-450.
36. Ha YC, Barter PJ: Differences in plasma cholesteryl ester transfer activity in sixteen vertebrate species. Comp Biochem Physiol 1982; 71B: 265-269.
37. Howard B: Lipoprotein metabolism in diabetes mellitus. J Lipid Res 1987; 28: 613-628.
38. Haffner SM: Cardiovascular risk factors in confirmed prediabetic individuals: does the clock for coronary heart disease start ticking before the onset of clinical diabetes. JAMA 1990; 263: 2893-2898.
39. Hartung GH, Foreyt JP: The effect of alcohol intake on high density lipoprotein cholesterol and coronary heart disease. Cardiovasc Rev Rep 1990; 11: 27-36.

40. Ma Y, Henderson HE, Ven Murthy MR, et al: A mutation in the human lipoprotein lipase gene as the most common cause of familial chylomicronemia in French Canadians. N Engl J Med 1991; 324: 1761-1766.
41. Mahley RW, Weisgraber KH, Innerarity TL, et al: Genetic defects in lipoprotein metabolism. JAMA 1991; 265: 78-83.
42. Wilson ED, Wardell MR, Weisgraber KH, et al: The three- dimensional structure of the LDL receptor-binding domain of human apoprotein E. Science 1991; 252: 1817-1822.
43. Berg K: A new serum type system in man: the Lp(a) system. Acta Pathol Microbiol Scand 1963; 59: 369-382.
44. Utermann G: The mysteries of lipoprotein(a). Science 1989; 246: 904-910.
45. Utermann G: Lipoprotein(a): a genetic risk for premature coronary artery disease. Curr Opin Lipid 1990; 1: 404-410.
46. Hajjar KA, Gavish D, Breslow JL, et al: Lipoprotein(a) modulation of endothelial cell surface fibrinolysis and its potential role in atherosclerosis. (Letter) Nature 1989; 339: 303-305.
47. Scanu AM: Lipoprotein(a): a potential bridge between the fields of atherosclerosis and thrombosis. Arch Pathol Lab Med 1988; 112: 1045-1047.
48. Genest J, Jenner JL, McNamara JR, et al: Prevalence of lipoprotein(a) [Lp(a)] excess in coronary artery disease. Am J Cardiol 1991; 67: 1039-1045.
49. Makino K, Abe A, Maeda S, et al: Lipoprotein(a) in nonhuman primates. Atherosclerosis 1989; 78: 81-85.
50. Utermann G, Hoppichler F, Dieplinger H, et al: Defects in the low density lipoprotein receptor gene affect lipoprotein(a) levels: multiplicative interaction of two gene loci associated with premature atherosclerosis. Proc Natl Acad Sci 1989; 86: 4171-4174.
51. Rhoads GC, Dahlen GH, Berg K, et al: Lp(a) lipoprotein as a risk factor for myocardial infarction. JAMA 1986; 256: 2540-2544.
52. Sandkamp M, Funke H, Schulte H, et al: Lipoprotein(a) is an independent risk factor for myocardial infarction at a young age. Clin Chem 1990; 36: 20-23.
53. Seed M, Hoppichler F, Reaveley D, et al: Relation of serum lipoprotein(a) concentration and apolipoprotein (a) phenotype to coronary heart disease in patients with familial hypercholesterolemia. N Engl J Med 1990; 322: 1494-1499.
54. Scott J: Lipoprotein(a): Thrombogenesis at last? Nature 1989; 341: 22-23.
55. Sundell IB, Nilsson TK, Hallmans G, et al: Interrelationships between plasma levels of plasminogen activator inhibitor, tissue plasminogen activator, lipoprotein(a) and established cardiovascular risk factors in a North Swedish population. Atherosclerosis 1989; 80: 9-16.
56. Maeda S, Abe A, Seishima M, et al: Transient changes of serum lipoprotein(a) as an acute phase protein. Atherosclerosis 1989; 78: 145-150.
57. Qiu S, Theroux P, Genest J, et al: Lipoprotein(a) blood levels in unstable angina pectoris, acute myocardial infarction, and after thrombolytic activity. Am J Cardiol 1991; 67: 1175-1179.
58. Gavish D, Breslow JL: Lipoprotein(a) reduction by N-acetyl-cysteine. Lancet 1991; 1: 203-204.

59. Ross R: The pathogenesis of atherosclerosis - an update. N Engl J Med 1986; 314: 488-500.

60. Atherosclerosis Study Group: Optimal resources for primary prevention of atherosclerotic diseases. Circulation 1984; 70: 157A-205A.

61. Grundy SM: Cholesterol and coronary heart disease: a new era. JAMA 1986; 256: 2849-2858.

62. Hulley SB, Rhodes GG: The plasma lipoproteins as risk factors: comparison of electrophoretic and ultracentrifugation results. Metabolism 1982; 31: 773-777.

63. Kannel WB, Neaton JD, Wentworth D, et al: Overall and CHD mortality rates in relation to major risk factors in 325,348 men screened for the MRFIT. Am Heart J 1986; 112: 825-836.

64. Consensus Development Conference: Treatment of hypertriglyceridemia. JAMA 1984; 251: 1196-1200.

65. Myers LH, Phillips NR, Havel RJ: Mathematical evaluation of methods for estimation of the concentration of the major lipid components of human serum lipoproteins. J Lab Clin Med 1976; 88: 491-505.

66. Kukita I, Hiwada K, Kokubu T: Serum apolipoprotein A-I, A-II and B levels and their discriminative values in relatives of patients with coronary artery disease. Atherosclerosis 1984; 51: 261-267.

67. National Center for Health Statistics: Total serum cholesterol levels of adults 20 to 74 years of age: United States, 1976-1980, Vital and Health Statistics, Ser. II, No. 236. Dept. Health & Human Services publication (PHS) 86-1686. Government Printing Office, May 1986.

68. A Report from the Laboratory Standardization Panel of the National Cholesterol Education Program. Improving cholesterol measurement. National Heart Lung & Blood Institute. National Institutes of Health, Bethesda, Maryland 1990 (NIH Publication 90-2964).

69. Koerselman HB, Lewis B, Pilkington TRE: The effect of venous occlusion on the level of serum cholesterol. J Atheroscler Res 1961; 1: 85-88.

70. Hagan RD, Upton SJ, Avakian EV, et al:: Increases in serum lipid and lipoprotein levels with movement from the supine to standing position in adult men and women. Prev Med 1986; 15: 18-27.

71. Central Patient Registry and Coordinating Center for the Lipid Research Clinics: Reference Manual for the Lipid Research Clinics Program Prevalence Study, I and II. Chapel Hill, North Carolina: Department of Biostatistics, University of North Carolina at Chapel Hill, February 1974.

72. Manual of Operations, Lipid Research Clinics Program I: Lipid and lipoprotein analysis. National Heart, Lung & Blood Institute, National Institutes of Health, Bethesda, Maryland, 1974. U.S. Department of Health Education and Welfare publication (NIH 75-628).

73. Laboratory Methods Committee of the Lipid Research Clinics Program: Cholesterol and triglyceride concentrations in serum/ plasma pairs. Clin Chem 1977; 23: 60-63.

74. Warwick G, Packard CJ, Shepherd J: Plasma lipid measurement. Curr Sci 1990; 1: 500-507.

75. Naito HK: Reliability of lipid and lipoprotein testing. Am J Cardiol 1985; 56: 6J-9J.

76. Kaufman HW, McNamara JR, Anderson KM, et al: How reliably can compact chemistry analyzers measure lipids? JAMA 1990; 263: 1245-1249.
77. Laker MF: Cholesterol screening as an indicator of coronary risk. Curr Sci 1990; 1: 536-540.
78. Davis CE, Rifkind BM, Brenner H, et al: A single cholesterol measurement underestimates the risk of coronary heart disease. An empirical example from the Lipid Research Clinics Mortality Follow-Up Study. JAMA 1990; 264: 3044-3046.
79. Friedewald WT, Levy RI, Fredrickson DS: Estimation of the concentration of low-density lipoprotein cholesterol in plasma, without use of the preparative ultracentrifuge. Clin Chem 1972; 18: 499-502.
80. Rosseneu MY, Labeur C: Apolipoprotein structure, function and measurement. Curr Sci 1990; 1: 508-513.
81. Grundy SM, Vega GL: Role of apolipoprotein levels in clinical practice. Arch Intern Med 1990; 150: 1579-1582.
82. Sniderman AD, Silberberg J: Is it time to measure apolipoprotein B? Arteriosclerosis 1990; 10: 665-667.
83. Lauer RM, Clarke WR: Use of cholesterol measurements in childhood for the prediction of adult hypercholesterolemia. The Muscatine Study. JAMA 1990; 264: 3034-3038.
84. Newman TB, Browner WS, Hulley SB: The case against childhood cholesterol screening. JAMA 1990; 264: 3039-3043.
85. Phillips NR, Havel RJ, Kane JP: Levels and interrelationships of serum and lipoprotein cholesterol and triglycerides: association with adiposity and the consumption of ethanol, tobacco, and beverages containing caffeine. Arteriosclerosis 1981; 1: 13-34.
86. Taskinen M-R: Hyperlipidemia in diabetics. Clin Endocrinol Metab 1990; 4: 743-775.
87. Garg A, Grundy SM: Management of dyslipidemia in NIDDM. Diabetes Care 1990; 13: 153-169.
88. Lerner DJ, Kannel WB: Patterns of coronary heart disease morbidity and mortality in the sexes: a 26 year follow-up of the Framingham population. Am Heart J 1986; 111: 383-390.
89. Feinlieb M, Gillum RF: CHD in the elderly: the magnitude of the problem in the US. In Wenger NK, Furberg CD, Pitt E (eds): CHD in the Elderly. New York, Elsevier, 1986; 29-59.
90. Report of the National Cholesterol Education Program Expert Panel on Blood Cholesterol Levels in Children and Adults. J Pediatr 1992; (in press).
91. Gordon DJ, Rifkind BM: Treating high blood cholesterol in the older patient. Am J Cardiol 1989; 63: 48H-52H.
92. Rubin SM, Sidney S, Black DM, et al: High blood cholesterol in elderly men and the excess risk for coronary artery disease. Ann Intern Med 1990; 113: 916-920.
93. Working Group on Management of Patients with Hypertension and High Blood Cholesterol: National Education Programs Working Group Report on the Management of Patients with Hypertension and High Blood Cholesterol. Ann Intern Med 1991; 114: 224-237.

94. Bonaa KH, Thelle DS: Association between blood pressure and serum lipids in a population. Circulation 1991; 83: 1305-1314.

95. Cohen MV, Byrne MJ, Levine B, et al: Low rate of treatment of hypercholesterolemia with suspected and proven coronary artery disease. Circulation 1991; 83: 1294-1304.

96. Pekkanen J, Linn S, Heiss G, et al: Ten-year mortality from cardiovascular disease in relation to cholesterol level among men with and without preexisting cardiovascular disease. N Engl J Med 1990; 322: 1700-1707.

97. Rossouw JE, Lewis B, Rifkind BM: The value of lowering cholesterol after myocardial infarction. N Engl J Med 1990; 323: 1112-1118.

98. Campeau L, Enjalbert M, Lesperance J, et al: The relation of risk factors to the development of atherosclerosis in saphenous vein bypass grafts and the progression of disease in the native circulation: a study 10 years after aortocoronary bypass surgery. N Engl J Med 1984; 311: 1329-1332.

99. Leimgruber PP, Roubin GS, Hollman J, et al: Restenosis after successful coronary angioplasty in patients with single vessel disease. Circulation 1986; 73: 710-717.

100. Mata LA, Bosch X, David PR, et al: Clinical and angiographic assessment 6 months after double vessel percutaneous coronary angioplasty. J Am Coll Cardiol 1985; 6: 1239-1244.

101. Dehmer GJ, Popma JJ, Van Den Berg EK, et al: Reduction in the rate of early restenosis after coronary angioplasty by a diet supplemented with N-3 fatty acids. N Engl J Med 1988; 319: 733-740.

102. Austin GE, Ratliff NB, Hollman J, et al: Intimal proliferation of smooth muscle cells as an explanation for recurrent coronary artery stenosis after percutaneous transluminal coronary angioplasty. J Am Coll Cardiol 1985; 6: 369-375.

103. Ross R, Bowen-Pope D, Raines EW: Platelets, macrophages, endothelium and growth factors: their effects upon cells and their possible roles in atherogenesis. Ann NY Acad Sci 1985; 454: 254-260.

104. Whiteworth HB, Roubin GS, Hollman J, et al: Effect of nifedipine on recurrent stenosis after percutaneous transluminal coronary angioplasty. J Am Coll Cardiol 1986; 8: 1271-1276.

105. Schwartz L, Bourassa MG, Lesperance J, et al: Failure of antiplatelet agents to reduce restenosis after PTCA in a double blind placebo controlled trial. (abstr) J Am Coll Cardiol 1988; 11: 236A.

106. Gellman J, Ezekowitz MD, Sarembock IJ, et al: Effect of lovastatin on intimal hyperplasia after balloon angioplasty: a study in an atherosclerotic hypercholesterolemic rabbit. J Am Coll Cardiol 1991; 17: 251-259.

107. Sahni R, Maniet AR, Voci G, et al: Prevention of restenosis by lovastatin after successful coronary angioplasty. Am Heart J 1991; 121: 1600-1608.

108. Keogh A, Simons L, Spratt P, et al: Hyperlipidemia after heart transplantation. J Heart Transplant 1988; 7: 171-175.

109. Butman S: Hyperlipidemia after cardiac transplantation: be aware and possibly wary of drug therapy for lowering of serum lipids. Am Heart J 1991; 121: 1585-1590.

110. O'Neill BJ, Pflugfelder PW, Singh NR, et al: Frequency of angiographic detection and quantitative assessment of coronary arterial disease one and three years after cardiac transplantation. Am J Cardiol 1989; 63: 1221-1226.
111. Ballantyne CM, Podet EJ, Patsch WP, et al: Effects of cyclosporine therapy on plasma lipoprotein levels. JAMA 1989; 262: 53-56.
112. Gao SZ, Schroeder JS, Alderman EL, et al: Clinical and laboratory correlates of accelerated coronary artery disease in the cardiac transplant patient. Circulation 1987; 76 (Suppl V): V56-6l.
113. Olivari MT, Homans DC, Wilson RF, et al: Coronary artery disease in cardiac transplant patients receiving triple-drug immunosuppressive therapy. Circulation 1989; 80 (Suppl III): III-111-115.
114. Johnson DE, Gao SZ, Schroeder JS, et al: The spectrum of coronary artery pathological findings in human cardiac allografts. J Heart Transplant 1989; 8: 349-359.
115. Burke GL, Sprafka JM, Folsom A, et al: Trends in serum cholesterol levels from 1980 to 1987. The Minnesota Heart Survey. N Engl J Med 1991; 324: 941-946.

Part II

Nonpharmacological Approaches

Chapter 2

Dietary Therapy for Hyperlipidemia

Lynn Edlen-Nezin, M.A., Judith Wylie-Rosett, Ed.D., R.D.,
William H. Frishman, M.D.

In 1913, Anitschkow demonstrated production of arterial lesions in rabbits in response to a high cholesterol diet.[1] Since then, there has been extensive research on the relationship between diet and atherosclerosis. Evidence of a "diet-heart" connection has been supported by numerous studies conducted with animal models,[2,3] and proof in human beings has been provided by cross-sectional, retrospective, and prospective epidemiologic studies.[4,5]

Evidence that Diet Causes Atherosclerosis in Animal Models

It has been recognized that the etiology of atherosclerosis is multifactorial and serum cholesterol levels are affected by genetic and environmental influences.[6] Extensive animal research has provided valuable insights into possible mechanisms and effects of dietary intake on serum cholesterol.[7] Extrapolation to humans must, as always, be undertaken with caution. The majority of data that support the diet-heart connection are the result of large-scale observational studies of various populations.[8]

A diet high in saturated fat and cholesterol has induced atherosclerosis in rhesus monkeys.[9] Diets of cholesterol plus corn oil, hydrogenated corn oil, and butter have proved atherogenic in Japanese quail.[10] Vervet monkeys fed an atherogenic diet of normal foods for westernized

From *Medical Management of Lipid Disorders: Focus on Prevention of Coronary Artery Disease,* edited by William H. Frishman, M.D. © 1992, Futura Publishing Inc., Mount Kisco, NY.

people developed increased levels of LDL-cholesterol and atherosclerotic lesions in comparison to monkeys fed a more prudent, lower fat Western diet.[11]

Animal research indicates that "metabolic training" may occur, such that early exposure to an atherogenic diet seems to impact on serum cholesterol response later in life. The effect of a 6-week feeding period of a high cholesterol diet in rabbits was different in animals exposed to the diet for the first time when compared to animals fed a similar diet at an earlier age.[12] Animals fed the high-fat diet early in life exhibited quantitative and qualitative differences in intestinal transport of fats, showing less responsiveness to dietary fat during rechallenge with the atherogenic diet.

The magnitude and duration of hypercholesterolemia have been shown to be related to the extent of atherosclerotic process in rabbits,[13] with lesions becoming more severe over time in response to a high cholesterol diet. Jayakody et al[14] found evidence of continued impairment of endothelium-dependent relaxant factor in rabbits fed an atherogenic diet even after the diet was replaced by a standard lab diet.

Although discrepancies exist among species in response to dietary cholesterol as opposed to saturated fat, the majority of studies support the existence of an atherogenic diet. Long-term feeding of small amounts of cholesterol has been shown to lead to atherosclerosis in rabbits, chickens, and monkeys,[15] despite negligible rises in serum total cholesterol.

Epidemiologic Evidence Linking Diet To Atherosclerosis

Dietary Risk Factors in Coronary Heart Disease (CHD)

Observational studies of diverse populations have provided support for the connection among dietary patterns, serum cholesterol levels, and atherosclerosis. In 1970, Keys et al[16] published results from the Seven Countries Study, comparing the frequency of hypercholesterolemia (defined as cholesterol levels greater than 6.47 mm/L [250 mg/dl]) in samples of middle-aged men from Finland, the United States, Japan, the Netherlands, Greece, Italy, and Yugoslavia. Keys, a physiologist whose earlier work examined the effects of starvation, noted that similar rankings were obtained when countries were ordered according to (1) heart disease death rates and (2) percentage of total calories in the national diet provided by fat.[17] Highly significant positive correlations were demonstrated among median serum cholesterol levels, saturated fat intake, and 5- and 10-year mortality rates from coronary heart disease with Finland ranking the highest and Japan the lowest.

There is concern that Italy may be losing its "Mediterranean advantage"[18] due to departures from traditional dietary patterns. The Mediterranean diet is rich in fish, beans, fruit, and vegetables and low in both saturated fat and cholesterol.[19] In a study in the northern hill town of Gubbio,[18] 1983-1985 serum cholesterol levels were considerably higher (5.77 mm/L [223 mg/dl] versus 5.09-5.33 mm/L [197-206 mg/dl]) than those reported in the 1960 Italian population of the Seven Countries study. Dietary analyses conducted showed that animal fat intake had increased almost 50% and saturated fat intake by 18% in just 10 years.

A health practice score based on six different habits, including the amounts consumed of fruits/vegetables, daily bread, and potatoes, was constructed based on two postal interviews of a random sample of Norwegian men.[20] Scores showed a strong inverse relationship with total mortality as well as the death rate from cancer and cardiovascular diseases. Higher intakes of vegetables, fruit, potatoes, and bread were associated with lower mortality.

In a Nigerian population sample,[21] low serum lipids (3.92-4.25 mm/ L [151.7-164.4 mg/dl]) were determined to be related to a low dietary fat intake. Palm oil, considered to be atherogenic, is the major source of fat in this diet, but the quantity ingested is quite small. Rates of CHD are also correspondingly low in this population.

A randomized study designed to examine the relationship between diet and serum lipids was conducted in a Belgium sample of 5,485 men and 4,856 women.[22] The data obtained supported a highly significant positive relationship between intake of saturated fat and regional mortality from all causes and cardiovascular disease. A negative relationship was found between mortality and polyunsaturated fat intake.

The influence of migratory status on dietary composition, serum cholesterol levels, and risk of CHD and stroke was investigated in the prospective Ni-Hon-San study.[23] Dietary analyses were made of more than 10,000 middle-aged men of Japanese ancestry living either in Japan, Hawaii, or California. In all age groups where data were available, fat consumption was higher in the mainland United States and Hawaii than in Japan. More importantly, dietary saturated fat was inversely related to unsaturated fat intake in the three cohorts. Japanese subjects had lower total fat intake, and the majority of fat was derived from unsaturated sources, such as fish. Differences in nutrient intake paralleled differences in body weight and serum cholesterol. Prevalence, incidence, and mortality rates for CHD increased positively and significantly with migratory status, with Japanese subjects living in California showing the highest rates followed by the Hawaiian and Japanese cohort, respectively. Increase in risk status was correlated with adoption of an increasingly "westernized diet." In contrast to these data, migratory status was not associated with increased mortality from CHD in the Ireland-Boston Diet-Heart Study[24] in which dietary practices were not substantially altered in response to immigration.

Aggregate dietary data from three different prospective studies of cardiovascular disease[25] were used to determine the relationship between fat intake and CHD. Intake was assessed by 24-hour dietary recall in men from the Puerto Rico Heart Health Program, the Honolulu Heart Study, and the Framingham study in 1965 who were then followed for up to 6 years for first appearance of CHD or death. In all three studies, intake of a larger percentage of calories as fat was predictive of development of CHD.

Analyses of data from over 24 years in the Framingham study[26] describe a positive linear relationship between serum cholesterol levels and atherosclerotic disease in men. In women, the cholesterol distribution curve most closely resembled that of men only in the 40- to 49-year-old decade, and it was in this group that the relative risk of disease increased in similar magnitude to that observed in men.

Dietary intake of the Framingham subjects was quite similar within the cohort and resembled the "typical" American diet, high in animal fat and cholesterol. Data from other countries in which national diets are significantly lower in saturated fat intake produce curves for serum cholesterol distribution that are markedly lower than those seen in the Framingham study.[27]

The Zutphen Study[28] followed a cohort of 829 Dutch men for 25 years. Survival analysis showed that serum cholesterol level in 1960 was independently related to the 25-year incidence of myocardial infarction, and low serum cholesterol was not associated with increased long-term mortality from other diseases.

The Western Electric Study[29] evaluated diet, serum cholesterol, and other variables in 1900 middle-aged men. Serum cholesterol concentration varied positively with dietary saturated fat and cholesterol and tended to vary inversely with polyunsaturated fatty acid intake. After adjustment for serum cholesterol concentration, dietary cholesterol was significantly associated with death from CHD, based on 20-year follow-up of the initial cohort.

Data on over 356,000 middle-aged American men screened for the Multiple Risk Factor Intervention Trial (MRFIT) provided support for the contention that the relationship between serum cholesterol and CHD is continuous and graded.[30] These data were instrumental in the eventual formulation of national dietary guidelines.

The Cooperative Lipoprotein Phenotyping Study, known as the Pooling Project,[31] was a large multicenter investigation in the United States devoted to uniform assessment of risk and standardization of cholesterol measurement and cardiovascular endpoints. This study demonstrated the increasing risk of CHD with rising levels of serum cholesterol.[27] The Lipid Research Clinics Program, conducted in the United States during the 1970s, produced distributions for both total serum cholesterol and LDL-cholesterol values that increased with age.[32]

Autopsy Evidence

A review of autopsy data[33] from both retrospective and prospective studies found conclusive evidence that elevated serum cholesterol is associated with increased atherosclerosis. Factors leading to increased total serum cholesterol and decreased HDL-cholesterol levels were implicated in the acceleration or development of atherosclerosis, but it was observed that the effect of a particular risk factor may not be consistent across all arterial segments. Individual response to risk factors, at the level of the arterial wall, seems to depend on multifactorial response to both type and intensity of risk factors, and variation occurs among even the most homogeneous group of subjects.

The Honolulu Heart Program,[34] which provided the Hawaiian cohort for the Ni-Hon-San Study, is a prospective study of cardiovascular disease incidence in middle-aged men of Japanese ancestry. Atherosclerosis scores were determined at autopsy for 198 men free of cardiovascular disease at entry examination. Scores for large arteries were consistently and positively associated with age, diastolic blood pressure, serum cholesterol, and inversely with height. Scores for the small arteries were higher for men who reported low intakes of fat and animal protein and high intakes of vegetable protein and total carbohydrates. In the

Ni-Hon-San study, saturated fat intake was also determined to be inversely correlated with stroke incidence in the Japanese subjects living in Japan,[35] suggesting that serum cholesterol may exert a differential effect on large versus small vessels. Lesions of coronary arteries were compared at autopsy in middle-aged Norwegian and Japanese men.[36] Large differences were seen between the samples, which were positively correlated with serum cholesterol levels. The increased atherosclerosis in the Norwegian sample was attributed in part to dietary factors.

The Effect of Dietary Cholesterol on Serum Cholesterol Levels in Human Studies

Despite numerous investigations, establishment of the role of dietary cholesterol in the promotion of atherosclerosis has yet to be conclusively defined. Only about 40% of ingested cholesterol is absorbed. Exogenous cholesterol does not enter directly into hepatic formation of VLDL-cholesterol and LDL-cholesterol, but sufficient intake can down-regulate hepatic LDL-cholesterol receptor activity and subsequently increase plasma levels of LDL-cholesterol.[19]

It has been shown that doubling or tripling amounts of dietary cholesterol will not necessarily increase plasma levels, if there has been a previous, established high intake of dietary cholesterol.[19] Average American intake of dietary cholesterol, based on dietary surveys, has been estimated at about 400 mg/d for women and 500 mg/d for men[37] or the dietary equivalent of about two eggs per day. Evidence of a threshold effect for dietary cholesterol estimates the level to be about 100 mg/d, therefore most people would respond significantly to a decrease in dietary cholesterol from current levels to 100 mg/d or less.[19]

Research on response to dietary cholesterol has determined the existence of subgroups of hypo- and hyper-responders to dietary challenge.[9] Characteristics of human response to dietary cholesterol were examined in a Dutch study of three controlled dietary trials.[38] Serum total and HDL-cholesterol concentrations were on the average higher in the hyper- than in the hypo-responders on the controlled diets. Subjects reporting a habitual high cholesterol intake relative to energy intake were less reactive to dietary cholesterol variation. Results showed that a high HDL concentration, low habitual cholesterol intake, and low percent body fat do not make one less susceptible to dietary cholesterol-induced hypercholesterolemia.

Effects of Dietary Manipulation on Serum Cholesterol

In pursuit of the optimal lipid-lowering, heart-protective diet, research has focused on both the quantity and quality of dietary composition. Total calories; amount and type of calories derived from fat, carbohydrate, protein, cholesterol; and alcohol consumption are dietary components that influence levels of lipids and lipoproteins.[39] The effects of dietary fiber, plant sterols, lecithin, and certain vitamins and minerals has also been investigated in relation to serum cholesterol.

Animal Studies

Modification of elevated serum cholesterol levels (as well as component lipoprotein subfractions) by dietary manipulation has been well documented in animal studies.[40] Induction and then regression of atherosclerosis has been demonstrated in rhesus monkeys subjected to an atherogenic diet followed by a trial of a low-fat, lipid-lowering diet.[41] Regression of lesions has also been achieved in fowl and dogs, but regression has not been consistently reproducible in rabbits.[41]

In both normotensive and hypertensive rabbits fed an atherogenic diet, reduction of aortic lesions and significant reversal of luminal narrowing was observed when the animals were returned to a normal lab diet.[42] Hypertension was seen to aggravate the severity and extent of both aortic and coronary atherosclerosis.

Human Studies

Studies conducted on metabolic wards demonstrated that serum cholesterol concentration can be experimentally altered in men.[43] Keys et al[44] developed equations to calculate the predicted effect of altering the lipid ratio of polyunsaturated to saturated fat (P:S) in the diet. Reducing saturated fat by a specific amount lowers cholesterol to approximately the same degree as supplementing the diet with twice that amount of polyunsaturated fat. Hegsted et al[45] developed similar equations with comparable results.

Subsequent dietary trials have continued to provide support for the relationship of the P:S ratio to serum cholesterol. The multicenter National Diet-Heart Study[46] compared responses of middle-aged men to three concomitant dietary modifications: (1) moderate reduction of percent calories derived from total fat and/or saturated fat; (2) increase in percent calories from polyunsaturated fat and in P:S ratio; and (3) moderate reduction in dietary cholesterol. The largest drop in serum cholesterol was experienced by men with the largest decrease in weight from the baseline period, providing evidence for the connection between body weight and serum cholesterol levels. In addition, percent reduction in cholesterol was positively related to initial cholesterol levels, with the more hypercholesterolemic men showing the greatest decrease with intervention. At the 6-month follow-up evaluation, participants' serum cholesterol values had reverted to baseline, suggesting subjects had failed to maintain dietary changes of lowered fat intake.

Evidence That Lowering Serum Cholesterol Lowers CHD Morbidity

Drug treatment trials have demonstrated that CHD mortality and morbidity can be decreased by altering blood lipids.[47] Administration of lovastatin to genetically hyperlipidemic rabbits reduced plasma cholesterol by 60% due to reduced levels of LDL-cholesterol.[48] Arterial disease was profoundly less in treated versus untreated animals.

The Lipid Research Clinics Coronary Primary Prevention Trial (LRC-CPPT)[49] was a 7-year randomized, double-blind study of cholystyramine versus placebo in 3,806 asymptomatic men. The treatment group demonstrated significant differences in myocardial infarction rates as well as other cardiac endpoints, such as angina and positive exercise stress test results when compared to control subjects.

The Helsinki Heart Study[50] conclusively demonstrated the benefits of lowering serum cholesterol. In a 5-year double-blind placebo-controlled primary prevention trial of gemfibrozil in 4081 asymptomatic middle-aged men with primary dyslipidemia, increases in HDL-cholesterol and decreases in LDL-cholesterol were associated with risk reduction in the gemfibrozil versus the placebo treated group. These data confirmed and strengthened findings by the LRC-CPPT study.

Data from the Los Angeles Veterans Administration Study[51] demonstrated a 20% mean reduction in serum cholesterol in a sample of middle-aged and elderly men receiving a diet low in cholesterol and saturated fat. Overall incidence of fatal and nonfatal atherosclerotic events was significantly less (-31%, p < 0.05) in the intervention group versus the control group which received a conventional diet.

The Oslo Study[52] was a nondrug trial designed to assess the effect of diet and nonsmoking advice on the first CHD event in 1232 normotensive, hyperlipidemic middle-aged men. Subjects experiencing the greatest reduction in serum cholesterol were shown by dietary interview to consume more fish and vegetables, skimmed versus whole milk, and more polyunsaturated and less saturated fat. The total number of CHD events was 47% lower in the intervention versus the control group. In contrast to the Diet-Heart Study, the Oslo Study found at both 5- and 8-year follow-up that subjects who had modified dietary fat intake had maintained the dietary changes.

Hyperaggregability of platelets has been related to increased levels of serum cholesterol and CHD risk.[53] Platelet aggregability was significantly reduced in hyperlipidemic men following a 2-week trial of a low-fat, low-cholesterol diet.[54]

A meta analysis of lipid-lowering trials permits direct comparability of data that would otherwise be compromised by differences in study populations and protocols.[55] Using this method, Peto et al[56] found that cholesterol lowering was associated with reduction in CHD incidence. The reduction in CHD was directly correlated with the magnitude and duration of the cholesterol reduction. These relationships held whether the reduction in serum cholesterol was achieved through diet or drug treatment.

Evidence for Regression of CHD

Prevention of CHD has been considered to be dependent on the magnitude and duration of cholesterol reduction, and not upon the means.[57] It is generally accepted that the cornerstone of dietary therapy for both primary and secondary prevention of hyperlipidemia is the reduction of saturated fat intake.[58-60] Increased saturated fat consumption is related to down-regulation of LDL-cholesterol receptors in the liver, which may be precursory to dyslipidemia. The typical American diet derives approximately 40% of its energy from calories supplied as a mix of fats of various saturations, with the majority in a saturated form.

During the period of semi-starvation in Germany at the end of World War I, diminution in the amount of aortic atherosclerosis was observed at autopsy in soldiers.[61] Varainen and Kanerva[62] reported similar findings in a corresponding sample after World War II. Animal experiments have provided models for the reversibility of atherosclerosis.[41] Evidence of stabilization of the atherosclerotic process in humans has been obtained in the Leiden Intervention Trial.[63] This trial studied the impact of a vegetarian diet on serum cholesterol and the progression of coronary lesions in 39 patients with stable angina pectoris. Coronary angiography performed before intervention in all subjects had shown at least one vessel with 50% obstruction. Analyses of subsequent angiography at 24 months post-intervention indicated progression of disease in 21 of 39 patients, but no lesion growth in 18 patients. Patients who exhibited no lesion growth either had lower total/HDL-cholesterol values throughout the trial or had high initial values that were significantly lowered by dietary intervention. The results of this trial provide further support for individual variation in response to dietary manipulation.

The Cholesterol Lowering Atherosclerosis Study,[64,65] a prospective, placebo-controlled trial of combined colestipol- niacin therapy, demonstrated significant benefit with therapy on angiographic progression and regression of coronary lesions. Each quartile of increased consumption of fat, as determined by 24-hour dietary recall, was associated with a significant increase in risk of new coronary lesions. New lesions did not develop in subjects who increased dietary protein in compensation for reduced intake of fat by substitution of low-fat meats and dairy products for high-fat meats and dairy products.

The Lifestyle Heart Trial[66] assessed the effects of comprehensive changes in lifestyle over one year on the status of coronary artery lesions. In this randomized study, 48 patients with angiographically documented coronary lesions received either a low-fat vegetarian diet (10% total fat, 15%-20% protein, 70%-75% predominantly complex carbohydrates) or a control diet (30% fat). The experimental group could eat unlimited amounts of fruits, vegetables, grains, legumes, and soybean products. However, no animal products except egg whites and 1 cup of nonfat yogurt or milk were permitted, limiting cholesterol intake to 5 mg per day. Caffeine and smoking were eliminated, and alcohol was limited to no more than 2 ounces per day. The diet was supplemented with vitamin B12. In addition, subjects performed individually tailored moderate aerobic exercises and underwent stress management. Angiographic findings showed that the average percent diameter stenosis regressed from 40% to 37.8% in the experimental group, but progressed from 42.7% to 46.2% in the control group. Overall, 82% of the subjects in the experimental group had lesion change scores in the direction of regression, while 53% of the control group had change in the direction of progression. Those in the experimental group lost an average of 10 kg and showed significant improvement in their lipid levels. The authors concluded that nonpharmacological approaches could bring about associated regression of coronary atherosclerosis after 1 year.

There was a dose-response relationship between adherence and regression, and it was noted that the most severely stenosed lesions showed the greatest improvement. The adherence to this very stringent dietary plan was excellent in the experimental group, however the feasibility of acceptance of such a restrictive diet by most patients is questionable. The exceptions to the general findings were the change scores of the five women in the trial. Although all five made only moderate lifestyle changes, all showed overall regression. The four women in the control group showed greater improvement than any of the men in that group, despite greater lifestyle changes by some of the men. This is further evidence that gender may differentially affect progression and regression of atherosclerosis.[66]

The results of three recently reported studies have also shown regression and attenuated rates of progression of atherosclerosis produced by different lipid-lowering therapies in patients with coronary artery disease.[67-69] In the first study,[67] 120 men at high risk for cardiovascular events were studied by quantitative coronary angiography at entry and $2\frac{1}{2}$ years of therapy for elevated LDL-cholesterol levels. Treatment consisted of a conventional cholesterol-lowering diet, and, if necessary, treatment with colestipol, lovastatin and colestipol, or niacin and colestipol. Levels of LDL-cholesterol decreased to a greater extent in patients receiving the combination drug treatments. These patients also had a reduced frequency of progression of coronary artery lesions and an increased frequency of regression. A reduction in apoprotein B levels, a reduction in systolic blood pressure, and an increase in HDL-cholesterol levels each correlated independently with the occurrence of regression. Clinical events such as death, myocardial infarction, recurrent symp-

toms, or need for coronary revascularization occurred less in those patients receiving combination drug treatments.

In the second study,[68] 72 patients with heterozygous familial hypercholesterolemia were studied in a controlled trial to test whether reducing plasma low-density lipoprotein levels by diet and combined drug
regimens could induce regression of coronary artery lesions. The drugs
used as monotherapy or in combination therapy were niacin, colestipol,
and lovastatin. Using computer-based quantitative angiography, 457
lesions were measured before and after a 26-month interval. The primary outcome variable was within-patient mean change in percent area
stenosis. Significant reductions in mean LDL-cholesterol were observed.
Control subjects showed progression of their lesions while the treatment
group showed regression. Of note was the observation that women on
drug treatment also showed regression of their lesions. The change
in percent area stenosis was correlated with low-density lipoprotein
changes.

In the third study,[69] the long-term effects of partial ileal bypass
surgery for the treatment of hyperlipidemia were assessed in survivors
of a first myocardial infarction over a 10-year period. Significantly less
progression of coronary artery lesions was observed in those patients
who had partial ileal bypass compared to those who did not, according
to a semiquantitative assessment of coronary angiograms obtained 3, 5,
7, and 10 years after study entry. Ileal bypass surgery was shown to
produce a greater reduction in total and LDL-cholesterol levels and a
significant increase in HDL-cholesterol levels compared to the control
group. Also reported was a lower incidence of death from coronary
heart disease and recurrent nonfatal myocardial infarction in the surgical
group.

Although not directly comparable, these latter three studies[67-69]
present complementary information about the dynamic evolution of
coronary atherosclerosis and its lipid determinants.[70] The studies suggest that lowering of lipid levels can reduce clinical cardiovascular
events and that these benefits are associated with less progression and
more regression of coronary artery lesions.[70]

Recent studies have also demonstrated that LDL-apheresis in the
management of familial hypercholesterolemia could reverse and prevent
atherosclerotic lesions in blood vessels.[71]

Dietary Clinical Trials to Lower Serum Cholesterol

The National Cholesterol Education Program[72] has identified dietary treatment as the first step in the treatment of elevated serum cholesterol, recognizing that not all patients will be responsive to such treatment. Dietary therapy is designed to reduce elevated cholesterol levels without sacrificing a nutritionally adequate eating pattern. High intake of saturated fat, cholesterol, and calories in excess of body requirements are implicated as contributing to elevated plasma cholesterol. Rationale for current recommendations for dietary modification are based to a large extent on extrapolation of data from population-based observational studies as well as results from smaller, controlled dietary trials.

Composition of Fatty Acids: Effect on Serum Cholesterol

Saturated, polyunsaturated, and monounsaturated fats are thought to raise, lower, and have no effect on serum cholesterol, respectively. Grundy[73] has postulated that monounsaturated fats (such as olive and rapeseed oil), consisting mainly of oleic acid, lower serum cholesterol as much as polyunsaturated fats, which consist mainly of lineolic acid, with the added benefit of maintaining heart-protective HDL-cholesterol levels. In a test of this hypothesis, healthy men and women were randomly assigned to a diet high in monounsaturated or polyunsaturated fat that had been preceded by an induction diet high in saturated fat.[74] The monounsaturated diet lowered LDL-cholesterol as effectively as the polyunsaturated diet in both men and women. In men only, both diets slightly lowered HDL-cholesterol.

A recent study by Mensink and Katan[75] examined the effect of dietary trans fatty acids on high-density and low-density lipoprotein cholesterol levels in healthy subjects. These fatty acids are formed by commercial hydrogenation processes in which polyunsaturate-rich marine and vegetable oils are hardened. In the United States, consumption of dietary trans fatty acids averages about 8 to 10 g per day or approximately 6% to 8% of total daily fat intake, much of it in the form of margarine. When normocholesterolemic men and women consumed 3-week cycles of mixed natural diets of identical nutrient composition

(10% of daily energy intake was supplied either as oleic acid, trans isomers of oleic acid, or saturated fatty acids) lipid profiles were shown to be affected adversely by the trans fatty acid diet. The trans fatty acid diet depressed mean HDL-cholesterol level and elevated mean LDL-cholesterol level in comparison to the oleic acid diet. HDL-cholesterol level on the saturated fat diet was the same as when subjects consumed the oleic acid diet. The investigators concluded that since trans fatty acids affected the serum lipid profiles of subjects at least as unfavorably as the cholesterol-raising saturated fatty acids, patients at increased risk of atherosclerosis should consider limiting intake of this type of fat.

The American Heart Association Step-one diet (30% total calories from fat, supplied as 10% saturated, 10% monounsaturated, and 10% polyunsaturated fats with 250 mg cholesterol/d) was compared with a monounsaturated-enriched Step-one diet (38% total calories from fat, supplied as 10% saturated, 18% monounsaturated, and 10% polyunsaturated fats with 250 mg cholesterol/d) in a randomized double-blind trial with healthy young men.[76] Plasma total cholesterol level was reduced in both groups, with parallel reductions in LDL cholesterol levels. Plasma triglyceride and HDL-cholesterol levels remained unchanged with both diets.

Stearic acid contributes substantially to the fatty acid composition in beef and other animal products. In a metabolic ward study in men,[77] stearic acid was found to be as effective as oleic acid in lowering plasma cholesterol, when either replaced palmitic acid. These findings have implications for the use of lean beef as a meat choice in a lipid-lowering diet.[78]

The favorable effects of polyunsaturated fat on serum cholesterol have been counterbalanced by evidence that high intake not only tends to lower HDL levels but may promote gallstone formation.[79] Animal studies have also shown suppression of the immune system and enhancement of tumor formation to be associated with increases in dietary polyunsaturates.[79]

Clearly, research remains equivocal on certain key issues, e.g., (1) the most effective macronutrient composition of a lipid-lowering diet and (2) the relationship of exogenous cholesterol to serum lipid levels. The influence of additions to the diet of such substances as fish oil and fiber will be discussed in the following sections.

Omega-3 Polyunsaturated Fatty Acids: The Effects of Fish Oil on CHD

Investigation into therapeutic properties of dietary fish oils originated from observational studies in Greenland Eskimos[80] that reported decreased disease rates from CHD despite a high-fat diet. This traditional diet was determined to contain a high intake of dietary fish oils, rich in omega-3 fatty acids, including eicosapentaenoic (EPA) and docosahexaenoic (DHA) acids. Hopes have been raised for these oils as potential preventive or therapeutic agents in CHD.[81]

The reduction of circulating triglyceride levels[82] seen with addition to the diet of omega-3 fatty acids may be due to (1) inhibition of synthesis of VLDL-triglyceride, (2) suppression in VLDL-cholesterol apolipoprotein B and VLDL-cholesterol formation, (3) reduction of hepatic VLDL-cholesterol secretion, or (4) enhanced fecal steroid excretion. These mechanisms are thought to increase peripheral VLDL-cholesterol triglyceride clearance.[19,82] Moderate or large doses of dietary fish oil prolong bleeding time in normal subjects, which may be due to inhibition of platelet aggregation.[82]

Animal Studies

Suppression of atherosclerosis with omega-3 fatty acid supplementation has been reported in a number of species. In a study investigating the progression of atherosclerosis,[83] fish oil was fed to rhesus monkeys in combination with diets of proven atherogenicity. Fish oil markedly reduced serum cholesterol levels and inhibited atherosclerosis, despite diet-induced depression of HDL levels, compared to animals fed the same diet without supplementation.

The addition of cod liver oil to a highly atherogenic butter diet in swine drastically reduced atherosclerotic lesion development.[84] Overall plasma cholesterol levels were only modestly reduced, but distribution of cholesterol in the various lipoprotein classes was substantially altered. In contrast to human studies, plasma triglycerides were not remarkably reduced, and although overall LDL-cholesterol levels increased, there was still a marked retardation of atherogenesis.

Human Studies

Comparison of men from a fishing village to those from a farming village in rural Japan[85] revealed a lower incidence of thrombotic cardiovascular disorders in the fishing village. Diets of fishing village residents were significantly higher in EPA and DHA. Platelet aggregability was also markedly reduced in relation to high fish intake.

Consumption of as little as two fish dishes per week was related to decreased death from CHD during 20 years of follow-up of the Zutphen cohort of the Seven Countries Study.[86] Mortality from CHD was lower by more than 50% in men who ate at least 30 g of fish per day compared to those who did not.

A dose-response relationship between consumption of fish and blood lipids was demonstrated by Hanninen et al.[87] In a study with healthy young men, consumption of as little as 1.5 fish-containing meals per week favorably modified lipid and prostanoid metabolism.

In patients with type IIb (hypercholesterolemia and moderately elevated triglycerides) and type V hyperlipidemia (hyperchylomicronemia), a fish oil supplemented diet led to decreases in plasma cholesterol and triglycerides. In the type V patients, a vegetable oil diet rapidly and significantly raised plasma triglyceride levels.[88]

Data from studies of diabetic subjects raise concerns about the advisability of fish oil supplementation for certain patients. In type II (NIDDM) diabetic patients not treated with insulin or sulfonylurea agents, supplementation at the dose of 8 g/d significantly improved plasma triglyceride levels, but increased both fasting and meal-stimulated glucose concentrations.[89] In a double-blind, placebo-controlled trial,[89] dietary supplementation with MaxEPA capsules (a commercial formulation of omega-3 fatty acids) was associated with improvement in hypertriglyceridemia, but deterioration in glycemic control. In their review of 10 published studies of fish oil supplementation in diabetic subjects, Hendra et al[90] conclude that fish oil cannot be recommended to NIDDM subjects as an aid to reducing cardiovascular risk.

At this time, there is no consensus advocating fish oil supplementation to the general diet. Some studies have demonstrated adverse lipid changes, and spontaneous or excessive bleeding, vitamin E deficiency, and with some preparations, Vitamin A and D toxicity have been reported.[82] There is also concern about contamination of fish products secondary to environmental pollution.[72] Commercial availability, combined with questionable health benefit claims on the part of manufacturers, have led to recent restrictions on the advertising of these products,[84] but use of fish as a lean meat is recommended as part of the Step-one dietary plan.

Increased restriction on the advertising of omega-3 fatty acid supplements may decrease self-medication by patients. However, research suggests that fish oils may favorably modulate aspects of the atherogenic process,[82] and therefore may prove to be clinically useful in averting myocardial infarction. In addition, patients with elevated triglyceride levels and a secondary elevation in cholesterol values may derive benefit from this type of supplementation.

Lipid-Lowering Properties Of Dietary Fiber

Dietary fiber may be divided into two major categories, water-insoluble and water-soluble (see Chapter 9). Insoluble fiber is the primary fiber in vegetables, wheat, and most grain products. Fruits, oats, barley, and legumes are high in soluble fiber, and oat bran and dried beans are particularly high sources.

Insoluble fiber has been shown to decrease intestinal transit time, increase fecal bulk, and delay glucose absorption and starch hydrolysis. Soluble fiber delays gastric emptying, increases intestinal transit time, slows glucose absorption, and lowers serum cholesterol. The cholesterol-lowering properties seem to be related to the binding of bile-acids in the intestine, which reduces cholesterol available for lipid synthesis. Soluble fiber is fermented in the colon into short-chain fatty acids, which are thought to inhibit cholesterol synthesis in the liver and increase clearance of LDL-cholesterol.[91]

Short-term studies of soluble fiber supplementation usually result in decreases of 11% to 19% of serum cholesterol.[91] In a metabolic ward study,[92] 100 g daily of oat bran lowered serum cholesterol in hypercholesterolemic men by 25% in 7 to 11 days. LDL-cholesterol was selectively lowered without significantly affecting HDL concentrations. Beans tended to lower HDL-cholesterol more than did oat bran, but the differences were not statistically significant. Oat bran supplemented diets have been associated with a decreased intake of calories, fat, and cholesterol. Significant decreases in total serum cholesterol of 10% to 17% were reported in hypercholesterolemic men and women in response to a low-fat, low-cholesterol diet supplemented with processed or unprocessed oat bran.[93]

In a study comparing the effects of high-fiber oat bran with a low-fiber refined wheat product in healthy subjects, Swain et al[94] found no evidence for specific cholesterol-lowering properties of oat bran. It was concluded that dietary grain supplements result in lowered cholesterol probably because they replace dietary fats.

Pectin, a water-soluble fiber derived from fruit, has also been shown to have hypocholesterolemic effects. In a review of 11 dietary studies[95] where subjects received at least 20 g of pectin per day, serum cholesterol levels were reduced 12% to 15%.

Guar gum has been shown to attenuate the postprandial rise in plasma triglycerols in rats[96] as well as diminishing ad libitum food intake, resulting in lower body weight. In hyperlipidemic men, 30 g/d of guar gum decreased mean LDL- cholesterol levels by 11.5% and mean total serum cholesterol by 9.6% over a 6-week trial period,[97] but considerable intersubject variability was noted. Following 4 weeks of guar therapy, supplied either in solid or liquid form, men with moderate hypercholesterolemia achieved significant reductions in total and LDL-cholesterol with no changes in triglyceride and HDL-cholesterol levels.[98]

Dietary fiber is thought to have a beneficial effect in the metabolic control of NIDDM. A high-fiber diet has been shown to significantly reduce fasting blood glucose levels and plasma cholesterol levels in comparison to a low-fiber diet in subjects with NIDDM.[99]

The current popularity of fiber supplementation is partially attributable to increased emphasis on high-fiber products by the media and advertising industry. Unfortunately, many commercial products advertised as "high fiber" also contain appreciable amounts of added fat. Increasing soluble fiber may modestly decrease cholesterol levels, but is not an alternative to a modified fat intake.

Alcohol

Moderation in alcohol consumption has been counseled by the Surgeon General.[100] Current evidence suggests that consumption of up to one to two drinks per day has not been associated with disease among healthy male and nonpregnant female adults. Data from population studies[101,102] suggest that light to moderate drinkers (based on self-report data) compared to those who abstain from alcohol are at reduced risk for coronary artery disease as well as nonfatal myocardial infarction.

Alcohol intake tends to increase HDL-cholesterol, however recent evidence suggests that alcohol has little effect on the HDL_2 subfraction, which is thought to confer protection against coronary artery disease. Hypertriglyceridemia is associated with alcohol abuse and alcoholism, and patients presenting with this lipid abnormality should be evaluated accordingly.

Diabetes, Glucose Tolerance, and Hyperlipidemia

Diabetes and hyperlipidemia frequently coexist, but the frequency of their coexistence is not related to genetic coinheritance.[103] Untreated or poorly controlled diabetes mellitus can result in hyperlipidemia. The associated lipid abnormalities include increased serum triglyceride and VLDL-cholesterol as well as VLDL-triglyceride values. HDL-cholesterol usually is decreased. These abnormalities appear to be related to the decrease in lipoprotein lipase activity associated with insulin deficiency. The elevation of triglycerides is directly related to reduced chylomicron clearance which is reversed with insulin therapy.

Hyperglycemia can cause nonenzymatic binding of glucose to LDL B apoprotein or apolipoprotein B. The excess production of apo B associated with diabetes may be independent of metabolic control. However, insulin deficiency has been directly related to decreased LDL-cholesterol catabolism. HDL-cholesterol levels are found to be decreased in noninsulin-dependent diabetes mellitus (NIDDM) but not in insulin-dependent diabetes mellitus (IDDM). Whether this difference is due to inherent factors or the coexistence of other risk factors in NIDDM such as obesity, inactivity, or medical treatment is not known.

In IDDM, diabetic ketoacidosis, acute insulin withdrawal, and elevated glycosylated hemoglobin levels have been associated with elevated triglyceride levels. Improving glycemic control with appropriate insulin therapy will reverse the lipid abnormalities associated with acute insulin deficiency. Individuals with insulin-dependent diabetes are eight-times more likely to have coronary disease than age- and sex-matched peers,[104] but this increased prevalence does not appear to be directly related to lipid abnormalities. Rather, the excess rate of coronary disease appears to be related to a combination of risk factors including hypertension and clotting abnormalities.

Coronary artery disease is reported as the cause of death in one third of all individuals with NIDDM. Obesity is present in an estimated 60%-90% of individuals with NIDDM, and the presence of obesity is closely linked to elevated triglyceride levels and lower HDL-cholesterol levels.[105] The exact cause of the high death rate from coronary disease in individuals with NIDDM is unknown. Possible mechanisms include glucose elevation, the coexistence of lipid abnormalities, and/or factors related to insulin.

Glucose intolerance has been associated with an increased risk of cardiovascular (coronary) mortality.[26] Elevated insulin levels have been associated with increased CHD.[106-108] This may be an indication that insulin itself or insulin resistance may be atherogenic. The elevated insulin levels may merely serve as a marker for some other unknown factor. Further investigation is required to determine the exact relationship between elevated endogenous insulin levels and atherosclerosis. It is not known whether use of high doses of exogenous insulin in treating diabetes increases atherosclerosis.

Changing Trends in American Dietary Habits

The trend toward increasing fat consumption in the United States appears to have reached its peak in the 1970s.[109] During the 1980s increased press coverage of nutritional issues made the American public more aware of the important relationship of fat intake with respect to disease. The National Institutes of Health conducted surveys of the American public[110] and physicians[111] regarding the importance of blood cholesterol in the development of heart disease. A large proportion of the public was concerned about lowering blood cholesterol even before the release of the data from the Lipid Research Clinics Coronary Primary Prevention Trial (LRC-CPPT),[49] but relatively few individuals knew their own cholesterol level. Physicians were considerably more skeptical about the importance of higher blood cholesterol levels before the release of the LRC-CPPT study that proved definitely that a 1% reduction in serum cholesterol reduced cardiovascular risk by 2%. When the surveys were repeated after the results of the LRC-CPPT trial were known, both physicians and the public were much more likely to be concerned about serum cholesterol levels. The National Cholesterol Education Program[72] has intensified the interest in cholesterol.

Consumer Concerns in Modifying Fat Intake

There has been a proliferation of product claims with respect to lowering serum cholesterol and/or cardiovascular risk. Foods laden with saturated fat have been promoted with label and advertising claims that such products were cholesterol free. Misinformation in many of these claims has made selection of prepared food suitable for a cholesterol-lowering diet virtually impossible.

Information about the fat content of foods tends to be confusing. Traditionally, food producers have listed the percentage of fat by volume. Consumers trying to select food items to achieve a total intake of less than 30% of calories from fat are forced to make several calculations at either the point of purchase and/or preparation. For example, whole milk contains less than 4% fat by volume, but approximately half of the calories are supplied as fat. Cheese and meat products are often promoted as containing only 20% or 30% fat (by volume) when actually 70% to 90% of the calories are derived from fat.

The Food and Drug Administration (FDA) has developed new labeling guidelines for food products[112] to facilitate consumer comparison of products. Labels with the total fat content, grams of saturated fat and cholesterol, and calorie information will be required on all food products. Standardization of portion sizes will also aid consumers in making product comparisons. Meat products will be exempt from these labeling regulations because meat labeling and inspection is regulated by the United States Department of Agriculture rather than the FDA. Fortunately, consumer trends have prompted the meat industry to develop leaner strains of cattle as well as to increase trimming of visible fat from packaged meat.[78]

Labels produced according to the new regulations should provide important nutritional information for a number of additional products. In addition, manufacturers have had restrictions imposed on making health claims for fish oil supplements and products containing oat bran.

Patient Education and Educational Resources

Nutritional Counseling

Increasing numbers of patients are expecting their physicians to provide nutrition education to aid them in achieving lower blood cholesterol levels. The NCEP[72] guidelines indicate that physicians should provide the first step of nutrition education for patients with borderline or high blood cholesterol levels who are at increased risk for cardiovascular disease. In some clinical practices, this role may be assumed by a nurse educator. Patients with more complex dietary problems or who need to progress to the NCEP[72] Step-two diet (total fat < 30% of total calories; saturated fatty acids < 7% of total calories) should be referred to a registered dietitian for more in-depth nutrition counseling and education.

An overview of the food patterns used in the NCEP Step-one program is presented in Table 1. For most patients with elevated blood cholesterol levels, providing a "diet instruction sheet" is inadequate. Physicians need to learn how to provide patients with a basic understanding of how to modify current intake to achieve a food pattern consistent with the NCEP Step-one plan. Conducting a brief dietary history is essential. Physicians can obtain an overview of current saturated fat intake by asking the patient to complete the dietary history outlined in Figure 1. A computerized version of a similar dietary history has been developed.[113] Issues related to the importance of assessing current dietary intake are reviewed in this chapter in the sections on indvidualizing dietary treatment goals and on adherence. If a patient reports daily consumption of several high fat items, setting specific goals for the weekly frequency of each item may be more realistic that trying to eliminate all such foods from the diet.

There are many common misperceptions about how to select foods low in saturated fat and/or cholesterol. An assessment of basic patient knowledge can be obtained using the test listed in Figure 2. Correction of knowledge deficits should include the rationale for the correct answers. Long-standing misconceptions may be easily corrected or may require a more in-depth educational effort. Educational materials containing terms in the text with multiple syllables such as cholesterol, saturated, and/or hydrogenated require a relatively high reading level. Preparation of low-literacy patient education materials may be necessary for utiliza-

How often do you eat:	Seldom or never ↓	1 or 2 times a week ↓	3 to 5 times a week ↓	Almost Daily ↓
1. Fried, deep-fat fried, or breaded foods?	☐	☐	☐	☐
2. Fatty meats such as bacon, sausage, luncheon meats, and heavily marbled steaks and roasts?	☐	☐	☐	☐
3. Whole milk, high-fat cheeses, and ice cream?	☐	☐	☐	☐
4. High-fat desserts such as pies, pastries, and rich cakes?	☐	☐	☐	☐
5. Rich sauces and gravies?	☐	☐	☐	☐
6. Oily salad dressings or mayonnaise?	☐	☐	☐	☐
7. Whipped cream, table cream, sour cream, and cream cheese?	☐	☐	☐	☐
8. Butter or margarine on vegetables, dinner rolls, and toast?	☐	☐	☐	☐

Figure 1: *Quick assessment of fat intake. (From United States Department of Agriculture Human Nutrition Information Service Home and Garden Bulletin Number 232-3, April 1986.)*

Please mark the following statement true or false	TRUE	FALSE
1. Fruits, vegetables, and most breads and cereals have little fat.	☐	☐
2. Fruits contain cholesterol.	☐	☐
3. Chicken without skin contains less fat than chicken with skin.	☐	☐
4. Cholesterol is found in both the lean and fat of meat.	☐	☐
5. Skim milk has almost no fat.	☐	☐
6. Cholesterol is found in both egg yolk and egg white.	☐	☐
7. Mozzarella cheese (part skim milk) has less fat than natural Cheddar cheese.	☐	☐
8. Chicken is a better choice than lean beef or pork to moderate dietary cholesterol.	☐	☐

Figure 2: *Patient test of nutritional knowledge. (From United States Department of Agriculture Human Nutrition Information Service Home and Garden Bulletin Number 232-3, April 1986.)*

Table 1.
Dietary Modifications for Hyperlipidemia Based on Step-One Diet Plan

Food Group	Choose	Recommended Daily Portions	Decrease
Eggs	Egg white or cholesterol-free egg substitute	Egg whites/substitutes may be used as required in recipes	Egg yolks limited to 2 or less per week
Dairy products and substitutes	Skim or 1% fat milk (liquid, powdered, or evaporated)	2 servings of nonfat or low-fat products (1 cup)	Whole (4%) milk, cream, half-and-half, 2% milk, most nondairy creamers, whipped toppings, whole-milk yogurt, regular cottage cheese (4% fat), natural cheeses (e.g., blue, roquefort, camembert, Swiss, cheddar, muenster, etc.), cream cheeses, sour cream, Ice cream, whole-milk frozen zogurt
	Buttermilk		
	Nonfat or low-fat yogurt		
	Low-fat (1% Or 2%) cottage cheese	Should contain no more than 2–6 g fat/oz	
	Farmer or pot cheese		
	Low-fat or "light" cream cheese	Limit to 2 times/week (1 tbs/serving)	
	Low-fat or "light" sour cream		
	Sherbert, sorbet, nonfat or low-fat frozen yogurt	Amount determined by weight control requirements	
Fish, poultry, meats	Fish and poultry without skin	6 oz or less	Fatty cuts of beef, lamb, pork spare ribs; organ meats; regular cold cuts; bacon; sausage; hot dog, sardines; roe.
	Lean cuts of beef, lamb, pork, veal		Fried foods should be avoided
	Shellfish		
	Prepare by broiling or baking with a minimum of added fat		

Meat alternatives	Beans, tofu (bean curd) Meatless meals should be used as often as possible, but should be prepared with a minimum of fat	Amount determined by weight control requirements	Avoid high-fat preparation, such as addition of cheese to recipes
Fats and oils	Polyunsaturated or monounsaturated vegetable oils; reduced cholesterol margarines; low-fat dressings; seeds and nuts; mayonnaise made with unsaturated oils	2–4 tbls	Butter and hydrogenated shortening, tropical fats (palm, coconut), bacon fat; chocolate; dressings made with egg yolk; coconut meat
Bread, cereals, grains	Whole grain products prepared without additional eggs or fat; rice; pasta Homemade baked goods with reduced oil	4 or more servings	Cereals with added tropical fats, most commercial baked goods, egg noodles
Fruits and vegetables	Fresh, frozen, canned, or dried Prepared with minimal or preferably no added fat	4 or more servings	Avoid fried vegetables, butter, or cream sauces

Table 2.
NCEP Step-one and Step-two Diet Plan

Calories/d	30% Total Fat (g)	Step-one 10% Saturated Fat (g)	Step-two 7% Saturated (g)
1200	40	13	9
1500	50	17	12
1800	60	20	14
2100	70	23	16
2400	80	27	19

tion in some clinical practices. For many patients, general guidance in food preparation may significantly alter dietary composition. Table 2 lists the number of grams of fat for various calorie levels based on NCEP guidelines for Step-one and Step-two diets.

Implementation of a diet plan should be preceded by assessment of overall goals for nutritional education, with special attention paid to adequacy of caloric intake and macronutrient distribution. Teaching begins once assessment is completed and the practitioner has decided on the most appropriate educational approach for the patient. Diet counseling can often be accomplished in three sessions, with the first devoted to history taking and goal setting and the next two to assessing progress. Patients who need to lose weight may require more time, support, and reinforcement over a longer period.

Assessing Adherence to Dietary Modification

Practitioners engaged in patient counseling should periodically evaluate the patient for "predictors of adherence,"[114,115] which include external obstacles to and support for dietary change, as well as patient strengths and weaknesses that may affect ability to achieve desired goals. Questions about involvement of others in food selection, preparation, and consumption should be included in the dietary history, as this may impact on a patient's ability to adhere to a diet plan. Structural obstacles such as work schedules should also be considered.

Information on food composition and methods of behavior modification should form the basis of counseling sessions. Adherence to dietary plan is assessed with a variety of tools, including the diet record, 24-hour dietary recall, and a behavioral diary. Patient progress is monitored through achievement of treatment objectives such as target

Table 3.
Techniques for Assessing Dietary Adherence

Sources of Information	Pros	Cons
Self-Report		
24-hour recall	Easily obtained; involves	Subject to participant
Food records	patient in assessment	bias; social desirability
Food frequency		of trying to please
questionnaire		practitioner
Self-reported deviations		
from dietary plan		
Collateral Information		
Questionnaire or	Can reveal	Subject to similar bias as
interview with	inconsistencies in	above; may create
significant other or care	self-report and focus on	conflict if not consistent
providers	forgotten or omitted	with patient self-report
	items	
Objective Data/		
** Physiological**		
** Outcome Measures**		
Blood tests	Theoretically not subject	Measures may not
Body weight	to perceptual biss;	accurately reflect dietary
	objective measure may	intake or behavior
	be a marker for risk or	
	represent a goal by	
	which patient and	
	provider measure	
	success	

weight, lipid levels, blood pressure, etc., which are then used to reinforce desirable behaviors (see Table 3).

When home preparation of foods traditionally or habitually includes a large proportion of fried and other high fat items, guidance in food preparation is needed. Table 4 lists food preparation tips to reduce total and saturated fat and cholesterol.

Individualization of Dietary Prescription

In clinical practice, the results of dietary instruction to patients with hypercholesterolemia may appear to vary widely. Some of the variability may be due to physiological responsiveness to dietary modification, but much of the variability may be predictable based on lipid

---

Table 4.
Tips to Reduce Fat in The Diet

Eat Less Fat

Eat smaller servings of meat. Eat fish and poultry more often. Choose lean cuts of red meat.

Prepare all meats by roasting, baking, or broiling. Trim off all fat. Be careful of added sauces or gravy. Remove skin from poultry.

Avoid fried foods. Avoid adding fat in cooking.

Eat fewer high-fat items such as cold cuts, bacon, sausage, hot dogs, butter, margarine, nuts, salad dressing, lard, and solid shortening.

Drink skim or low-fat milk.

Eat less ice cream, cheese, sour cream, whole milk, and other high-fat dairy products.

Eat More High-Fiber Foods

Choose dried beans, peas, and lentils more often.

Eat whole grain breads, cereals, and crackers.

Eat more vegetables—raw and cooked.

Eat whole fruit in place of fruit juice.

Try other high-fiber foods, such as oat bran, barley, bulgur, brown rice, wild rice.

Adapted from "Healthy Food Choices" Copyright 1986 American Diabetes Association, Inc.; The American Dietetic Association.

profile, dietary history, and the ability and willingness of the patient to make dietary changes. Table 5 lists the potential impact of effects of nutrition intervention on plasma lipoproteins, lipids, and glucose levels.

Consideration of Lipid Profile in Dietary Modification

The controversy about the relative merits of polyunsaturated versus monounsaturated fatty acids in the diet is far from resolved.[116] Clinical recommendations may need to be partially based on the lipid profile of the patient. The patient with an elevated LDL-cholesterol value and normal to high HDL may respond well to increasing intake of oil, nuts, or margarine rich in polyunsaturated fat. However, the patient with a low HDL-cholesterol level may experience a further decrease.

Table 5.
Effects of Nutrition Intervention on Plasma Lipids and Lipoproteins

Dietary Manipulation	VLDL Lipoprotein	LDL Lipoprotein	HDL Lipoprotein	Total Triglycerides	Total Cholesterol	Blood Glucose
Reducing calorie intake	Decrease	Possible secondary decrease	Increase with weight loss	Decrease	Variable	Probable decrease, especially in insulin resistance
Reducing proportion of fat	Effect depends on other macronutrients	Possible decrease	Possible decrease	Possible increase / Decrease in type I, III and V lipid disorders	Variable	Possible decrease fasting level NIDDM; Possible increase postprandial
N-3 Fatty acid supplementation	Probable decrease	Possible secondary decrease	Possible transient increase	Probable decrease if elevated	Possible secondary decrease	Probable increase with > ideal body weight
Increasing proportion monounsaturates	No direct effect	Moderate decrease	No direct effect	No direct effect	No direct effect	No direct effect
Increasing proportion polyunsaturates	No direct effect	Moderate to major decrease	Possible decrease	No direct effect	Decrease	No direct effect

Table 5.—Continued
Effects of Nutrition Intervention on Plasma Lipids and Lipoproteins

Increasing carbohydrate intake	Possible increase	No direct effect	Equivocal effect	Possible increase	No direct effect	May increase postprandial; Possible decrease fasting NIDDM
Increasing dietary fiber	May modulate effect of increasing carbohydrate intake	(Soluble) Possible modest decrease	No direct effect	No direct effect	(Soluble) Possible modest decrease	(Soluble) Decrease postprandial; possible second effect
Alcohol	Increase	No direct effect	Possible increase with moderate intake	Possible increase	No direct effect	May increase if insulin-deficient; May induce hypoglycemia if glucose is normal

When dietary fat is decreased the proportion of calories from carbohydrate usually increases. For patients with moderate triglyceridemia increasing carbohydrate intake may further elevate triglyceride levels. If the hypertriglyceridemia is severe, as is found in type V hyperlipoproteinemia, decreasing dietary fat and concomitantly increasing carbohydrate intake may help correct the lipid disorder. Table 6 summarizes dietary recommendations for different forms of hyperlipidemia.

Obesity

NCEP[72] guidelines include reduction of excess body weight as part of the Step-one plan. Increase in body fat has been associated with the observed age-related increase in total cholesterol and decrease in HDL-cholesterol.[117] For the obese patient with elevated cholesterol associated with hypertriglyceridemia, reducing calorie intake is likely to decrease VLDL production, in turn reducing VLDL-cholesterol and secondarily impacting on LDL-cholesterol and HDL-cholesterol levels. In the patient with normal triglyceride values, the impact on cholesterol may not be clinically significant. More important, decreasing fat intake often leads to weight loss which tends to improve the lipid profile.

Dietary Treatment Issues in Diabetes

Achieving metabolic control in diabetes involves normalization of lipid levels as well as glucose levels. The dietary management of diabetes has evolved from an emphasis on restricting carbohydrates to an emphasis on the quality of fat and carbohydrates. In 1971 the American Diabetes Association[118] recommended that the emphasis of dietary treatment of diabetes shift from the previous prescription of 40% of calories from carbohydrates and 40% of calories from fat to a focus on modifying fat intake in order to reduce atherosclerosis. Current recommendations[119] are consistent with the Step-one diet of the NCEP[72] and the dietary recommendations of the American Heart Association. Increasing carbohydrate intake may increase postprandial glucose levels. Focusing foods rich in fiber and with a relatively low glycemic impact will help modulate the potential negative effect.

In 1986 the American Diabetes Association[119] recommended that dietary treatment goals be tailored to the individual patient profile.

Table 6.
Dietary Therapy for Different Types of Hyperlipidemia

Primary or Polygenic (Nonfamilial) Hypercholesterolemia
Cholesterol > 240 mg/dl–300 mg/dl; LDL level > 160 mg/dl
Reduce intake of total fat to 30% calories
Reduce saturated fat to < 10% calories
Reduce dietary cholesterol to > 200 mg/d
Aim of dietary therapy: reduction of LDL level to at least 140 mg/dl
Failure of dietary therapy may indicate addition of drug therapy, especially if
    other risk factors are present

Familial Hypercholesterolemia
Heterozygous: patient inherits only half normal number of LDL receptors
LDL concentration approx. twice normal CHD often develops in young adults
Patients usually respond to dietary therapy
Reduce saturated fat < 10% and preferably < 7% total calories
Reduce dietary cholesterol < 200 mg/d
Keep polyunsaturated fats < 10% total calories
Complementary drug therapy needed in most patients

Homozygous: No Functioning LDL Receptors (Extremely Rare)
Cholesterol levels about four times normal
Severe disease frequently occurs in teenage patients
Patients essentially unresponsive to dietary modification

Dietary Hypercholesterolemia
Total cholesterol > 200 mg/dl but < 240 mg/dl
Reduce saturated fat to < 10% calories
Reduce dietary cholesterol to < 300 mg/d
Overweight individuals should try to achieve desirable body weight
Drug therapy rarely indicated

Familial Combined Hyperlipidemia
Occurs in about 10% of patients with CHD
May occur in about 1% of entire population
Characterized by multiple lipoprotein phenotypes within single family
Many affected patients are obese and weight reduction can reduce
    circulating lipids in these patients
Decreased intake of saturated fat and cholesterol considered prudent, but bene-
    fit in disorder has not been proved
Patients with hypertriglyceridemia should avoid diets high in carbohydrates
    and alcohol

Familial Hypertriglyceridemia
Plasma triglycerides range from 250–500 mg/dl; may be up to 1000 mg/dl
Plasma VLDL usually elevated

Table 6.—Continued
Dietary Therapy for Different Types of Hyperlipidemia

Total cholesterol levels frequently < 240 mg/dl, unless triglyceride levels are
substantially > 500 mg/dl
Weight reduction indicated if overweight
Avoid excessive intake of carbohydrates and alcohol
Drug therapy not required

Primary Hyperchylomicronemia
Type I hyperlipoproteinemia of "fat-induced" hyperlipidemia:
Severe hypertriglyceridemia and chylomicronemia with relatively normal VLDL
Very rare; usually manifests clinically in infancy or childhood
Primary purpose of therapy to prevent pancreatitis
Total fat should be reduced to < 10% total calories
Drug therapy not useful

Type V Hyperlipoproteinemia
Chylomicrons and VLDL are increased
Occurs most often in adults
Primary purpose of therapy to prevent pancreatitis
Total fat should be reduced to < 15% total calories
Drug therapy often indicated

Adapted from Grundy SM: Dietary therapy for different forms of hyperlipoproteinemia. Circulation 1987;
76; 3: 523–528.

Conversion factor for cholesterol is 0.02586 mm/L for 1 mg/dl. Conversion factor for triglycerides is
0.01129 mm/L for 1 mg/dl.

Unfortunately, there may be many individuals with diabetes and elevated lipid levels for whom dietary treatment has only targeted carbohydrate restriction rather than addressed comprehensive medical needs.

Dietary Modification for Women

Although it has been concluded that risk factors predicting CHD
in women are essentially the same as those for men,[120] the epidemiology
and biology of CHD in women requires further study to understand
the large gender differential seen in most westernized countries. There
is a paucity of clinical trials of women and dietary modification. This
has raised concerns that the decreases in HDL-cholesterol observed with

low-fat diets may undermine what seems to be a sex-specific advantage women currently enjoy and consequently increase risk.[121] A multicenter 2-year trial[122] of a very low-fat diet (20% of calories) studied the relationship of dietary fat to incidence of breast cancer in one of the few studies to exclusively use women as subjects. Average total cholesterol was significantly reduced in the intervention group with no reports of any serious health effects. However, CHD endpoints were not evaluated. Evidence of strong motivation on the part of subjects was seen in the high attendance rates during the extended trial.

Older Patients

Data from the aging Framingham cohort[123] indicate that cholesterol levels continue to predict CHD incidence and mortality in older men and women, but the relationship diminishes in strength with age. It has been suggested that active medical management of older hypercholesterolemic patients be restricted to those most likely to benefit from long-term therapy, the first step of which should be dietary modification.[124] Men aged 50 to 89 were placed on either a diet high in polyunsaturated and low in saturated fatty acids or a control diet.[51] Mean serum cholesterol levels were significantly reduced on the low-fat diet, and men with high initial values showed significant reduction in coronary clinical events when compared with controls. This benefit was not seen in subjects with initial low levels of serum cholesterol during 8 years of observation.

Although a smaller percentage of CHD cases may be amenable to prevention by cholesterol reduction in older versus younger patients, the short-term potential benefit of treatment (expressed in terms of number of events prevented annually per 1000 treated) tends to be greater in older than in younger patients.[125]

The addition of fiber to the diets of older patients may help protect against disorders of the colon, including constipation, diverticulosis, diverticulitis, and cancer, which are common in the elderly.[126] Attention should also be given to energy balance, and reduction of excess weight should be encouraged.[72]

Children and Adolescents

The recent report of the Expert Panel on Blood Cholesterol Levels in Children and Adolescents[127] reviewed the evidence that atherosclerosis or its precursors begin in young people; that elevated cholesterol levels early in life play a role in the development of adult atherosclerosis; that eating patterns and genetics affect blood cholesterol levels and CAD risk; and that lowering levels in children and adolescents will be beneficial. Cholesterol was the focus of the report, but the panel also emphasized that attention be given to cigarette smoking, hypertension, obesity, diabetes mellitus, and exercise.[127]

The panel recommended an approach for cholesterol lowering in all children and adolescents through population-wide changes in nutrient intake and eating patterns.[127] In children and adolescents, it was recommended that nutritional adequacy be achieved by eating a wide variety of foods that are adequate to support growth and development and to reach or maintain desirable body weight. A pattern of nutrients was recommended (Table 7).[127]

The panel's recommendations were not intended for infants from birth to 2 years of age where a higher percentage of calories from fat is required.[127]

Diet therapy is the primary approach to treating children and adolescents with high cholesterol (Chapter 1).[127] Diet therapy is prescribed in two steps that progressively reduce the saturated fatty acid and cholesterol intake. The Step-one diet calls for the same nutrient intake shown in Table 7. Instruction on the Step-one diet requires detailed assessment of current eating patterns and instruction by a physician, dietician, or nurse.[127] If the minimal goals of therapy are not reached with careful adherence to this diet for at least 3 months (Chapter 1), then a Step-two diet should be prescribed. This entails further reduction of the saturated fatty acid intake to less than 7% of calories, and of the cholesterol intake to less than 200 mg a day. Adoption of the Step-two diet requires careful nutritional planning by a registered dietician or other qualified nutrition professional.[127]

Table 7.
Recommended Nutrient Intake in Children and Adolescents

Saturated	Fatty	< 10% calories
Acids		Average no more than
Total Fat		30%
	Polyunsaturated	Up to 10%
	Monounsaturated	10–15%
Cholesterol		< 300 mg/day

Adapted from Reference 125 with permission.

Referral to a Dietitian

Utilization of a dietitian may be necessary to effect constructive changes in patient diets.[128,129] Some patients find it difficult to modify long-standing food preferences and need consultation with a nutritional specialist to address specific issues. Varying degrees of competence can be found among individuals who offer nutritional counseling, and many physicians face the problem of determining whether a person practicing "nutrition" has the appropriate qualifications and expertise.

A registered dietitian (R.D.) will have at least a bachelor's and sometimes a master's degree, with course work in biochemistry, physiology, food science, and counseling techniques. The candidate must pass a written qualifying examination after prerequisite credentials have been reviewed by the Commission of Dietetic Registration of the American Dietetic Association. In addition, a minimum of 6 months of clinical experience under supervision of a registered dietitian is required.

Many hospital-based dietitians also offer outpatient dietary consultation and may be contacted through a hospital dietary department or nutrition support service. Fees vary widely, but consultations may sometimes be provided free of charge. Written referral is usually required, and services may be limited to patients referred by physicians on staff. In general, third-party reimbursement is not available for nutritional counseling, but some insurance companies may cover services if the physician provides a letter indicating such services are a "medical necessity."

Increasing numbers of dietitians maintain private practices in addition to hospital positions, offering services during evenings or weekends. Fees often are higher than hospital-based consultations in the same area, although the fee often includes a two-visit initial consultation. Once a qualified dietitian has been found, techniques should be discussed to determine if there is a compatible approach to patient counseling. A physician who is most comfortable with exchange lists, for example, may not wish to refer patients to a dietitian who exclusively uses behavior modification as a counseling method.

Effective communication between medical staff and the dietitian is critical, and the dietitian should be provided with current lipid level information on each patient in counseling. A written consultation report should be provided to the referring physician once evaluation has been completed by the dietitian, which can then become part of the patient's permanent medical record.

It should be emphasized that for many patients, modification of dietary practices may occur very slowly and change may be barely perceptible to the clinician. On the positive side, even seemingly insignificant dietary changes may have considerable impact on a patient's health status. Desirable behavior should be consistently reinforced with positive feedback, and treatment goals should be negotiated in a supportive framework. Successful dietary modification can avert the need for pharmacological therapy in a substantial number of hypercholesterolemic patients,[130] as well as serving as primary prevention for normolipidemic patients currently consuming a "traditional American diet."

References

1. Anitschkow NN: A history of experimentation on arterial atherosclerosis in animals. In Blumenthal HT (ed): Cowdry's Arteriosclerosis. Second edition. Springfield, Illinois, CC Thomas, 1967; 21-44.
2. Wissler RW, Vesselinovitch D: Evaluation of animal models for the study of the pathogenesis of atherosclerosis. In Hauss WH, Wissler RW, Lehmann R (eds): International Symposium: State of Prevention and Therapy in Human Arteriosclerosis and in Animal Models. Germany, Westdeutscher Verlag, 1977; 13-29.
3. Yamori Y, Horie R, Nara Y, et al: Nutritional causation and prevention of cardiovascular disease: experimental evidence in animal models and man. In Lovenberg W, Yamori Y (eds):Nutritional Prevention of Cardiovascular Disease. Orlando, Academic Press, 1984; 37-51.
4. Miller GJ: The epidemiology of plasma lipoproteins and atherosclerotic disease. In Miller NE, Lewis B (eds): Lipoproteins, Atherosclerosis and Coronary Heart Disease. The Netherlands, Elsevier, 1981; 59-71.
5. Blackburn H: Epidemiologic evidence for the causes and prevention of atherosclerosis. In Steinbeg D, Olefsky JM (eds): Hypercholesterolemia and Atherosclerosis: Pathogenesis and Prevention. Contemporary Issues in Endocrinology and Metabolism; 3. New York, Churchill Livingstone, 1987; 53-98.
6. Stokes J: Cardiovascular risk factors. In Frohlich E (ed): Preventive Aspects of Coronary Heart Disease. Cardiovascular Clinics 20;3: Philadelphia, FA Davis, 1990; 3-20.
7. Vesselinovitch D, Wissler RW: Prevention and regression in animal models by diet and cholestyramine. In Hauss WH, Wissler RW, Lehmann R (eds): International Symposium: State of Prevention and Therapy in Human Arteriosclerosis and in Animal Models. Germany, Westdeutscher Verlag, 1977; 127-134.

8. Gordon T: The diet-heart idea: outline of a history. Am J Epidemiol 1988; 2: 220-225.
9. Manalo-Estrella P, Cox GE, Taylor CB: Atherosclerosis in rhesus monkeys. VII. Mechanism of hypercholesterolemia: hepatic cholesterolgenesis and the hypercholesterolemic threshold of dietary cholesterol. Arch Pathol 1963; 76: 413-423.
10. Toda T, Fukuda N, Sugano M: Morphological evaluation of the atherogenicity of corn oil, hydrogenated corn oil and butter fat in quail. J Nutr Sci Vitaminol 1988; 34: 615-626.
11. Benade AJ, Fincham JE, Smuts CM, et al: Plasma low density lipoprotein composition in relation to atherosclerosis in nutritionally defined vervet monkeys. Atherosclerosis 1988; 74: 157-168.
12. Thomson ABR, Keelan M: Rechallenge following an early life exposure to a high-cholesterol diet enhances diet-associated alterations in intestinal permeability. J Pediatr Gastroenterol 1989; 9: 98-104.
13. McCormack Nolte CJ, Tercyak AM, Wu HM, et al: Chemical and physico-chemical comparison of advanced atherosclerotic lesions of similar size and cholesterol content in cholesterol-fed New Zealand white and Watanabe heritable hyperlipidemic rabbits. Lab Invest 1990; 62: 213-222.
14. Jayakody L, Senaratne MP, Thomson AB, et al: Persistent impairment of endothelium-dependent relaxation to acetylcholine and progression of atherosclerosis following 6 weeks of cholesterol feeding in the rabbit. Can J Physiol Pharmacol 1989; 67: 1454-1460.
15. Stamler J, Shekelle R: Dietary cholesterol and human coronary disease. The epidemiologic evidence. Arch Pathol Lab Med 1988; 112: 1032-1040.
16. Keys A, ed: Coronary heart disease in seven countries. Circulation 1970; 41 (Suppl.I): 211.
17. Keys A: Seven Countries: Death and Coronary Heart Disease in Ten Years. Cambridge, Harvard University, 1979.
18. Laurenzi M, Stamler R, Trevisan M, et al: Is Italy losing the 'Mediterranean advantage?" Report on the Gubbio population study: cardiovascular risk factors at baseline. Prev Med 1989; 18: 35-44.
19. Connor WE, Connor SL: Diet, atherosclerosis and fish oil. Adv Intern Med 1990; 35: 139-172.
20. Rotevatn S, Akslen LA, Bjelke E: Lifestyle and mortality among Norwegian men. Prev Med 1989; 18: 433-443.
21. Kesteloot H, Obasohan AO, Olomu A, et al: Serum lipid and apolipoprotein levels in a Nigerian population sample. Atherosclerosis 1989; 78: 33-38.
22. Kesteloot H, Geboers J, Joosens JV: On the within-population relationship between nutrition and serum lipids: the B.I.R.N.H. study. Eur Heart J 1989; 10: 196-202.
23. Tillotson JL, Hiroo Kato MA, Nichaman MZ, et al: Epidemiology of coronary heart disease and stroke in Japanese men living in Japan, Hawaii and California: methodology for comparison of diet. Fam J Clin Nutr 1973; 26: 177-184.
24. Kushi LH, Lew RA, Stare FJ, et al: Diet and 20-year mortality from coronary heart disease. The Ireland-Boston diet-heart study. N Engl J Med 1985; 312: 811-818.

25. Gordon T, Kagan A, Garcia-Palmieri M, et al: Diet and its relation to coronary heart disease and death in three populations. Circulation 1981; 63: 500-515.
26. Kannel WB, Castelli WP, Gordon T, et al: Serum cholesterol, lipoproteins and risk of coronary heart disease: the Framingham study. Ann Intern Med 1971; 74: 1-12.
27. Wilson WF: The epidemiology of hypercholesterolemia: a global perspective. Am J Med 1989; 87: S-13S.
28. Kroumhout D: Bosschieter EB, Drijver M, et al: Serum cholesterol and 25-year incidence of mortality from myocardial infarction and cancer: the Zutphen study. Arch Intern Med 1988; 148: 1051-1055.
29. Shekelle RB, MacMillan Shryock A, Paul O, et al: Diet, serum cholesterol and death from coronary heart disease: the Western Electric study. N Engl J Med 1981; 304: 65-70.
30. Stamler J, Wentworth D, Neaton JD: Is relationship between serum cholesterol and risk of premature death from coronary heart disease continuous and graded? Findings in 356,222 primary screenees of the Multiple Risk Factor Intervention Trial (MRFIT) JAMA 1986; 256: 2823-2828.
31. Pooling Project Research Group: Relationship of blood pressure, serum cholesterol, smoking habit, relative weight and ECG abnormalities to incidence of major coronary events: final report of the Pooling Project. J Chron Dis 1978; 31: 201-306.
32. Lipid Research Clinics population studies data book, Vol.1. The Prevalence Study 1980 (National Institutes of Health publication no.80-1527) Washington: United States Government Printing office, 1980. 1-134.
33. Solberg LA, Strong JP: Risk factors and atherosclerotic lesions: a review of autopsy studies. Arteriosclerosis 1983; 3: 187-198.
34. Reed DM, Resch JA, Hayashi T, et al: A prospective study of cerebral artery atherosclerosis. Stroke 1988; 19: 820-825.
35. Shimamoto T, Komachi Y, Inada H, et al: Trends for coronary heart disease and stroke and their risk factors in Japan. Circulation 1989; 79: 503-515.
36. Solberg LA, Ishii T, Strong JP, et al: Comparison of coronary atherosclerosis in middle-aged Norwegian and Japanese men. An autopsy study. Lab Invest 1987; 56: 451-456.
37. Gordon T, Fisher M, Ernst N, et al: Relation of diet to LDL cholesterol, VLDL cholesterol, and plasma total cholesterol and triglycerides in white adults. The Lipid Research Clinics prevalence study. Arteriosclerosis 1982; 2: 502-512.
38. Katan MB, Beynen AC: Characteristics of human hypo- and hyperresponders to dietary cholesterol. Am J Epidemiol 1987; 125: 387-399.
39. Ernst ND, Levy RI: Diet and cardiovascular disease. In Nutrition reviews' present knowledge in nutrition. Washington, D.C.: The Nutrition Foundation, 1984:724-739.
40. Armstrong ML, Heistad DD, Megan MB, et al: Reversibility of atherosclerosis. In Frohlich E (ed): Preventive Aspects of Coronary Heart Disease. Cardiovascular Clinics 20;3: Philadelphia: FA Davis, 1990; 113-126.
41. Armstrong ML, Warner ED, Connor WE: Regression of coronary atheromatosis in rhesus monkeys. Circ Res 1970; 27: 59-67.

42. Hirata M, Watanabe T: Regression of atherosclerosis in normotensive and hypertensive rabbits. A quantitative analysis of cholesterol-induced aortic and coronary lesions. Acta Pathol Jpn 1988; 38: 559-575.
43. Gotto AM: Cholesterol intake and serum cholesterol level. N Engl J Med 1991; 324: 912-913.
44. Keys A, Anderson JT, Grande F: Serum cholesterol response to changes in the diet. IV. Particular saturated fatty acids in the diet. Metabolism 1963; 14: 776-787.
45. Hegsted DM, McGrandy RB, Myers MI, et al: Quantitative effects of dietary fat on serum cholesterol in man. Am J Clin Nutr 1965; 17: 281-295.
46. National Diet-Heart Study Research Group: The national diet-heart study final report. Circulation 1968; 37 (Suppl 1): 3-419.
47. Blankenhorn DH: Prevention or reversal of atherosclerosis: review of current evidence. Am J Cardiol 1989; 63: 38H-41H.
48. La Ville AE, Seddon AM, Shaikh M, et al: Primary prevention of atherosclerosis by lovastatin in a genetically hyperlipidemic rabbit strain. Atherosclerosis 1989; 78: 205-210.
49. The Lipid Research Clinics Coronary Primary Prevention Trial Results. 1. Reduction in Incidence of Coronary Heart Disease. JAMA 1984; 251: 351.
50. Manninen V, Huttunen JK, Heinonen OP, et al: Relation between baseline lipid and lipoprotein values and the incidence of coronary heart disease in the Helsinki heart study. Am J Cardiol 1989; 63: 42H-47H.
51. Dayton S, Pearce ML, Hashimoto S, et al: A controlled clinical trial of a diet high in unsaturated fat in preventing complications of atherosclerosis. Circulation 1969; 40 (Suppl II): 163.
52. Hjermann I: Strategies for dietary and anti-smoking advice. Practical experiences from the Oslo study. Drugs 1988; 36: 105-109.
53. Tada M, Kuzuya T, Hoshida S, et al: Significance of thromboxane A2 and prostaglandin I2 in coronary artery disease. In Lovenberg W, Yamori Y (eds): Nutritional Prevention of Cardiovascular Disease. Orlando, Academic Press, 1984; 331-337.
54. Barnard RJ, Hall JA, Chaudhari A, et al: Effects of a low-fat, low-cholesterol diet on serum lipids, platelet aggregation and thromboxane formation. Prostaglandins Leukot Med 1987; 26: 241-252.
55. Tyroler HA: Overview of clinical trials of cholesterol lowering in relationship to epidemiologic studies. Am J Med 1989; 87 (Suppl 4A):14S-19S.
56. Peto R, Yusuf S, Collins R: Cholesterol-lowering trials results in their epidemiological context. Circulation 1985; 72 (Suppl 3): 451.
57. Tikkanen MJ, Pyorala K: Cholesterol reduction and coronary artery disease. An overview of clinical trials up to 1986. Drugs 1988; 36 (Suppl 3): 27-31.
58. O'Keefe JH, Lavie CJ, O'Keefe JO: Dietary prevention of coronary artery disease. Postgrad Med 1985; 6: 243-261.
59. Stein EA: Management of hypercholesterolemia. Approach to diet and drug therapy. Am J Med 1989; 87 (Suppl 4A): 20S-27S.
60. Grundy SM: Cholesterol and coronary heart disease. A new era. JAMA 1986; 256: 2849-2858.

61. Aschoff L: Lectures in pathology. Atherosclerosis, Lane lecture, San Francisco. New York, Hoeber, 1924.
62. Varainen I, Kanerva K: Arteriosclerosis and wartime. Ann Med Experimentalis et Biologiae Fenniae 1947; 36: 748.
63. Arntzenius AC, Kromhout D: Barth JD: et al: Diet, lipoproteins, and the progression of coronary atherosclerosis. The Leiden intervention trial. N Eng J Med 1985;312;13:805-810.
64. Blankenhorn DH, Johnson RL, Nessim SA, et al: The cholesterol lowering atherosclerosis study (CLAS): design, methods, and baseline results. Controlled Clin Trials 1987; 8: 356-387.
65. Cashin-Hemphill L, Mack WJ, Pagoda JM, et al: Beneficial effects of colestipol-niacin on coronary atherosclerosis. JAMA 1990; 264: 3013-3017.
66. Ornish D., et al: Can lifestyle reverse coronary heart disease? Lancet 1990; 336: 129-133.
67. Brown G, Albers JJ, Fisher LD, et al: Regression of coronary artery disease as a result of intensive lipid lowering therapy in men with high levels of apolipoprotein B. N Engl J Med 1990; 323: 1289-98.
68. Kane JP, Malloy MJ, Ports TA, et al: Regression of coronary atherosclerosis during treatment of familial hypercholesterolemia with combined drug regimens. JAMA 1990; 264: 3007-3012.
69. Buchwald H, Varco RL, Matts PJ, et al: Effects of partial ileal bypass surgery on mortality and morbidity from coronary heart disease in patients with hypercholesterolemia: report of the Program on the Surgical Control of the Hyperlipidemias (POSCH) N Engl J Med 1990; 323: 946-955.
70. Loscalzo J: Regression of coronary atherosclerosis. N Engl J Med 1990; 323: 1337-1339 (editorial).
71. Mabuchi H: Use of LDL-apheresis in the management of familial hypercholesterolemia. Curr Sci 1990; 1: 43-50.
72. Report of the National Cholesterol Education Program Panel on Detection, Evaluation, and Treatment of High Blood Cholesterol in Adults. Arch Intern Med 1988; 148: 36-69.
73. Grundy SM, Florentin L, Nix D, et al: Comparison of monounsaturated fatty acids and carbohydrates for reducing raised levels of plasma cholesterol in man. Am J Clin Nutr 1988; 47: 965-969.
74. Mensink RP, Katan MB: Effect of a diet enriched with monounsaturated or polyunsaturated fatty acids on levels of low-density and high-density lipoprotein cholesterol in healthy men and women. N Engl J Med 1989; 321: 436-441.
75. Mensink RP, Katan MB: Effect of dietary trans fatty acids on high-density and low-density lipoprotein cholesterol levels in healthy subjects. N Engl J Med 1990; 323: 439-445.
76. Ginsberg HN, Barr SL, Gilbert A, et al: Reduction of plasma cholesterol levels in normal men on an American Heart Association step 1 diet with added monounsaturated fat. N Engl J Med; 322; 9: 574-579.
77. Bonanome A, Grundy SM: Effect of dietary stearic acid on plasma cholesterol and lipoprotein levels. N Engl J Med 1988; 318: 1244-1248.
78. Sweeten MK, Cross HR, Smith GC, et al: Lean beef: impetus for lipid modifications. J Am Diet Assoc 1990; 90: 87-92.

79. Grundy SM, Brown WV, Dietschy JM, et al: Workshop III. Basis for dietary treatment. Circulation 1989; 80: 729-734.
80. Bang HO, Dyerberg J, Hyorne N: The composition of foods consumed by Greenlandic Eskimos. Acta Med Scand 1973; 200: 69-74.
81. Zhu BQ, Parmley WW: Modification of experimental and clinical athero-sclerosis by dietary fish oil. Am Heart J 1990; 119: 168-178.
82. Goodnight SH: Effects of dietary fish oil and omega-3 fatty acids on platelets and blood vessels. Semin Thromb Hemost 1988; 14: 285-289.
83. Davis HR, Bridenstine RT, Vesselinovitch D et al: Fish oil inhibits develop-ment of atherosclerosis in monkeys. Arteriosclerosis 1987; 7: 441-449.
84. Kim DN, Ho HT, Lawrence DA, et al: Modification of lipoprotein patterns and retardation of atherogenesis by a fish oil supplement to a hyperlipid-emic diet for swine. Atherosclerosis 1989; 76: 35-54.
85. Hirai A, Terano T, Tamura Y, et al: Eicosapentaenoic acid and adult dis-eases in Japan: epidemiological and clinical aspects. J Intern Med 1989; 225 (Suppl)1: 69-75.
86. Kromhout D, Bosschieter EB, Coulander CDL: The inverse relation be-tween fish consumption and 20-year mortality from coronary heart dis-ease. N Engl J Med 1985; 312: 1205-1209.
87. Hanninen OO, Agren JJ, Laitinen MV, et al: Dose response relationships in blood lipids during moderated freshwater fish diet. Ann Med 1989; 21: 203-207.
88. Phillipson BE, Rothrock DW, Connor WE, et al: Reduction of plasma lipids, lipoproteins, and apoproteins by dietary fish oils in patients with hypertriglyceridemia. N Engl Med 1985; 312: 1210-1216.
89. Friday KE, Childs MT, Tsunehara CH, et al: Elevated plasma glucose and lowered triglyceride levels from omega-3 fatty acid supplementation in type II diabetics. Diabetes Care 1989; 12: 276-281.
90. Hendra TJ, Britton ME, Roper DR, et al: Effects of fish oil supplements in NIDDM subjects: controlled study. Diabetes Care 1990; 13: 821-829.
91. Anderson JW, Gustafson NJ: High-carbohydrate, high-fiber diet: is it practical and effective in treating hyperlipidemia? Postgrad Med 1987; 82: 40-50.
92. Anderson JW, Gustafson NJ: Hypocholesterolemic effects of oat and bean products. Am J Clin Nutr 1988; 48: 749-753.
93. Demark-Wahnefried W, Bowering J, Cohen PS: Reduced serum choles-terol with dietary change using fat-modified and oat-bran supplemented diets. J Am Diet Assoc 1990; 90: 223-229.
94. Swain JF, Rouse IL, Curley CB, et al: Comparison of the effects of oat bran and low-fiber wheat on serum lipoprotein levels and blood pressure. N Engl J Med 1990; 322: 147-152.
95. Kay RM, Truswell AS: Dietary fiber: effects on plasma and biliary lipids in man. In Spiller GA, Kay RM (eds): Medical Aspects of Dietary Fiber. New York, Plenum, 1980; 153-173.
96. Deshaies Y, Begin F, Savoie L, et al: Attenuation of the meal-induced increase in plasma lipids and adipose tissue lipoprotein lipase by guar gum in rats. J Nutr 1990; 120: 64-70.

97. Turner PR, Tuomilehto J, Happonen P, et al: Metabolic studies on the hypolipidaemic effect of guar gum. Atherosclerosis 1990; 81: 145-150.

98. Superko HR, Haskell WL, Sawrey-Kubicek L, et al: Effects of solid and liquid guar gum on plasma cholesterol and triglyceride concentrations in moderate hypercholesterolemia. Am J Cardiol 1988; 62: 51-55.

99. Hagander B, Asp NG, Efendic S, et al: Dietary fiber decreases fasting blood glucose levels and plasma LDL concentration in noninsulin-dependent diabetes mellitus patients. Am J Clin Nutr 1988; 47: 852-858.

100. The Surgeon General's report on nutrition and health. U.S. Department of Health and Human Services public health service DHHS (PHS) publication no. 88-50210, 1988, 629-670.

101. Blackwelder WC, Yano K, Rhoads GG, et al: Alcohol and mortality; the Honolulu heart study. Am J Med 1980; 68: 164-169.

102. Yano KM, Rhoads GG, Kagan A: Coffee, alcohol and risk of coronary heart disease among Japanese men living in Hawaii. N Engl J Med 1977; 297: 405-409.

103. Dorman JS, LaPorte RE, Kuller LH, et al: The Pittsburgh insulin-dependent diabetes mellitus (IDDM) morbidity and mortality study: mortality results. Diabetes 1984; 33: 271-276.

104. Barrett-Connor E, Orchard T: Diabetes and heart disease. In Diabetes in America, National Diabetes Data Group, NIH publication no. 85-1468, August 1985.

105. National Diabetes Data Group: Classification and diagnosis for diabetes mellitus and other categories of glucose intolerance. Diabetes 1979; 28: 1039-1057.

106. Welborn TA: Coronary heart disease incidence and cardiovascular mortality in Busselton with reference to glucose and insulin concentrations. Diabetes Care 1979; 2: 154-162.

107. Grant N: Insulin and atherosclerosis. N Engl J Med 1979; 300: 679-680.

108. Pyorala K: Relationship of glucose tolerance and plasma insulin to the incidence of coronary heart disease: results from two population studies in Finland. Diabetes Care 1979; 2: 131-141.

109. Kahn HA: Changes in serum cholesterol associated with changes in the United States civilian diet, 1909-1965. Am J Clin Nutr 1970; 23: 879-882.

110. Schucker B, Bailey K, Heimbach JT, et al: Change in public perspective on cholesterol and heart disease. Results from two national surveys. JAMA 1987; 258: 3527-3529.

111. Schucker B, Wittes JT, Cutler JA, et al: Change in physician perspective on cholesterol and heart disease. Results from two national surveys. JAMA 1987; 258: 3521-3531.

112. Position of the American Dietetic Association: nutrition and health information on food labels. J Am Diet Assoc 1990; 90: 583-585.

113. Smucker R, Block G, Coyle L, et al: A dietary and risk factor questionnaire and analysis system for personal computers. Am J Epidemiol 1989; 129: 445-449.

114. Wylie-Rosett J, Wassertheil-Smoller S, Elmer P: Assessing dietary intake for patient education planning and evaluation. Pat Educ Counseling 1990; 15: 217-227.

115. Kristal AR, Shattuck AL, Henry HJ: Patterns of dietary behavior associated with selecting diets low in fat: reliability and validity of a behavioral approach to dietary assessment. J Am Diet Assoc 1990; 90: 214-220.
116. Willett W, Sacks FM: Chewing the fat. N Engl J Med 1991; 324: 121-123 (editorial).
117. Berns MAM, de Vries JHM, Katan MB: Increase in body fatness as a major determinant of changes in serum total cholesterol and high density lipoprotein in young men over a 10-year period. Am J Epidemiol 1989; 130: 1109-1122.
118. Wylie-Rosett J, Rifkin H: History of nutrition and diabetes. In Jovanovic L, Peterson CM (eds): Nutrition and Diabetes. New York, Alan Liss, 1985; 1-14.
119. American Diabetes Association: Nutritional recommendations for individuals with diabetes mellitus. Diabetes Care 1987; 10: 126-132.
120. Eaker ED, Packard B, Thom TJ: Epidemiology and risk factors for coronary heart disease in women. In Eaker ED, Packard B, Wenger NK, et al (eds): Coronary Heart Disease in Women. New York, Haymarket Doyma, 1987; 129-145.
121. Crouse JR: Gender, lipoproteins, diet, and cardiovascular risk. Sauce for the goose may not be sauce for the gander. Lancet 1989; Feb 11: 318-320.
122. Insull W, Henderson MM, Prentice R, et al: Results of a randomized feasibility study of a low-fat diet. Arch Intern Med 1990; 150: 421-427.
123. Cupples Al, D'Agostino RD: Some risk factors related to the annual incidence of cardiovascular disease and death using pooled repeated biennial measurements: Framingham heart study, 30-year follow-up: Section 34. In Kannel WB, Gordon T (eds): The Framingham study: An Epidemiologic Investigation of Cardiovascular Disease: Section 30, Washington D.C., U.S. Department of Health and Human Services, 1978 (DHHS publication (NIH) 87-2703).
124. Denke MA, Grundy SM: Hypercholesterolemia in elderly persons: resolving the treatment dilemma. Ann Intern Med 1990; 112: 780-792.
125. Gordon DJ, Rifkind BM: Treating high blood cholesterol in the older patient. Am J Cardiol 1989; 63: 48H-52H.
126. Cummings JH: Dietary fibre. Gut 1973; 14: 69-81.
127. National Cholesterol Education Program: Report of the Expert Panel on Blood Cholesterol Levels in Children and Adolescents. J Pediatr 1992; (in press).
128. Lorber D, Anastasio P: Integrating nutrition and medical practice. In Wassertheil-Smoller S, Alderman MH, Wylie-Rosett J (eds): Cardiovascular Health and Risk Management. The Role of Nutrition and Medication in Clinical Practice. Littleton, MA, PSG Publishing, 1989; 183-201.
129. Frank GC: Nutritional therapy for hyperlipidemia and obesity: office treatment integrating the roles of the physician and the registered dietitian. JACC 1988; 12: 1098-1101.
130. Carleton RA, Dwyer J, Finberg L, et al: Report of the Expert Panel on Population Strategy for Blood Cholesterol Reduction: A Statement from the National Cholesterol Education Program. Circulation 1991; 83: 2154-2232.

Chapter 3

Effects of Exercise on Lipid and Lipoprotein Levels

Marjorie F. Dannis M.D., William H. Frishman M.D.,
Eliot J. Lazar M.D.*

The complications of coronary artery disease (CAD) are the major causes of adult mortality and morbidity in the United States.[1] Evidence exists from both epidemiologic and prospective studies that a relationship exists between the occurrence of CAD and lipid and lipoprotein concentrations in the blood.[2,3] Favorable changes in lipids and lipoproteins have been shown to reduce the incidence of complications from CAD,[4,5] as well as retard the progression of atherosclerosis in patients with documented disease.[6-10]

From the results of epidemiologic studies, a strong inverse relationship between physical exercise and the prevalence and incidence of clinical CAD has been demonstrated.[1,5,11-17] This relationship has been thought to be independent of other risk factors for CAD, such as cigarette smoking, hypertension, obesity, and family history.[18] Both endurance and resistive exercise training have been implicated as important factors that can favorably affect serum lipid and lipoprotein levels.[18-24] It has been suggested, therefore, that some of the benefit of physical exercise on coronary heart disease risk might be influenced through activity-induced changes in lipids and lipoproteins.[18,19] Exercise can also cause improved glucose tolerance with increased insulin receptor

* Dr. Lazar contributed to this chapter prior to his appointment as a consultant to the Department of Health and Human Services. No official support or endorsement by HHS is intended or should be inferred.

From *Medical Management of Lipid Disorders: Focus on Prevention of Coronary Artery Disease*, edited by William H. Frishman, M.D. © 1992, Futura Publishing Inc., Mount Kisco, NY.

sensitivity,[18,25,26] a lowering of blood pressure,[14] and a reduction in blood hypercoagulability.[14,27]

The mechanism by which physical exercise affects plasma lipids and lipoproteins is not known. Some investigators have suggested that physical exercise may have a direct effect on the enzyme lipoprotein lipase, causing an increase in the activity of skeletal muscle and adipose tissue lipoprotein lipase (Fig. 1).[18] Exercise may also increase lipoprotein lipase activity through its effects on insulin receptor sensitivity.[18,19] The consequences of these actions on lipoprotein lipase activity would be

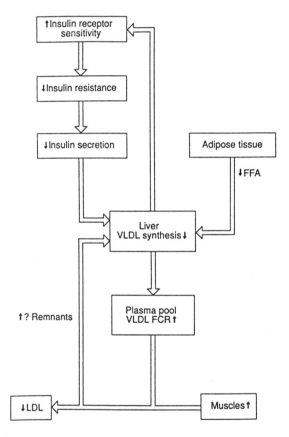

Figure 1: *Effects of endurance training on very-low density lipoprotein (VLDL) metabolism in relation to insulin and the pathogenesis of hypertriglyceridemia. FCR = fractional catabolic rate; LDL = low-density lipoprotein; LPLA = lipoprotein lipase activity. (Adapted from Julius and Hanefeld,[18] with permission.)*

to decrease very low-density lipoprotein (VLDL) levels and to increase high-density lipoprotein (HDL) concentrations.

In this chapter, the effects of physical exercise on lipids and lipoproteins in human beings are discussed.

Total and LDL-Cholesterol

Neither epidemiologic nor prospective studies have shown conclusively a direct relationship between exercise and cholesterol levels (Table 1), although individual studies have demonstrated a trend towards reduced levels of LDL.

Rauramaa and his associates[28] studied 60 males over a period of 8 weeks, and demonstrated a significant decrease in plasma LDL compared to a matched untrained control group. Ballantyne et al[29] studied the effects of exercise in 42 post-infarction patients, and in their controlled study were able to demonstrate a significant decrease in LDL levels with exercise compared to a control population. Other investigators also observed significant reductions in LDL after exercise[20,30] and have reported that those individuals with the highest initial pretraining LDL levels experienced the largest decreases in LDL following aerobic training.[30]

Some studies reported differences between sexes in the effects of aerobic training on LDL. Brownell et al[31] described a significant decrease in LDL of 6% in males following their exercise regimen, whereas the females failed to attain any significant reduction. In a controlled study of 70 individuals recruited from exercise fitness classes, the investigators reported significant increases in LDL values for males and females in the exercise groups, as well as in the control groups.[32]

Overall, the effects of exercise on total and LDL-cholesterol appear to be variable and inconsistent. Probable explanations include the fact that investigators did not always consider the effects of body fat and diet in their analyses. The use of medication and the intensity and duration of exercise training also may have influenced the results.

HDL-Cholesterol

HDL-cholesterol has been reported to have cardioprotective value,[14] and many investigators have reported correlations in population

Table 1.
Effects of Exercise on Lipids and Lipoproteins

Author/Year	No. of Pts.	Control Subjects	Duration of Study	TC	HDL-C	LDL-C	TG	Comments
Huttunen et al 1979[20]	100 M	yes	4 mos	↓*	↑*	↓*	↓*	
Rauramaa et al 1984[28]	60 M	yes	8 wks		HDL2/HDL3 ↑*/↓*	↓*		
Ballantyne et al 1982[29]	42 M	yes	6 mos	→	HDL/HDL2 ↑*/↑*	↓*	↑*	–all <65 years and post-MI
Heath et al 1983[30]	10 M		29±7 wks	↓*	↑*	↓*	↓*	–all with CAD
Brownell et al 1982[31]	24 M / 37 F		10 wks	↓* / ↓*	↑* / ↓	↓* / →	↓* / ↑*	
Allison et al 1981[32]	70	yes	8 wks		↓*	↑*		–aged 17–26, recruited from fitness class
Reaven et al 1990[33]	2292		3 yrs		↑*		↓*	–Older population (50–89 yrs) –Self-reported exercise
Kavanagh et al 1983[34]	62		1 yr	→	↑**	→		–all post MI
Blumenthal et al 1988[35]	45 M		3 mos		↑*			–all post MI
Streja et al 1979[36]	32 M		13 wks	↑*	↑*	↑	→	–all with CAD

Study	N	Exercise	Duration	TC	TG	HDL-C	LDL-C	Comments
Erkelens et al 1979[37]	369 M	Yes	6 mos	↑*	↑*	↑*		–all >65 years and post-MI
	18 F			→	↑*	↑*		–all post-MI
Hartung et al 1981[38]	18 M		3 mos	→	↑*	↑*	→	–all with CAD and normal baseline HDL values
Thompson et al 1991[40]	20 M	Yes	6 wks	→	→	↑		–young males without known CAD
LaRosa et al 1982[42]	223 M	Yes	1 yr	↑f	↑f	↑f		–all post MI
Lipson et al 1980[43]	5 F		6 wks	↓*	→	→		–ages 19–22 –inpatient study with strict diet control
Hill et al 1989[44]	9 F		10 wks	↓* / No	No / ↑*			
Oscai et al 1972[46]	7 M		15 days	No		↓*		–all hyperlipidemic
Farrell & Barboriak 1980[49]	7 M / 9 F		8 wks	↑ / ↓	↑*	↓*		–average age 23 years

TC = total cholesterol; HDL-C = high-density lipoprotein-cholesterol; LDL-C = low-density lipoprotein-cholesterol; TG = triglyceride; M = male; F = female; MI = myocardial infarction; CAD = coronary artery disease; * = statistically significant (p < 0.05); ** = not a statistically significant increase in members of jogging group, but significant in others; f = change from baseline similar in control and exercise group. Results are of exercise group except when indicated otherwise.

studies between concentrations of HDL and level of physical activity. Most of the studies reviewed in this chapter (Table 1) have described a significant increment in HDL following mild, moderate, and intense exercise programs having durations of 6 weeks to 3 years. The studies vary in design (cross sectional and longitudinal, controlled and noncontrolled) and include subjects of varying age and sex, healthy individuals, and those with documented CAD.

Reaven et al[33] studied a group of 1113 older subjects (aged 50-89 years) and reported significantly increased HDL levels in males and females who participated in strenuous exercise. The HDL levels were even higher than those observed in a similar study of younger subjects. The same investigators also described significant increments in HDL levels for females who participated in a lower-intensity exercise program, when compared to their male counterparts. These results could imply that elderly subjects could benefit substantially from participation in aerobic exercise programs, and that women could reap benefit even with minimal exertion.

Kavanagh and associates[34] followed 52 post-myocardial infarction patients and reported that HDL levels seemed to correlate directly with the weekly running distances of a 27-member jogging group observed over a 1-year period. They demonstrated increased HDL levels with increased mileage and lower levels with decreased mileage. The study also showed that the effect of exercise on HDL levels could only be maintained with continued distance running. There appeared to be a threshold dose of exercise necessary to increase HDL values above those observed in normal sedentary adults (20 km/week).

In contrast, Blumenthal et al[35] reported that patients who were post-myocardial infarction could benefit from either low-intensity or high-intensity aerobic exercise programs with significant increments in HDL with both physical activity regimens.

Streja and Mymin[36] studied 32 males with CAD who demonstrated significant elevations in HDL levels with exercise even when there was no evidence of a cardiovascular training effect.

Erkelens et al[37] reported that the HDL levels of exercising patients with histories of CAD were similar to healthy controls; both groups having higher HDL levels than a nonexercising group of patients with CAD. These same investigators studied the effects of exercise in a longitudinal study of 18 males who survived an acute myocardial infarction and showed a significant increase in HDL within 1 week of training.[37] The level remained elevated during the entire 6-week period of study. Similar observations were made by Hartung et al[38] in an uncontrolled study of 18 male patients with CAD. This finding was in contrast to the observation made in other studies that a significant increase in VO_2 max was necessary to see an increase in HDL.[34]

Herbert and his associates[39] demonstrated that endurance athletes have higher HDL concentrations than sedentary controls. In a more recent study, the mechanism for this effect was examined by Thompson et al in 10 endurance athletes and 10 sedentary men.[40] The investigators found that endurance training was associated with more efficient catabolism of plasma triglycerides and prolonged survival of the LDL lipoproteins. HDL apoprotein survival appears, in turn, to be directly related to HDL-cholesterol and, in particular, the levels of protective HDL_2-cholesterol.[40,41] In contrast, apoprotein-I and -II synthetic rates were not consistently related to HDL concentrations.[40]

Other investigators have failed to demonstrate significant increases in HDL among either healthy men or those with CAD engaged in moderate to vigorous physical activity. The National Exercise and Heart Disease Project reported on by LaRosa et al[42] found that neither changes in physical fitness nor regular aerobic exercise influenced HDL or any other lipid value, despite reductions of body fat in patients who had survived a myocardial infarction. This was a controlled study of 223 subjects with 1 year of follow-up. The exercise group underwent moderate aerobic activity for 35 minutes, three times a week. The limitations of the study were that the baseline levels of HDL were already at reasonable levels, which would leave less room for improvement. In addition, there was no control of diet in the trial, as compared to most other studies where dietary intake was prescribed and/or monitored.

In an attempt to remove the influence of diet and body weight, Lipson and associates[43] studied 10 subjects in a prospective 6-week exercise program. The participants were all maintained on a consistent diet and exhibited an exercise training effect. Although total cholesterol was reduced, HDL cholesterol was unaltered.

Allison et al[32] not only failed to find increased HDL concentrations but also noted a significant reduction of this lipoprotein among young, healthy men after endurance training. In this study, subjects were recruited from fitness classes and assigned to one of two exercise groups that varied only in the duration of training per day. Both exercise groups demonstrated an increase in VO_2 max and decreases in mean HDL concentrations. It might be concluded that aerobic activity at a greater intensity or for a longer duration is necessary to positively affect HDL levels in this group, in contrast to older, less fit individuals who may have lower baseline HDL values. This was suggested by the findings of Hill et al[44] and Leon et al[15] who noted that the largest increases in HDL with exercise training were observed in those individuals who were least fit and in those having the lowest initial HDL values. These findings suggest that those who could benefit the most from aerobic training are those who are at greater risk for developing CAD.

Overall, there does appear to be a positive effect of exercise training on the levels of HDL. However, covariables such as age, diet, body composition, smoking habits, medication, and alcohol use should be acknowledged before ascribing all HDL changes to exercise alone.

Triglycerides

Acute bouts of exercise have been shown to cause reductions in triglycerides in men with hypertriglyceridemia.[19,45,46] This effect may be related to enhanced peripheral uptake of triglycerides[47] and increased activity of lipoprotein lipase.[18,48] Although most studies have demonstrated a definite downward trend in triglyceride levels with exercise, controversy still exists when the effects of prolonged exercise training are assessed.

In the National Exercise and Heart Disease Project, a significant decrease in triglycerides were seen in the exercise group compared to the control group.[42] Similar observations were made by both Ballantyne et al[29] in males who were post-myocardial infarction, and by Huttunen et al[20] in asymptomatic middle-aged males, when exercising subjects were compared to those who were sedentary.

Conflicting results have been reported in studies comparing the effects of exercise on the triglyceride levels of males and females. Brownell et al[31] described a significant decrease (9.5%) in triglycerides for male subjects participating in their exercise protocol, whereas their female counterparts showed a significant increase in triglycerides (14.5%). In contrast, Reaven et al[33] demonstrated that in elderly individuals, males had to exercise more intensely to decrease their triglycerides; women less intensively to show a decrease in triglycerides. Finally, Farrell and Barboriak[49] studied 16 young individuals and reported that triglycerides were reduced in both males and females during an 8-week exercise program.

Oscai et al[46] studied seven hyperlipidemic males whose exercise regimen lasted for 15 days. The results demonstrated a significant reduction in triglyceride levels during exercise, with subsequent return to baseline values after exercise was discontinued. This study suggests that one must maintain aerobic fitness in order to sustain the resultant decrease in triglyceride levels.

Discussion

There is now good evidence to suggest, from cross-sectional and prospective studies, that increased physical activity might help reduce the risk of morbidity and mortality from CAD.[11-16] However, an independent relationship between exercise and fitness and the level of total cholesterol, HDL, LDL, and triglycerides has yet to be established definitively. The effects of training on plasma lipids and lipoproteins may occur only as a consequence of changes in body weight, diet, or medication use. At the same time, the studies that have looked at a direct relationship between exercise and lipids have, for the most part, not been well designed.

From the information that is available, it does appear that individuals with higher cholesterol, LDL, and triglyceride levels, as well as individuals with lower HDL levels can show favorable changes in these parameters[50] with physical training (both endurance and resistive[19]). The findings from studies using self-reports of increased physical activity and more favorable lipid profiles also suggest that regular physical activity alone rather than regimented aerobic training may be sufficient to achieve benefit.[19] What still needs to be learned is the exercise dose (intensity, duration, frequency) necessary to result in a benefit to the patients, as well as the metabolic mechanisms involved in lipid and lipoprotein change.

Since participation in some form of physical activity is one of the few measures one can control to provide better health, more studies should be encouraged as part of an overall risk reduction plan[51-53] in those individuals who are susceptible to complications of CAD.

References

1. American Heart Association. Heart Facts. New York, American Heart Association, 1982.

2. Stamler J, Wentworth D, Neaton J: Is the relationship between serum cholesterol and risk of death from coronary heart disease continuous and graded? JAMA 1986; 256: 2823-2828.
3. Gordon DJ, Probstfeld JL, Garrison RJ, et al: High-density lipoprotein cholesterol and cardiovascular disease: four prospective American series. Circulation 1989; 79: 8-15.
4. Lipid Research Clinics Program: The Lipid Research Clinics Coronary Primary Prevention Trial Results: I. Reduction in the incidence of coronary heart disease. JAMA 1984; 251: 351-364.
5. Frick MH, Elo MO, Haapa K, et al: Helsinki Heart Study: primary prevention trial with gemfibrozil in middle-aged men with dyslipidemia. N Engl J Med 1987; 317: 1237-1245.
6. Blankenhorn DH, Johnson RL, Nessim SA, et al: The cholesterol lowering atherosclerosis study (CLAS): design, methods and baseline results. Controlled Clin Trials 1987; 8: 356-387.
7. Kane JP, Malloy MJ, Ports TA, et al: Regression of coronary atherosclerosis during treatment of familial hypercholesterolemia with combined drug regimens. JAMA 1990; 264: 3007-3012.
8. Cashin-Hemphill L, Mack WJ, Pogoda JM, et al: Beneficial effects of colestipol-niacin on coronary atherosclerosis. JAMA 1990; 264: 3013-3017.
9. Brown G, Albers JJ, Fisher LD, et al: Regression of coronary artery disease as a result of intensive lipid-lowering therapy in men with high levels of apolipoprotein B. N Engl J Med 1990; 323: 1289-1298.
10. Buchwald H, Varco RL, Matts JP, et al: Effect of partial ileal bypass surgery on mortality and morbidity from coronary heart disease in patients with hypercholesterolemia. N Engl J Med 1990; 323: 946-955.
11. Paffenbarger Jr. RS, Hyde RT: Exercise in the prevention of +coronary heart disease. Prevent Med 1984; 13: 3-22.
12. Shaw LW: Effects of a prescribed supervised exercise program on mortality and cardiovascular morbidity in patients after a myocardial infarction. The National Exercise and Heart Disease Project. Am J Cardiol 1981; 48: 39-46.
13. O'Connor GT, Buring JE, Yusuf S, et al: An overview of randomized trials of rehabilitation with exercise after myocardial infarction. Circulation 1989; 80: 234-244.
14. Leon AS: Physical activity levels and coronary heart disease. Analysis of epidemiologic and supporting studies. Med Clin N Am 1985; 69: 3-20.
15. Leon AS, Connett J, Jacobs Jr. DR, et al: Leisure-time physical activity levels and risk of coronary heart disease and death. The Multiple Risk Factor Intervention Trial. JAMA 1987; 258: 2388-2395.
16. Berlin JA, Colditz GA: Meta-analysis of physical activity in the prevention of coronary heart disease. Am J Epidemiol 1990; 132: 612-618.
17. Pedoe DST: Exercise and heart disease: is there still a controversy? Br Heart J 1990; 64: 293-294.
18. Julius U, Hanefeld M: Environmental factors and serum lipoproteins. Curr Opin Lipidol 1990; 1: 255-261.
19. Goldberg L, Elliot DL: The effect of physical activity on lipid and lipoprotein levels. Med Clin N Am 1985; 69: 41-55.

20. Huttunen JK, Lansimies E, Voutilainen E, et al: Effect of moderate physical exercise on serum lipoproteins. A controlled clinical trial with special reference to serum high-density lipoproteins. Circulation 1979; 60: 1220-1229.

21. Haskell WL, Taylor HL, Wood PD, et al: Strenuous physical activity, treadmill exercise test performance and plasma high-density lipoprotein cholesterol. Circulation 1980; 62 (Suppl IV): IV-53-IV-61.

22. Kiens B, Lithell H: Lipoprotein metabolism influenced by training-induced changes in human skeletal muscle. J Clin Invest 1989; 83: 558-564.

23. Hanefeld M, Fischer S, Julius U, et al: More exercise for the hyperlipidaemic patients? Ann Clin Res 1988; 20: 77-83.

24. Wood PD, Haskell W, Klein H, et al: The distribution of plasma lipoproteins in middle-aged male runners. Metabolism 1976; 25: 1249-1257.

25. Seals DR, Hagberg JM, Hurley BF, et al: Effects of endurance training on glucose tolerance and plasma lipid levels in older men and women. JAMA 1984; 252: 645-649.

26. Leon AS, Conrad J, Hunninghake DB, et al: Effects of a vigorous walking program on body composition, and carbohydrate and lipid metabolism of obese young men. Am J Clin Nutr 1979; 32: 1776-1787.

27. Williams RS, Logue EE, Lewis JL, et al: Physical conditioning augments the fibrinolytic response to venous occlusion in healthy adults. N Engl J Med 1980; 302: 987-991.

28. Rauramaa R, Salonen JT, Kukkonen-Harjula E, et al: Effects of mild physical exercise on serum lipoproteins and metabolites of arachidonic acid: a controlled randomised trial in middle aged men. Br Med J 1984; 2818: 603-606.

29. Ballantyne FC, Clark RS, Simpson HS, et al: The effect of moderate physical exercise on the plasma lipoprotein sub-fractions of male survivors of myocardial infarction. Circulation 1982; 65: 913-917.

30. Heath GW, Ehsani AA, Hagberg JM, et al: Exercise training improves lipoprotein lipid profiles in patients with coronary artery disease. Am Heart J 1983; 105: 889-895.

31. Brownell KD, Bachorik PS, Ayerle RS: Changes in plasma lipid and lipoprotein levels in men and women after a program of moderate exercise. Circulation 1982; 63: 477-484.

32. Allison TG, Iammarino RM, Metz KF, et al: Failure of exercise to increase high density lipoprotein cholesterol. J Cardiac Rehab 1981; 1: 257-265.

33. Reaven PD, McPhillips JB, Barrett-Connor EL, et al: Leisure time exercise and lipid and lipoprotein levels in an older population. J Am Geriatr Soc 1990; 38: 847-854.

34. Kavanagh T, Shephard RJ, Lindley LJ, et al: Influence of exercise and lifestyle variables upon high density lipoprotein cholesterol after myocardial infarction. Arteriosclerosis 1983; 3: 249-259.

35. Blumenthal JA, Rejeski J, Walsh-Riddle M, et al: Comparison of high- and low-intensity exercise training early after acute myocardial infarction. Am J Cardiol 1988; 61: 26-30.

36. Streja D, Mymin D: Moderate exercise and high-density lipoprotein-cholesterol. JAMA 1979; 242: 2190-2192.

37. Erkelens DW, Alberts JJ, Hazzard WR, et al: High-density lipoprotein-cholesterol in survivors of myocardial infarction. JAMA 1979; 242: 2185-2189.
38. Hartung GH, Foreyt JP, Mitchell RE, et al: Relation of diet to high-density-lipoprotein cholesterol in middle-aged marathon runners, joggers, and inactive men. N Engl J Med 1980; 302: 357-36l.
39. Herbert PN, Bernie DN, Cullinane EM, et al: High-density lipoprotein metabolism in runners and sedentary men. JAMA 1984; 252: 1034-1037.
40. Thompson PD, Cullinane EM, Sady SP, et al: High density lipoprotein metabolism in endurance athletes and sedentary men. Circulation 1991; 84: 140-152.
41. Salonen JT, Salonen R, Seppanen K, et al: HDL, HDL_2 and HDL_3 subfractions, and the risk of acute myocardial infarction. Circulation 1991; 84: 129-39.
42. LaRosa JC, Cleary P, Muesing RA, et al: Effect of long-term moderate physical exercise on plasma lipoproteins. Arch Intern Med 1982; 142: 2269-2274.
43. Lipson LC, Bonow RO, Schaefer EJ, et al: Effect of exercise conditioning on plasma high density lipoproteins. Atherosclerosis 1980; 37: 529-538.
44. Hill JO, Thiel J, Heller PA, et al: Differences in effects of aerobic exercise training on blood lipids in men and women. Am J Cardiol 1989; 63: 254-256.
45. Gyntelberg F, Brennan R, Holloszy JO, et al: Plasma triglyceride lowering by exercise despite increased food intake in patients with type IV hyperlipoproteinemia. Am J Clin Nutri 1977; 30: 716-720.
46. Oscai LB, Patterson JA, Bogard DL, et al: Normalization of serum triglycerides and lipoprotein electrophoretic patterns by exercise. Am J Cardiol 1972; 30: 775-780.
47. Havel RJ, Pernow B, Jones NL: Uptake and release of free fatty acids and other metabolites in the legs of exercising men. J Appl Physiol 1967; 23: 90-99.
48. Nikkila EA, Taskinen MR, Ruhunen S, et al: Lipoprotein lipase activity in adipose tissue and skeletal muscle of runners - relation to serum lipoproteins. Metabolism 1978; 27: 1661-1671.
49. Farrell PA, Barboriak J: The time course of alterations in plasma lipid and lipoprotein concentrations during eight weeks of endurance training. Atherosclerosis 1980; 37: 231-238.
50. Wood PD, Haskell WL: The effect of exercise on plasma high density lipoproteins. Lipids 1979; 14: 417-426.
51. Johnson C, Greenland P: Effects of exercise, dietary cholesterol, and dietary fat on blood lipids. Arch Intern Med 1990; 150: 137-141.
52. Horton ES: Exercise and decreased risk of NIDDM. N Engl J Med 1991; 325: 196-198.
53. Barnard RJ: Life-style modification on serum lipids. Arch Intern Med 1991; 151: 1389-1394.

Part III

Pharmacological Approaches

Chapter 4
Bile-Acid Sequestrants

William H. Frishman M.D., Martin Ast M.D.

The bile-acid binding resins, cholestyramine and colestipol, are the drugs of first choice for hypercholesterolemia in patients without concurrent hypertriglyceridemia. Cholestyramine originally was used for treatment of pruritus caused by elevated concentrations of bile-acids secondary to cholestasis. Attention recently has been focused on the bile-acid sequestrants' (BAS) ability to lower LDL-cholesterol plasma concentration. The resins have been extensively tested in large-scale, long-term, follow-up clinical trials to explore their efficacy for such an application.[1,2] These drugs are not absorbed in the gastrointestinal (GI) tract, and therefore have a limited range of systemic side effects. For this reason they are particularly useful for treatment of pregnant women with hypercholesterolemia, and are the only drugs to be considered safe for use in children with heterozygous familial hypercholesterolemia.[3] The disadvantage of the sequestrants lie in their mode of administration and the frequency of GI side effects.

Chemistry

Cholestyramine (Questran powder) is the chloride salt of a basic anion exchange resin. The ion-exchange sites are provided by the presence of trimethylbenzylammonium groups in a large copolymer of styrene and divinyl benzene. Cholestyramine's average polymeric molecular weight is $> 10^6$.[4] The resin is hydrophilic yet insoluble in water. It is given orally after being suspended in water or juice. It is not absorbed

From *Medical Management of Lipid Disorders: Focus on Prevention of Coronary Artery Disease,* edited by William H. Frishman, M.D. © 1992, Futura Publishing Inc., Mount Kisco, NY.

in the GI tract and is not altered by digestive enzymes, permitting it to remain unchanged while traversing the intestines. Cholestyramine is also available as chewable flavored bars (Cholybar®) each containing 4 g of anhydrous resin.

Colestipol (Colestid), supplied as the powder colestipol hydrochloride, is a basic anion exchange copolymer made up of diethylenetriamine and 1-chloro-2,3-epoxypropane. It has approximately 1 out of its 5 amine nitrogens protonated (chloride form). Like cholestyramine, colestipol is not altered by digestive enzymes, nor is it absorbed in the digestive tract. It is supplied in powder form and is taken orally after it is suspended in liquid.

Pharmacology

Bile-acids are synthesized in the liver from cholesterol, their sole precursor. They are then secreted into the GI tract where they interact with fat-soluble molecules, thereby aiding in the digestion and subsequent absorption of these substances. Bile-acids are absorbed along with the fat-soluble molecules and are subsequently recycled by the liver via the portal circulation for resecretion into the GI tract. The bile-acids remain in the enterohepatic circulation and never enter the systemic circulation.

Both cholestyramine and colestipol bind bile-acids in the intestine. The complex thus formed is then excreted in the feces. By binding the bile-acids, the resins deny the bile-acids entry into the blood stream, and thereby remove a large portion of the acids from the enterohepatic circulation. The decrease in hepatic concentrations of bile-acids allows a disinhibition of cholesterol 7 α-hydroxylase, the rate-limiting enzyme in bile- acid synthesis.[5,6] Also seen is an increase in activity of phosphatidic acid phosphatase, an enzyme responsible for the conversion of α-glycerol phosphate to triglyceride. The increased activity of this enzyme causes a shift away from phospholipid production and ultimately, an increase in the triglyceride content and size of very low density lipoprotein particles (VLDL).[7] Recent evidence suggests that the BAS also cause an increase in the activity of 3-hydroxy-3-methyl glutaryl-coenzyme A (HMG-CoA reductase), the rate-limiting enzyme in the hepatic cholesterol synthesis pathway.[8] Although cholesterol synthesis is increased when BAS are used, there is no rise in plasma cholesterol, presumably due to the immediate shunting of the newly formed cholesterol into the bile-acid synthesis pathway. The apparent shortage of cholesterol causes the hepatocyte cell surface receptors for LDL particles to be altered either quantitatively by increasing in number or qualitatively by increasing in affinity for the LDL particle.[9,10] By sequestering the cholesterol-rich LDL particles, the liver decreases the plasma concentration of cholesterol.

Pharmacokinetics

Cholestyramine and colestipol bind bile-acids in the intestines forming a chemical complex which is excreted in the feces. There is no chemical modification of the resins while in the GI tract, however the chloride ions of the resins may be replaced by other anions with higher affinity for the resin. Colestipol is hydrophilic but is virtually insoluble in water (99.75%). Neither the high molecular polymer of cholestyramine or colestipol is absorbed in the GI tract. Less than 0.05% of 14C-labeled colestipol is excreted in the urine.

Since the resins are not absorbed into the systemic circulation, any interactions that occur between the resins and other molecules occur in the intestines and usually occur with substances ingested with or near the time of resin ingestion. Interaction between resins and fat-soluble substances, such as the fat-soluble vitamins, cause a decrease in absorption of these substances. Malabsorption of Vitamin K, for instance, has been associated with a hypoprothrombinemia. It is therefore recommended that vitamins K and D be supplemented in patients on long-term resin therapy. Likewise, medications taken with or near the time of resin ingestion may be bound by the resin and not be absorbed. Drugs at risk include phenylbutazone, warfarin, chlorothiazide (acidic), propranolol (basic), penicillin G, tetracycline, phenobarbital, thyroid, and thyroxine preparations, and digitalis.

The dose-response curves for the bile-acid resins are nonlinear with increases in the antihypercholesterolemic effect minimal for doses > 30 g/d. Furthermore, there tends to be compliance problems when large doses of resin are used, making doses > 15 g two times daily inefficacious.[11]

Since the BAS are polymeric cations bound to chloride anions, continued ingestion of the resins places a chloride load on the body. This chloride load may cause a decrease in the urine pH and an increase in the urinary excretion of chloride, which can reach 60% of the ingested resin load. Furthermore, there may be an increase in excretion of calcium ions that is dependent on the extent of chloride ion excretion. Due to this increase in calcium ion excretion, care should be taken, especially when treating a person at risk for osteoporosis, to limit the extent of calcium excretion by controlling the chloride dietary load.[12]

Clinical Experiences

Numerous studies have shown the BAS cholestyramine and colestipol to be efficacious in lowering LDL- and total cholesterol levels in the plasma. Studies have further correlated the decreased levels of LDL-cholesterol with the slowing of progression of coronary atherosclerosis and a lowered incidence of coronary events. Furthermore, studies of lipoprotein content in resin-treated individuals have detected a qualitative effect that may have a contributory role in the antiatherosclerotic effects of the drug. Sequestrants are limited to use in those patients with hypercholesterolemia not associated with severe hypertriglyceridemia. Therefore, unless the use of bile-acid resins are combined with other antihyperlipidemic drugs, their use is limited to treatment of individuals with type II hyperlipoproteinemia.

Early Use of Resins

Ileal exclusion has long been a treatment for hypercholesterolemia.[13-15] Its mechanism of action appears to be via the interruption of the ileal absorption of dietary cholesterol and its subsequent lowering of the plasma cholesterol levels. Subsequently, it was discovered that along with the effect of the procedure on dietary cholesterol, there was a decreased absorption of bile-acid from the gut that disrupted the normal enterohepatic circulation of the bile-acids. This physiological change proved to be the primary antihypercholesterolemic effect of the procedure. Bile-acid binding resins, in effect, achieve a chemical ileal exclusion with similar effects on the plasma cholesterol levels.

In a study comparing the relative efficacy of bile-acid resins and the ileal exclusion procedure for lowering serum cholesterol, nine patients with type IIa hyperlipoproteinemia were treated with either the ileal exclusion procedure or cholestyramine.[5] Results showed that both groups had similar decreases in bile-acid absorption and plasma cholesterol concentration, and also had similar increases of cholesterol synthesis in hepatocytes and intestinal cells. These results supported the view that cholestyramine treatment is as effective as the ileal exclusion procedure in lowering cholesterol.[5]

Another early study examined 25 patients with type IIa hyperproteinemia.[16] These subjects were randomized into two groups consisting of a low-cholesterol diet plus placebo group, and a diet plus colestipol group. The dose of colestipol used was 30 mg and the study lasted 7 to $7\frac{1}{2}$ years. The colestipol group had a decrease in total plasma cholesterol from a mean of 10.65 ± 0.59 to 6.98 ± 0.28 mm/L (412 ± 22.8 to 270 ± 11.0 mg/dl). They also had a decrease in LDL-cholesterol from 8.56 ± 0.59 to 4.86 ± 0.36 mm/L (331.1 ± 22.8 to 188.1 ± 13.8 mg/dl). The diet plus placebo group showed no significant changes. Although there were no significant changes in the HDL level, the HDL:LDL ratio increased in the treatment group. Twenty of the 25 patients had a decrease in pretreatment xanthoma size and stabilization of angiographically visualized atherosclerotic lesions. There was no significant change in triglyceride levels in these patients, which was attributed to the unusually close adherence of the patients to the low-fat, low-cholesterol diet.[16] Another early study done on a very small groups of patients (8 subjects) showed that colestipol's lipid-lowering ability was associated with increased cholesterol turnover and bile-acid loss.[17]

Heterozygous Familial Hypercholesterolemia: Effects on LDL-Cholesterol in Adults

The Lipid Research Clinics Coronary Primary Prevention Trial (LRC-CPPT)[1] represents the most extensive study of BAS and it's effects on lowering the incidence of symptomatic coronary artery disease. The study involved 3806 subjects with type II hyperlipoproteinemia with plasma cholesterol values > 6.85 mm/L (> 265 mg/dl). The subjects were either placed into a placebo group on a low-cholesterol diet or a treatment group consisting of cholestyramine therapy (24 g/d) plus diet. Results showed that diet accounted for a 5% decrease in total cholesterol in both groups. The cholestyramine-treated group experienced a decrease in mean total cholesterol and LDL-cholestereol of 13.4% and 20.3%, respectively. These decreases were 9% and 13% lower than the placebo group for total and LDL-cholesterol, respectively (placebo total cholesterol decreased 8.5% and LDL-cholesterol decreased

12.6%). The study then looked for correlations between lower cholesterol and the incidence of coronary heart disease. In order to do this,
the researchers defined two primary endpoints that would be used as
markers for coronary heart disease: death from coronary heart disease
and nonfatal myocardial infarction. The study found an overall 19%
reduction in the incidence of the primary endpoints for the treated
group over the placebo group. This included a 24% lower incidence of
death from coronary heart disease and a 19% reduction in nonfatal
myocardial infarction. Secondary endpoints, including the incidence of
new positive exercise stress tests, new onset angina, coronary bypass
surgery, and intermittent claudication, also showed a beneficial effect
of cholestyramine treatment (decreases of 25%, 20%, 21%, and 15%,
respectively). The cumulative incidence (over 7 years) of the primary
endpoints were 7% for subjects on cholestyramine and 8.65% for subjects on placebo. The favorable effects of cholestyramine were most
apparent in those patients with the highest initial cholesterol values.
Death from all causes was slightly decreased in the cholestyramine-
treated group but was not statistically significant. This was offset by
the higher incidence of violent deaths in the cholestyramine-treated
group, which was thought to be a coincidental finding. The results
of this study indicated that the extent of decrease in the total and
LDL-cholesterol was directly related to the fall in the incidence of the
coronary heart disease primary and secondary endpoints.[2] The participants who did not respond to cholestyramine treatment by lowering
their cholesterol did not experience the cardioprotective effects of the
drug, further implying that the lower cholesterol caused the decrease in
the incidence of the coronary heart disease endpoints. It was calculated
that a 1% lowering of total cholesterol concentration was associated with
a 2% decline in coronary risk.

A study was performed by the National Heart, Lung, and Blood
Institute (NHLBI) that examined the effects of cholestyramine on ana-
tomical coronary atherosclerosis.[18,19] The NHLBI study differed from
the LRC-CPPT study in size of study group (and endpoints evaluated).
The study looked at 116 people who had documented type II hyperlipoproteinemia and coronary artery disease. All subjects were assigned to
a low-fat, low-cholesterol diet and were randomized to placebo or 6 g
of cholestyramine four times daily. Progression of coronary artery disease was assessed via serial coronary angiography over 5 years, and was
correlated to the extent of LDL-cholesterol change. Results indicated
that diet alone decreased LDL-cholesterol levels 6% before randomiza-

tion and another 5% after randomization, while cholestyramine de-creased LDL-cholesterol 26% after randomization. In addition to the decrease in LDL-cholesterol with the drug, there was a decrease in total cholesterol and an increase in HDL-cholesterol. Coronary artery disease progressed in 49% (28/57) of subjects on placebo and 32% (19/59) of subjects on cholestyramine. When definite progression of a vascular lesion was considered, 35% (20/57) of subjects on placebo versus 25% (15/59) of subjects on cholestyramine showed changes, a difference which is not statistically significant. However, when individual differ-ences in baseline lesions were taken into account, there was a tendency toward statistically significant beneficial effects in the cholestyramine-treated group. The subgroups of lesions examined included progression of baseline lesion of > 50% stenosis (33% in placebo vs 12% in treated group), percent of baseline lesion progressed, lesions that progressed to total occlusion, lesions that regressed, and size of lesion change. None of these results reached statistical significance due to the small sample size in the study. Based on the above results, however, larger studies of BAS are warranted to examine the effects on coronary artery lesions.

It was found that when lipid values were studied independent of the treatment group, there was an inverse relationship between coronary artery disease progression and HDL-cholesterol concentration and a direct relationship between coronary artery disease and LDL-cholesterol concentration. The ratios of HDL-cholesterol to total cholesterol and HDL-cholesterol to LDL-cholesterol were the best predictors of coro-nary heart disease. These findings support the hypothesis that the cardi-oprotective effect of cholestyramine works via the lowering of LDL-cholesterol and the raising of HDL-cholesterol.

Effects on Intermediate Density (IDL)-Cholesterol

Recent evaluation of a subset of the NHLBI study group examined the effect of cholestyramine on IDL particles.[20] The study found that the drug-induced changes of IDL mass seen 2 years into treatment were the best predictors for progression of coronary heart disease 5 years into treatment. Based on these findings, it was hypothesized that the major antiatherosclerotic effect of cholestyramine may not be its LDL-lowering and HDL-raising effect but an IDL-lowering effect caused by the binding of the IDL particles to the upwardly regulated LDL receptors on the hepatocytes. This hypothesis is based on the fact that IDL particles are able to bind to LDL receptors.[20]

Pediatric Use of BAS

An early study looked at the effect of cholestyramine (12 g/d) in 36 children with type II hyperlipoproteinemia.[21] Of the 36 children, 11 had normal cholesterol after 6 months of pretreatment diet therapy. Of the 25 remaining children, 20 received cholestyramine treatment; only 10 of the 20 children had good drug compliance. Six of the 10 children on full treatment received treatment for 6 to 12 months, and their LDL-cholesterol levels were normalized. Ten of the 20 children received suboptimal treatment of 8 g/d, and none were found to have a sustained decrease in LDL and total cholesterol levels. Overall, the LDL-cholesterol was reduced to normal in 11 of 36 (31%) children on diet alone, and 6 of 11 (60%) of children on diet and cholestyramine. There were no reported changes in growth rate and no evidence of other major side effects.[21] The lipid-lowering action of cholestyramine in a pediatric population was again shown in a study of 35 children with heterozygous familial hyperlipoproteinemia.[22] But, as in the study cited above, compliance was low. Only 55% of the children were still on treatment at 6 years into the study, and only 48% after 8 years. Compliance was better when patients were started on therapy before their tenth birthday.[22] Compliance in the pediatric population is especially important since treatment with the antihypercholesterolemic drug will likely be lifelong.

In a more recent study done on 73 children with heterozygous familial hypercholesterolemia, diet plus cholestyramine was found to cause a significant decrease in total cholesterol when compared to the decrease seen in diet alone.[23] The study also followed developmental changes of the treated and untreated group and no significant differences in height or weight were found.[3,23] The early use of cholestyramine in the pediatric population may have unforeseen advantages based on a study on Watanabe rabbits.[24] In the study, those rabbits treated in early life with cholestyramine not only experienced an antihyperlipoproteinemic effect while on the drug, but also had a lower incidence of coronary artery disease even after drug treatment was stopped and the plasma cholesterol levels returned to pretreatment concentrations. The cause of this residual cardioprotective effect is thought to be linked to a sustained activation of the 7 α-hydroxylase enzyme along with a sustained inhibition of the acyl-CoA cholesterol acetyltransferase enzyme (responsible for the formation of cholesterol esters).[24] Despite the above evidence, the supposition that early use of cholestyramine by members of a high-risk pediatric population may produce a protracted cardioprotective effect is premature, and further investigation is warranted.

Effects on VLDL-Cholesterol and Triglycerides

Cholestyramine has the tendency to increase synthesis of triglycerides, which may contribute to the observed increases in VLDL particle concentration. In a study comparing normotriglyceride, hypertriglyceride, and obese patients, the observed increase in VLDL-triglyceride seen with resin treatment was shown to be due to increased synthesis of the lipoprotein and not decreased catabolism.[25] In order to better define those patients best suited for cholestyramine treatment, a study was done looking at the relative concentrations of cholesterol and triglycerides in 139 patients.[26] Results showed that < 5% of subjects with triglyceride levels 5.65 mm/L (> 500 mg/dl) had abnormally high LDL levels, and none of the patients with triglyceride levels 11.29 mm/L (> 1000 mg/dl) had high LDL levels. Five patients studied who initially had high triglyceride and cholesterol levels were treated with resins and subsequently had a substantial increase in their triglyceride levels. This seemed to imply that, in most cases, the cause of very high plasma triglyceride concentrations is not high LDL lipoprotein, and that patients with both high cholesterol and triglyceride levels may be refractory to resin therapy because the raised cholesterol would be caused by particles other than LDL. For the above reason, bile-acid binding resins should only be used in patients with triglyceride levels 3.39 mm/L (< 300 mg/dl), and it is therefore important to determine not only a patient's LDL level but also triglyceride level in order to distinguish hypercholesterolemia due to hyper-LDL and hyper-VLDL.[26]

Effects on HDL-Lipoprotein Concentration

In a study of 1907 patients enrolled in the LRC-CPPT trials, the HDL levels were found to be inversely proportional to the extent of coronary artery disease (as defined by the number of patients reaching the primary endpoint).[27] Each 0.03 mm/L (1 mg/dl) increase of HDL above the mean at baseline was associated with a 5.5% decrease in the chance of a definite coronary artery disease associated death or a nonfatal myocardial infarction. Furthermore, each 0.03 mm/L (1 mg/dl) increase of HDL from baseline during the course of the study was associated with a 4.4% risk reduction for the primary endpoints. There was a similar finding in the placebo group when diet appeared to induce an increase in HDL. Cholestyramine had its greatest antihypercholesterolemic effect in those patients with the highest HDL concentrations. It is important to keep in mind that the LRC-CPPT study was not designed to answer questions about HDL levels, and therefore the above suppositions are not conclusive.

Effects on Lipoprotein Composition

Not only has the absolute and relative amounts of lipoproteins in the plasma been looked at as risk factors for atherosclerosis, but the actual composition of the particles have been studied to better understand their role in coronary artery disease progression. Both LDL and VLDL particles have apoprotein B-100 as one of their major constituent lipoproteins, while HDL contains mostly apoprotein A-I and A-II. One study examined the correlation of apoprotein concentrations in the plasma to coronary artery disease.[28] This study found coronary artery disease to be directly related to apoprotein B-100 concentration and inversely related to apoprotein A-I and A-II. These correlations were more effective than plasma cholesterol levels in blindly discriminating between a control group and a group of post-myocardial infarction patients.[28] In addition, the actual subpopulations of HDL apoproteins may further be predictive of coronary artery disease. It has been suggested that apoprotein A-I levels are more inversely correlated to coronary artery disease than apoprotein A-II, and that high apoprotein A-I:A-II ratios have been found in people with a low incidence of coronary artery disease.[29] The mechanism by which the apoproteins affect the progression of atherosclerosis may lie in their ability to enzymatically modify the lipoprotein molecules and thereby change their binding specificity.[30] In fact, evidence now points to some form of oxidative modification of the LDL particle as being essential for the initiation of endothelial damage and fatty streak formation, the precursors of atherosclerotic plaque formation.[31]

For the above mentioned reasons, it is important to determine the extent and type of lipoprotein modification that occurs with antihyperlipidemic drugs. Theoretically, modification of an LDL particle may be just as effective in preventing coronary artery disease as its removal from the circulation. A study examined lipoprotein composition changes in 18 people with type II hyperlipoproteinemia treated with cholestyramine.[32] Results showed that with treatment, VLDL-triglyceride levels rose slightly, the extent dependent on pretreatment levels. LDL levels fell 28% compared to the diet-only group mean levels, LDL-triglyceride levels fell 13%, while apoprotein B levels fell 17%. The ratio of LDL-cholesterol:apoprotein B decreased as did the ratio of VLDL-cholesterol:apoprotein B. This indicated that all apoprotein B-containing particles contained less cholesterol relative to apoprotein B, implying that the LDL particle became cholesterol depleted. The concentration of HDL particles remained the same but the apoprotein A-I:A-II ratio increased due to a lowering of apoprotein A-II concentration; the concentration of A-I remained the same. In the LDL particles, the LDL-triglyceride:LDL-cholesterol ratio increased, suggesting a substitution of triglyceride for cholesterol.[32]

An animal study using guinea pigs was performed[33] to determine if the qualitative changes seen in LDL particles in animals treated with cholestyramine cause a change in the behavior of the lipoprotein when compared to the nonmodified molecules. Results of the study showed that after treatment with cholestyramine, the LDL-cholesterol of the guinea pig dropped by 55%. The LDL composition changed so that the LDL particle was smaller with decreased cholesterol ester and phospholipid content and a decreased cholesterol to protein ratio. LDL particles from treated and untreated animals were isolated and reinjected into both treated and nontreated animals to study the fractional catabolic rate (FCR) of the lipoprotein. Results indicated that the majority of LDL catabolism took place in the liver via the receptor-mediated pathway. There was a decrease in FCR when the resin modified LDL particle was injected into both the treated and untreated animals. The FCR for both the modified and unmodified LDL particles was greater when injected into the treated animal but to a greater extent for the unmodified LDL particle. These results suggest that there is a heterozygous population of LDL particles normally found in the body of the guinea pigs. When treated with bile-acid resins, there is an upregulation of the hepatocyte LDL receptor that has a higher affinity for high cholesterol LDL particles. The catabolism of these particles causes a relative increase in the concentration of the second member of the LDL population, the low-cholesterol, low lipoprotein LDL particle. This lipoprotein subset has a low affinity for LDL receptors on the hepatocyte, and therefore has a low FCR. These "light" LDL particles take over as the major constituent of the LDL population and may have a lower atherogenic potential than the "heavy" LDL particle.[33]

Effects on Human Coronary Vascular Lesions (Combination Therapy)

The LRC Trial[1] and the Helsinki Heart Study[34] provided evidence that lowering blood cholesterol levels with drugs could decrease the rate of myocardial infarction and death due to coronary artery disease. Similar to the previous NIH trial in patients with type II disease,[18,19] the Cholesterol Lowering Atherosclerosis Study (CLAS) investigated possible mechanisms underlying these benefits and examined whether cholesterol-lowering therapy could produce stabilization or even regression of atherosclerotic plaques in coronary venous bypass grafts and native coronary vessels.[35] A group of 188 nonsmoking men between 40 and 59 years of age who had undergone previous coronary bypass surgery were randomized to receive either placebo plus dietary intervention or diet plus drug therapy (30 g of colestipol and 3-12 g of niacin daily). Major entry criteria required patient cholesterol levels between 4.78-9.05 mm/L (185-350 mg/dl) and confirmed lipid-lowering response to the study and medications prior to randomization. A total of 162 men had baseline and 2-year angiograms. The combination drug regimen was significantly better than diet alone in lowering total cholesterol, LDL-cholesterol, triglycerides, and apoprotein B levels, and raising HDL-cholesterol and apoprotein A-I levels. At the end of 2 years, there was decreased atherosclerosis progression and increased regression by angiographic exam in the drug treatment group. A subgroup of 103 subjects were followed for 4 years (CLAS-II), with the results recently reported.[36] Changes in blood lipid, lipoprotein-cholesterol, and apolipoprotein levels were maintained. At 4 years, significantly more drug-treated subjects demonstrated nonprogression and regression in native coronary artery lesions. Significantly fewer drug-treated subjects developed new lesions in native coronary arteries. The authors concluded that coronary lesion regression can continue for 4 years with vigorous long-term lipid-lowering therapy in coronary bypass subjects.

Brown and associates[37] assessed the effects of intensive lipid-lowering therapy on the progression and regression of coronary atherosclerosis in men at high risk for cardiovascular events, using repeated quantitative arteriography. The men were 62 years of age or older, who had apoprotein B levels equal to or above 3.23 mm/L (125 mg/dl), documented coronary artery, and a family history of vascular disease. During the two and a half year study, 120 subjects completed the double-blind study that included arteriography at baseline and after treatment. Subjects were all given dietary counseling and were randomly assigned to one of three treatments: lovastatin 20 mg twice daily combined with colestipol 10 g three times daily; niacin 1 g four times daily combined with colestipol 10 mg three times daily; and placebo. Levels of LDL- and HDL-cholesterol changed only slightly in the placebo-dietary group, but more substantially in patients treated with lovastatin-colestipol or niacin-colestipol. Progression of coronary lesions was less common in those subjects receiving combination drug treatment, and regression more common with combination therapy. Multivariate analysis indicated that a reduction in the level of apoprotein B (or LDL-cholesterol) and in systolic blood pressure, and an increase in HDL-cholesterol correlated independently with regression of coronary lesions. Clinical events (death, myocardial infarction, or coronary revascularization for worsening symptoms) were significantly less in those patients receiving combination drug therapies. The authors concluded that intensive lipid-lowering therapy could reduce the progression of coronary lesions, increase the frequency of regression, and reduce the incidence of cardiovascular events.

In a third study, the effects of intensive dietary-drug therapy on coronary lesion regression were assessed in 72 patients with heterozygous familial hypercholesterolemia.[38] The effects of treatment on 457 coronary lesions were assessed over a 26-month period by repeated computer-based quantitative angiography. The control group received dietary treatment plus 15 g/d of BAS. Patients in the treatment group were initially given up to 30 g of colestipol and up to 7.5 mg of niacin daily, as tolerated. When lovastatin became available, it was added to the other drugs in binary or tertiary drug combinations. Mean LDL-cholesterol and total cholesterol were significantly reduced with intensive drug therapy, and HDL levels increased. Control subjects demonstrated evidence of coronary lesion progression, while the treatment group had significant regression. The change in percent area stenosis was correlated with LDL-cholesterol levels during the trial. These authors concluded that reductions in LDL-cholesterol with intensive drug therapy can induce regression of atherosclerotic lesions of the coronary arteries in patients with familial hypercholesterolemia. Benefit was seen in women and men.

Effects on Peripheral Vascular Lesions

Controlled atherosclerotic regression studies of peripheral arterial lesions are a recent development in clinical investigation.[39-41] In the CLAS study, the effects of combined colestipol-niacin therapy plus diet and diet alone on femoral atherosclerosis were assessed. The annual rate of change in computer-estimated atherosclerosis (CEA), a measure of lumen abnormality, was evaluated between treatment groups. A significant per segment therapy effect was found in subjects with moderately severe atherosclerosis and in proximal segments. When segmental CEA measures were combined into a per patient score using an adaptation of a National Heart, Lung and Blood Institute scoring procedure, a significant effect of diet-drug therapy was observed.[42] However, the therapy effect observed in the femoral arteries was less marked than the strong and consistent benefit reported for both native coronary arteries and aortocoronary bypass grafts,[35,36] specifically relating the benefit to effects on HDL-cholesterol.

Clinical Use of Resins

Bile-acid resins are indicated as adjunct therapy to diet for reduction of serum cholesterol in patients with primary hypercholesterolemia. Dietary therapy should precede resin usage, and should address both the specific type of hyperlipoproteinemia in the patient and the body weight of the patient, since obesity has been shown to be a contributing factor in hyperlipoproteinemia. Since resin use can cause a 5% to 20% increase in VLDL levels, its use should be restricted to hypercholesterolemic patients with only slightly increased triglyceride levels. The increase in VLDL seen with resin use usually starts during the first few weeks of therapy and disappears 4 weeks after the initial rise. It is thought that excessive increases in the VLDL particles may dampen the antihyper-LDL effect of the drug by competitively binding the upwardly regulated LDL receptors on the hepatocyte. The resins should, therefore, not be used in patients whose triglyceride levels exceed 3.5 mmol/L unless accompanied by a second drug that has antihypertriglyceride effects; some suggest not using resins if the triglyceride level exceeds 2.5 mmol/L. A general rule of thumb is that if the triglyceride level exceeds 7 mmol/L, the LDL concentration is seldom raised, and therefore, bile-acid resin treatment would not be effective.

Both cholestyramine and colestipol are powders that must be mixed with water or fruit juice before ingestion and are taken in two to three divided doses with or just after meals. BAS can decrease absorption of some antihypertensive agents, including thiazide diuretics and propranolol. As a general recommendation, all other drugs should be administered either 1 hour before or 4 hours after the BAS. The cholesterollowering effect of 4 g of cholestyramine appears to be equivalent to 5 g of colestipol. The response to therapy is variable in each individual, but a 15% to 30% reduction in LDL-cholesterol may be seen with colestipol 20 g/d or cholestyramine 16 g/d treatments. The fall in LDL concentration becomes detectable 4 to 7 days after the start of treatment, and approaches 90% of maximal effect in 2 weeks. Initial dosing should be 4 to 5 g of cholestyramine or colestipol, respectively, two times daily. In patients who do not respond adequately to initial therapy, the dosing can be increased to the maximum mentioned above. Dosing above the maximum dose does not increase the antihypercholesterolemic effect of the drug considerably but does increase side effects, and therefore decreases compliance. Since both resins are virtually identical in action, the choice of one over the other is based on patient preference, specifically taste and the ability to tolerate ingestion of bulky material. Recently, a new candy bar formulation of cholestyramine (Cholybar®) has been introduced, as well as a new low-calorie, low-volume formulation (Questran Light®), which has 1.4 calories per packet.[44]

If resin treatment is discontinued, cholesterol levels return to pretreatment levels within a month. In patients with heterozygous hypercholesterolemia who have not achieved desirable cholesterol levels on resin plus diet therapy, the combination therapy of colestipol hydrochloride and nicotinic acid has been shown to provide further lowering of serum cholesterol, triglycerides, and LDL, and cause an increase in serum HDL concentration.[44] Other drug combinations are now being studied, and the combination therapy of BAS and HMG-CoA reductase inhibitors shows particular promise[35-38,45] (see Chapter 6).

Adverse Effects of Resins

Since cholestyramine and colestipol are not absorbed in the body, the range of adverse effects is limited. A majority of patient complaints stem from the resin's effect on the GI tract and from subjective complaints concerning the taste, texture, and bulkiness of the resins. The most common side effect is constipation, which is reported in approximately 10% of patients on colestipol and 28% of patients on cholestyramine. This side effect is seen most commonly in patients taking large doses of the resin and most often in patients over 65 years of age. Although most cases of constipation are mild and self-limiting, progression to fecal impaction can occur. A range of 1/30 to 1/100 patients on colestipol and approximately 12% on cholestyramine experience abdominal distention and/or belching, flatulence, nausea, vomiting, and diarrhea. Peptic ulcer disease, GI irritation and bleeding, cholecystitis, and cholelithiasis have been reported in 1/100 patients taking colestipol, but has not been shown to be purely drug related.

Fewer than 1/1000 patients on colestipol experience hypersensitivity reactions such as uticaria or dermatitis. Asthma and wheezing were not seen with colestipol treatment but were reported with cholestyramine treatment in a small number of patients. In a small percentage of patients, muscle pain, dizziness, vertigo, anxiety, and drowsiness have been reported with both drugs. With cholestyramine treatment, hematuria, dysuria, and uveitis have also been reported. Resin therapy has been associated with transient and modest elevations of serum glutamic oxaloacetic transaminase and alkaline phosphatase. Some patients have shown an increase in iron binding capacity and serum phosphorus, along with an increase in chloride ions and a decrease in sodium ions, potassium ions, uric acid, and carotine.

Case reports have described hyperchloremic acidosis in a child taking cholestyramine suffering from ischemic hepatitis and renal insufficiency,[46] a child with liver agenesis and renal failure,[47] and in a patient with diarrhea due to ileal resection.[48] For these reasons, those patients at risk for hyperchloremia should have serum chloride levels checked during the course of resin treatment.

In the LRC-CPPT study, the incidence of malignancy in the cholestyramine treated group was equal to the control group, however, the incidence of GI malignancy in the treated group was higher than the nontreated group (21 vs 11, respectively), with more fatal cases in the treated group (8 deaths in the treated group vs 1 in the control group). In animal studies, cholestyramine was shown to increase the mammary tumerogenesis capabilities of 7,12 dimethylbenzanthracene (DMBA) in Wistar rats. In the cholestyramine plus DMBA treated rats, there was a fivefold increase in the incidence of mammary cancer over control.[49] Stemming from the resin's ability to disrupt normal fat-soluble vitamin absorption in the gut, there have been a number of reports concerning the occurrence of hypoprothrombinemic hemorrhage secondary to vitamin K malabsorption.[50,51] In both the above cited cases, the patients responded to vitamin K adjunct therapy.

An early study showed that colestipol can bind T_4 in the gut and in vitro. This binding can theoretically upset the normal reabsorption of T_4 from the gut and thereby disrupt normal T_4 recycling, causing hypothyroidism. However, a subsequent study showed that for euthyroid patients, thyroid function tests remained normal throughout resin treatment.[52] It is advisable that patients on thyroid replacement therapy avoid taking the replacement drug at the same time as ingesting the resin to avoid any malabsorption problems.

Conclusion

The bile-acid resins, cholestyramine and colestipol, have been extensively studied and have been proven effective in reducing cholesterol levels in patients with primary hypercholesterolemia caused by increases in LDL-cholesterol levels (type IIa and type IIb). Studies have shown that resins have the ability to slow the progression of atherosclerosis and limit the clinical consequences of the disease. Because of their effectiveness and safety, bile-acids will continue to be the drug of first resource for patients who have hypercholesterolemia unresponsive to diet therapy. Further use of resins will focus on combination therapy with other antihyperlipoproteinemic drugs, such as nicotinic acid or HMG CoA reductase inhibitors. The use of these combination therapies will increase the range of the antihyperlipoproteinemic effect of the agents and allow for a decrease in the dosage of the drugs used, thereby decreasing the incidence of side effects.

References

1. Lipid Research Clinics Program: The Lipid Research Clinics Coronary Primary Prevention Trial Results. I. Reduction in the incidence of coronary heart disease. JAMA 1984; 251: 351-364.
2. Lipid Research Clinics Program: The Lipid Research Clinics Coronary Primary Prevention Trial Results. II. The relationship in reduction of incidence of coronary heart disease to cholesterol lowering. JAMA 1984; 251: 365-374.
3. Glueck CJ: Pediatric primary prevention of atherosclerosis. N Engl J Med 1986; 314: 175-177.
4. Brown MS, Goldstein J: Drugs used in the treatment of hyperlipoproteinemias. In Gilman AGG, Rall TW, Nies AS, et al (eds): The Pharmacologic Basis of Therapeutics, 8th ed, New York, Pergamon Press, 1990; pp 874-894.
5. Grundy SM, Ahrens EH, Salen S: Interruption of the entero-hepatic circulation of bile acids in man: Comparative effects of cholestyramine and ileal exclusion on cholesterol metabolism. J Lab Clin Med 1971; 78: 94-121.
6. Packard CJ, Shepherd J: The hepatobiliary axis and lipoprotein metabolism: effects of bile acid sequestrants and ileal bypass surgery. J Lipid Res 1982; 23: 1081-1098.
7. Shepherd J: Mechanism of action of bile acid sequestrants and other lipid lowering drugs. Cardiology 1989; 76 (Suppl 1): 65-74.
8. Innis SM: The activity of HMG-CoA reductase and acyl-CoA cholesterol acyltransferase in hepatic microsomes in male, female and pregnant rats. The effect of cholestyramine treatment and the relationship of enzyme activity to microsomal lipid composition. Biochim Biophys Acta 1986; 875: 355-361.
9. Slater HR, Packard CJ, Bicker S, et al: Effects of cholestyramine on receptor-mediated plasma clearance and tissue uptake of human low density lipoproteins in the rabbit. J Biol Chem 1980; 255: 10210-10213.
10. Shepherd J, Packard CJ, Bicker S, et al: Cholestyramine promotes receptor-mediated low-density lipoprotein catabolism. N Engl J Med 1980; 302: 1219-1222.
11. Illingworth RD: Lipid lowering drugs: an overview of indications and optimum therapeutic use. Drugs 1987; 33: 259-279.
12. Runeberg L, Miettinen TA, Nikkils EA: Effect of cholestyramine on mineral excretion in man. Acta Med Scand 1972; 192: 71-76.
13. Buchwald H: Lowering of cholesterol absorption and blood levels by ileal exclusion. Experimental basis and preliminary clinical report. Circulation 1964; 296: 713-720.
14. Buchwald H, Varco R: Ileal bypass with hypercholesterolemia and atherosclerosis. JAMA 1966; 196: 627-630.
15. Buchwald H, Varco RL, Matts JP, et al: Effects of partial ileal bypass surgery on mortality and morbidity from coronary heart disease in patients with hypercholesterolemia. N Engl J Med 1990; 323: 946-955.
16. Kuo PT, Hayase K, Kostis JB, et al: Use of combined diet and colestipol in long term (7-7 1/2 years) treatment of patients with type II hyperlipoproteinemia. Circulation 1979; 59: 199-211.

17. Miller NE, Clifton-Bligh P, Nestel PJ: Effects of colestipol, a new bile acid sequestering resin on cholesterol metabolism in man. J Lab Clin Med 1973; 82: 876-890.

18. Brensike JF, Levy RI, Kelsey SF, et al: Effects of therapy with cholestyramine on progression of coronary arteriosclerosis: results of the NHLBI type II coronary intervention study. Circulation 1984; 69: 313-324.

19. Levy RI, Brensike JF, Epstein SE, et al: The influence of changes in lipid values induced by cholestyramine and diet on progression of coronary artery disease: results of the NHLBI type II coronary prevention study. Circulation 1984; 69: 325-336.

20. Krauss RM, Williams PT, Brensike J, et al: Intermediate-density lipoproteins and progression of coronary artery disease in hypercholesterolemic men. Lancet July 11, 1987; 62-66.

21. Glueck CJ, Fallat R, Tsang R: Pediatric familial type II hyperlipoproteinemia: therapy with diet and cholestyramine resin. Pediatrics 1973; 52: 669-679.

22. West RJ, Lloyd JK, Leonard JV: Long-term follow up of children with familial hypercholesterolemia treated with cholestyramine. Lancet 1980; October: 873-875.

23. Glueck CJ, Mellies MJ, Dine M, et al: Safety and efficacy of long-term diet and diet plus bile acid-binding resin cholesterol-lowering therapy in 73 children heterozygous for familial hypercholesterolemia. Pediatrics 1986; 78: 338-348.

24. Subbiah MTR, Yunker RL, Rymaszewski Z, et al: Cholestyramine treatment in early life of low-density lipoprotein deficient Watanabe rabbits: decreased aortic cholesterol ester accumulation and atherosclerosis in adult life. Biochim Biophys Acta 1981; 920: 251-258.

25. Beil U, Crouse JR, Einarsson K, et al: Effect of interruption of the enterohepatic circulation of bile acids on the transport of very low density lipoprotein triglycerides. Metabolism 1982; 31: 438-444.

26. Crouse JR: Hypertriglyceridemia: a contraindication for use of bile acid binding resins. Am J Med 1987; 83: 243-248.

27. Gordon DJ, Knoke J, Probstfield JL, et al for the Lipid Research Clinics Program: High-density lipoprotein cholesterol and coronary heart disease in hypercholesterolemic men: The Lipid Research Clinics Coronary Primary Prevention Trial. Circulation 1986; 74: 1217-1225.

28. Aogaro P, Bittolo Bon G, Cazzolato G, et al: Are apolipoproteins better discriminators than lipids for atherosclerosis? Lancet 1979; April: 901-903.

29. Brunzell JD, Sniderman AD, Albers JJ, et al: Apoprotein B and A-I and coronary artery disease in humans. Arteriosclerosis 1984; 4: 79-83.

30. Kottke BA: Apolipoprotein markers for coronary artery disease: a dissenting view. Drug Ther, October 1986; 151-171.

31. Steinberg D, Parthasarathy S, Carew TE, et al: Beyond cholesterol: modification of low-density lipoprotein that increase its atherogenicity. N Engl J Med 1989; 320: 915-924.

32. Witztum JL, Schonfeld G, Weidman JW, et al: Bile sequestrant therapy alters the composition of low-density and high-density lipoprotein. Metabolism 1979; 28: 221-229.

33. Witztum JL, Young SG, Elam RL, et al: Cholestyramine induced changes in low-density lipoprotein composition. I. Studies in the guinea pig. J Lipid Res 1985; 26: 92-103.
34. Frick MH, Elo O, Haapa K, et al: Helsinki Heart Study: Primary-prevention trial with gemfibrozil in middle-aged men with dyslipidemia: safety of treatment, changes in risk factors, and incidence of coronary heart disease. N Engl J Med 1987; 317: 1237-1245.
35. Blankenhorn DH, Nessim SA, Johnson RL, et al: Beneficial effects of combined colestipol-niacin therapy on coronary atherosclerosis and coronary venous bypass grafts. JAMA 1987; 257: 3233-3240.
36. Cashin-Hemphill L, Mack WJ, Pogoda JM, et al: Beneficial effects of colestipol-niacin on coronary atherosclerosis. JAMA 1990; 264: 3013-3017.
37. Brown G, Albers JJ, Fisher LD, et al: Regression of coronary artery disease as a result of intensive lipid lowering therapy in men with high levels of apolipoprotein B. N Engl J Med 1990; 323: 1289-1298.
38. Kane JP, Malloy MJ, Ports TA, et al: Regression of coronary atherosclerosis during treatment of familial hypercholesterolemia with combined drug regimens. JAMA 1990; 264: 3007-3012.
39. Olsson AG: Regression of femoral atherosclerosis. Circulation 1991; 83: 698-700.
40. Duffield RGT, Lewis B, Miller NE, et al: Treatment of hyperlipidaemia retards progression of symptomatic femoral atherosclerosis: a randomized controlled trial. Lancet 1983; 2: 639-642.
41. Olsson AG, Ruhn G, Erikson U: The effect of serum lipid regulation on the development of femoral atherosclerosis in hyperlipidaemia: a non-randomized controlled study. J Intern Med 1990; 227: 381-390.
42. Blankenhorn DH, Azen SP, Crawford DW, et al: Effects of colestipol-niacin therapy on human femoral atherosclerosis. Circulation 1991; 83: 438-447.
43. Kane JP, Malloy MJ, Tun P, et al: Normalization of low-density lipoprotein levels in heterozygous familial hypercholesterolemia with a combined drug regimen. N Engl J Med 1981; 304: 251-258.
44. Insull W, Marquis NR, Tsianco MC: Comparison of the efficacy of Questran Light, a new formulation of cholestyramine powder, to regular Questran in maintaining lowered plasma cholesterol levels. Am J Cardiol 1991; 67: 501-505.
45. Hoogerbrugge N, Mol M, VanDormaal JJ, et al: Efficacy and safety of pravastatin, compared to and in combination with bile acid binding resins in familial hypercholesterolemia. J Intern Med 1990; 228: 261-266.
46. Pattison M, Lee SM: Life-threatening metabolic acidosis from cholestyramine in an infant with renal insufficiency. Am J Dis Children 1987; 141: 479-480 (Letter).
47. Kleinman PA: Cholestyramine and metabolic acidosis. N Engl J Med 1974; 290: 861 (Letter).
48. Hartline JV: Hyperchloremia, metabolic acidosis, and cholestyramine. J Pediatrics 1976; 89: 155.
49. Melkem MF, Galoriet HF, Eskander ED, et al: Cholestyramine promotes 7,12 dimethylbenzanthracene induced mammary cancer in Wistar rats. J Cancer 1987; 56: 45-48.

50. Gross L, Brotman M: Hypoprothrombinemia and hemorrhage associated with cholestyramine therapy. Ann Intern Med 1970; 72: 95-96.
51. Shosania AM, Grewar D: Hypoprothrombinemic hemorrhage due to cholestyramine therapy. Can Med Assn J 1986; 134: 609-610.
52. Witztum JL, Jacobs LS, Schonfeld G: Thyroid hormone and thyrotropin levels in patients placed on colestipol hydrochloride. J Clin Endocrinol & Metab 1978; 46: 838-840.

Chapter 5

Effects of Gemfibrozil and Other Fibric Acid Derivatives on Blood Lipids and Lipoproteins

Peter Zimetbaum M.D., William H. Frishman M.D.,
Shoshonah Kahn M.D.

Fibric acid derivatives (FAD) are a class of drugs that have been shown to inhibit the production of VLDL, while enhancing VLDL clearance, due to stimulation of lipoprotein lipase activity. The drugs can reduce plasma triglycerides and concurrently raise HDL-cholesterol levels. Their effects on LDL-cholesterol are less marked and more variable.

In screening tests in rats in 1962 and 1963, a series of arloxyisobutyric acids reduced plasma concentrations of total lipid and cholesterol.[1-3] The compound that combined maximal effectiveness with relatively little toxicity was clofibrate. However, when the drug was used in the large World Health Organization Trial to determine its effect on primary prevention of coronary heart disease, problems with the agent were identified. Although a decline in the rate of nonfatal myocardial infarction was observed, an increase in the rates of noncardiac death and overall mortality were also reported.[4] Furthermore, there was also an observed increase in the frequency of gastrointestinal diseases with the drug, specifically cholelithiasis.[5] A twofold increase in the rate of cholelithiasis was also reported with clofibrate when compared to placebo in the Coronary Drug Project.[4,5]

From *Medical Management of Lipid Disorders: Focus on Prevention of Coronary Artery Disease,* edited by William H. Frishman, M.D. © 1992, Futura Publishing Inc., Mount Kisco, NY.

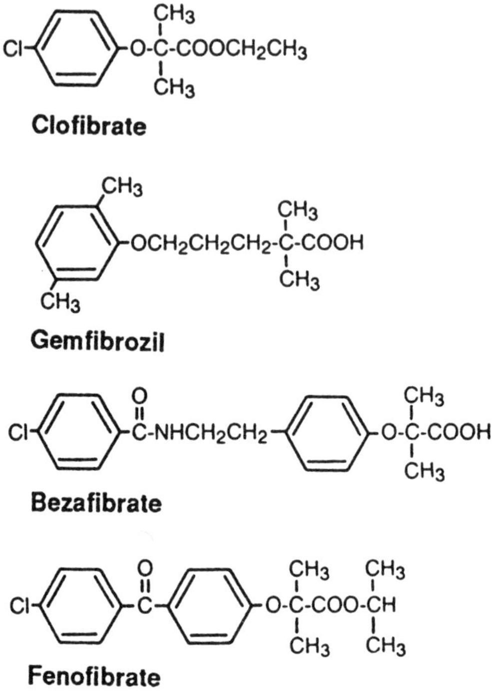

Figure 1: *Chemical structures of some fibric acid derivatives.*

During the 1960s and 1970s many analogues of clofibrate were developed and tested for their hypolipidemic potential (Fig. 1). Of these, gemfibrozil (Lopid®, Parke-Davis, Morris Plains, N.J.) currently is being marketed in the United States. The results of the Helsinki Heart Study[6,7] have demonstrated the safety and efficacy of gemfibrozil as a lipid-modifying agent, and its potential role for reducing the risk of coronary heart disease in patients with specific lipid and lipoprotein disorders.

Other FADs, including bezafibrate, ciprofibrate, and fenofibrate, are marketed in Europe and are actively being investigated in the United States.

This chapter reviews the clinical pharmacology of gemfibrozil and the other FADs, discusses the therapeutic experiences with these agents, and provides recommendations for their clinical use.

Pharmacokinetics

Gemfibrozil is well absorbed from the gastrointestinal (GI) tract with peak plasma levels seen 1-2 hours after administration.[8] The plasma half-life is 1.5 hours after single dose and 1.3 hours after multiple dose therapy.[8] The plasma drug concentration is proportional to dose and steady state, and is reached after 1-2 weeks of twice daily dosing.[9] Gemfibrozil undergoes oxidation of the ring methyl group in the liver to form hydroxymethyl and carboxyl metabolites[10] (in total, there are four major metabolites). No reports as yet have described distribution of the drug into human breast milk or across the placenta.[8] Two thirds (66%) of the twice daily dose is eliminated in the urine within 48 hours, 6% is eliminated in the feces within 5 days of dosing,[11] and less than 5% of the drug is eliminated unchanged in the urine. Regardless of the dosing schedule, there is no drug accumulation with normal or impaired renal function.[12]

In vitro, gemfibrozil is 98% bound to albumin at therapeutic levels.[10] There have been reports that gemfibrozil, in vitro, when administered concurrently with warfarin, leads to a doubling of the unbound warfarin fraction.[10] Similarly, clofibrate has been found to potentiate the anticoagulation activity of warfarin.[13]

The other FADs behave similarly to gemfibrozil. Of these, fenofibrate has been studied most extensively.[14] Fenofibrate is well absorbed after oral administration. It is hydrolyzed to fenofibric acid, subsequently undergoing carbonyl reduction, resulting in reduced fenofibric acid. Fenofibrate and reduced fenofibric acid are both active pharmacologically.[15] Sixty-five percent of fenofibrate is excreted into the urine, principally as fenofibryl glucoronide (< 20% is excreted through the bile).[16] Drug elimination is completed within 24-48 hours, and the half-life of the drug is approximately 4.9 hours. Steady-state equilibrium is established within 2 to 3 days. Unlike gemfibrozil, the newer FADs, particularly fenofibrate and bezafibrate, can accumulate in patients with renal failure, and dose adjustments may be necessary.[17] No pharmacokinetic interaction exists between fenofibrate and bile-acid sequestrants.[16]

Mechanism of Action of Gemfibrozil and Other FADs

Currently, it is impossible to delineate one clear mechanism of action of gemfibrozil and other FADs. However, observations have been made regarding the effects of the drugs on the individual lipoprotein components and the cholesterol-triglyceride metabolic pathways.

One direct action of FADs appears to be an increase in the level of plasma lipoprotein lipase (LPL).[18-20] LPL is deficient in type I hyperlipoproteinemia, type I and II diabetes mellitus, hypothyroidism, heart failure, and nephrotic syndrome. LPL is increased by insulin treatment of diabetes mellitus, aerobic exercise, and FADs. LPL is the rate-limiting enzyme governing the removal of triglycerides from lipoproteins in the plasma.[21] It functions at the luminal surface of the vascular endothelium and depends on the presence of apo C-II on chylomicrons, very low-density lipoproteins (VLDL), and high-density lipoproteins (HDL) to activate its hydrolytic capacity.[21] The level of LPL has been found to be increased after the addition of gemfibrozil for reasons that are not yet understood. Enhancement of LPL is also found with fenofibrate therapy.[22] Fenofibrate may alter apo C-II, a known activator of LPL.[23] Similarly, bezafibrate has been found to increase LPL activity, thus catabolism of VLDL is increased.[24]

VLDL is produced in the liver and circulates in the plasma where LPL hydrolyzes it to a VLDL remnant by removing triglycerides. The VLDL remnant is then either taken up by an apo E receptor- mediated process in the liver or converted to low-density lipoprotein (LDL). FADs have been shown to decrease the production of VLDL and to increase its fractional catabolic rate (FCR).[18] An increased FCR means an increased production of VLDL remnants that are then taken up by the liver or converted to LDL.

Gemfibrozil has been studied predominantly in subjects with hypertriglyceridemia. The newer FADs have been studied in subjects with hypertriglyceridemia and subjects with hypercholesterolemia. Although the FADs have similar triglyceride-lowering abilities, fenofibrate, bezafibrate, and ciprofibrate appear to have a greater cholesterol-lowering effect than gemfibrozil and clofibrate, which is allegedly related to additional HMG CoA reductase-inhibiting activity.[25]

In the hypertriglyceridemic state, there are alterations in the usual homogeneity of lipoprotein subtractions.[26,27] For instance, much of the LDL of hypertriglyceridemic patients contains a smaller amount of cholesterol ester and a greater amount of triglyceride than is usual.[18] Presumably, this aberration results from an exchange of triglyceride for cholesterol between VLDL and LDL. The triglyceride-enriched LDL is then hydrolyzed by hepatic triglyceride lipase leading to further reduction in size and increase in density of the LDL molecule. Thus, in the hypertriglyceridemic state, there are LDL fragments of normal composition coexisting with triglyceride-enriched and triglyceride-depleted forms. The clinical consequences of this heterogeneous LDL population are not yet apparent.

In the hypertriglyceridemic state, the production and fractional clearance of LDL are also increased.[26,28] Thus, patients with isolated hypertriglyceridemia may have low to normal LDL levels. Correction of the hypertriglyceridemic state with gemfibrozil restores the normal LDL population and reduces the production and catabolism of LDL. The result is often a slight increase in LDL levels. Similarly with fenofibrate or bezafibrate, when there are normal or low LDL levels, treatment will increase levels of LDL.[29] Grundy and Vega offer the explanation that during fibrate therapy, the increased lipolysis of VLDL-triglyceride promotes increased hepatic uptake of VLDL remnants, leaving fewer receptors for clearance of LDL and thus, increased plasma LDL.[18] Saku et al suggest that the short-term result of FAD therapy is an increased production of LDL-cholesterol secondary to increased VLDL catabolism and resultant down-regulation of hepatic LDL receptors.[20] As the VLDL levels decrease, the LDL-cholesterol content increases, establishing a more normal LDL particle. Regardless of the mechanism for changes in LDL levels, the importance of inhibiting production of VLDL, as well as enhancing catabolism, have been well documented.[30] Studies show that gemfibrozil, in the primary hypertriglyceridemic state, increases LDL less than clofibrate, a drug that enhances VLDL catabolism without altering production.[30] Fenofibrate treatment of hypertriglyceridemic patients causes LDL levels to increase by 25%, as VLDL levels decrease by 77%.[31] The drug also increases the clearance rate of apo B and causes a decrease in apo B levels of approximately 35%.[29] Similar observations have been made with bezafibrate treatment of hypertriglyceridemia.[32]

HDL composition is also altered in hypertriglyceridemia.[33] Normally, HDL_{2a}, the cholesterol ester-rich subfraction, predominates in the circulation. HDL_{2a} is transformed to HDL_{2b} when it acquires triglyceride. HDL_3 is formed from the removal of triglyceride from HDL_{2b} by hepatic TG lipase and LPL. HDL_3 then acquires new cholesterol ester via lecithin cholesterol acetyl transferase (LCAT) and forms HDL_{2a}. Hypertriglyceridemia markedly reduces HDL_{2a} concentration and increases HDL_{2b} concentrations. Essentially, hypertriglyceridemia decreases the cholesterol content of HDL. FAD therapy reverses this process, leading to increased cholesterol content of HDL.[18,20] Gemfibrozil has also been found to stimulate the synthesis of apo A-I, the major apoprotein on HDL without altering its catabolism. Similarly, fenofibrate and bezafibrate increase apo A-I levels during treatment of hypertriglyceridemia. However, the levels of apo A-I rarely increase to the extent that HDL rises.[34]

Finally, the hypertriglyceridemic state is felt to be associated with an increase in cholesterol synthesis.[35] One explanation for this is that hypertriglyceridemic LDL is altered and may present less cholesterol to the cells, thus leading to less effective down-regulation of LDL receptors and less inhibition of HMG-CoA reductase. Consequently, cholesterol synthesis is increased. There is some evidence that FADs inhibit cholesterol synthesis.[36] From comparison studies conducted by Hunninghake and Peters, it appears that the newer FADs, fenofibrate, bezafibrate, and ciprofibrate, are more effective than gemfibrozil and clofibrate in reducing cholesterol levels.[25] The results of animal studies appear to confirm that these new agents inhibit HMG CoA reductase.[37] Although the older agents may have some minimal HMG CoA reductase inhibition activity, the results of animal studies have shown much greater activity with the newer agent, i.e., bezafibrate versus clofibrate.[38] In vivo, fenofibrate has been shown to decrease HMG CoA activity on human mononuclear cells in type IIa and IIb patients.[39] Similarly, bezafibrate has been found to inhibit HMG CoA reductase activity from mononuclear cells of normal and hypercholesterolemic patients.[40] Other data suggest an increased peripheral mobilization of cholesterol from tissues with FADs and feedback inhibition of hepatic cholesterol synthesis.[18,41]

FADs are also known to increase the secretion of cholesterol into bile and to decrease the synthesis of bile acids.[42] This effect is modulated by LDL receptor activity, with FADs increasing hepatic uptake of cholesterol and subsequent secretion into the bile. In 1972, Grundy et al first noticed this increased lithogenicity of bile accompanying clofibrate therapy.[36] Since then, other investigators have reported decreased fecal bile-acid secretion and increased fecal excretion of neutral steroid with gemfibrozil therapy.[43-45] The net effect of decreased bile-acid concentration and increased cholesterol concentration is a cholesterol supersaturation of bile, providing the potential nidus for gallstone formation. Studies with the newer FADs, especially fenofibrate, have shown variable results in terms of total bile-acid synthesis, and subsequent bile-acid saturability.[46-48] European and American studies, so far, have shown no increase in gallstone formation in patients on fenofibrate therapy.[46] Thus, the newer FADs may have less potential for gallstone formation.

Patients with elevated cholesterol levels are believed to have increased platelet-mediated coagulation secondary to enhanced platelet reactivity and thromboxane A_2 production.[49] A suggested pathogenesis is the ability of elevated LDL and cholesterol to alter the lipid membranes of platelets. Hypertriglyceridemia has also been associated with platelet hyperaggregability; however, the postulated defect in this condition is abnormal fibrinolysis.[50]

Carvalho et al have demonstrated that type II hyperlipoproteinemia patients have a platelet abnormality causing increased aggregation in response to mediators such as adenosine diphosphate and epinephrine.[49] After the onset of aggregation, these platelets release factors that continue and accelerate the coagulation process and lead to increased fibrin formation. Data available thus far suggest that FADs might help correct the defective coagulation and fibrinolytic problems induced by hyperlipidemia.

Torstila et al studied the effects of gemfibrozil on type II patients and found that plasma prekallikrein and kininogen levels increased by 10.5% and 18.5%, respectively.[51] Laustiola et al observed that in patients with hypercholesterolemia who exercised, gemfibrozil caused a decrease in platelet reactivity and aggregability.[52] Sirtori et al[53] also studied gemfibrozil's effect on platelet function and found no statistically significant effect on aggregation or thromboxane A_2 levels. However, clofibrate and other FADs have been shown to decrease platelet aggregation in type II patients.

Fenofibrate and bezafibrate have been found to reduce platelet aggregation.[54] In a study of 62 patients with atherosclerotic vasculopathy and hyperfibrinogenemia, treatment with bezafibrate resulted in dose-dependent increases in fibrinolytic activity, with decreased fibrinogen, PG_4, blood filterability, and platelet aggregation when compared to placebo.[55] With regard to the myocardial microcirculation, Lesch et al[56] found that when 35 patients were treated with fenofibrate, there was a significant decrease in platelet viscosity and erythrocyte aggregation. Moreover, in 8 of 12 patients in this study selected for thallium myocardial scintigraphy after 8 weeks, 2 showed global and 6 showed regional improvement in myocardial blood flow.[56] Thus, a reduction in fibrinogen concentration may lead to an improved coronary microcirculation.

Additionally, fenofibrate has been shown to decrease platelet derived growth factor (PDGF) in vitro, which inhibits smooth muscle proliferation in rabbit aorta.[57] Thus, the FADs may directly inhibit atherosclerotic plaque formation.

An additional property unique to fenofibrate is the ability to decrease uric acid by 10% to 28% in 90% to 95% of all treated patients with an increase in renal uric acid secretion.[15,46] The exact mechanism and clinical significance of this observation is unclear.

Clinical Experience

The effects of FADs are largely dependent upon the pretreatment lipoprotein classification of the patient.[25] In short, most patients respond to therapy with a decrease in triglyceride levels and an increase in HDL levels. Hypertriglyceridemic patients without hypercholesterolemia often have a slight increase in cholesterol and LDL levels. However, patients with hypercholesterolemia often have a decrease in their cholesterol and LDL levels. The predominant difference between gemfibrozil and the newer FADs is that the newer FADs lower LDL to a greater degree than does gemfibrozil.[25] One explanation for this is that these new derivatives appear to inhibit HMG CoA reductase as well as enhance the action of LPL.[41]

The clinical data for FADs are best summarized according to their effect on hypertriglyceridemic patients, subjects with combined hypertriglyceridemia and hypercholesterolemia, and subjects with only hypercholesterolemia. Patients with type I chylomicronemia would not benefit from FADs because these individuals lack LPL, the enzyme upon which FADs presumably act.

Hypertriglyceridemic States

The Helsinki Heart Study, a 5-year double-blind intervention trial, used gemfibrozil on 2051 middle-aged men, 8.8% of whom had type IV hyperlipidemia. In this subgroup there was a 5% increase in LDL with gemfibrozil compared to a 7% increase with placebo.[6] There was a 10% increase in HDL and a significant decrease in total cholesterol. Type IV patients experienced the greatest drop in triglycerides compared to type IIa or IIb subjects. There was a 2% incidence in cardiovascular endpoints in this treated group compared to 3.3% in the placebo group. A relationship between the decreased triglyceride levels and the decreased cardiovascular morbidity was not observed.[7,57] Instead, it was proposed that the elevated HDL, perhaps resulting from triglyceride lowering, conferred protection.

Kasaniemi and Grundy[30] studied 14 patients with hypertriglyceridemia and mild hypercholesterolemia. They found that gemfibrozil caused a 51% decrease in triglycerides and a 31% increase in HDL and did not significantly change total cholesterol levels. LDL cholesterol levels increased by 11%. Furthermore, production of VLDL decreased by 28%, and catabolism increased by 92%. Similar findings have been observed with the newer FADs. The European experience with fenofibrate is extensive. Since 1975, there have been 82 trials and 6.5 million patient-years of experience treating hyperlipidemia.[46] Overall, European studies of hypertriglyceridemic patients treated with fenofibrate found mean triglyceride levels decreased by 57% after 6 months of treatment (baseline average 6.58 mm/L [583 mg/dl], and mean cholesterol decreased 21% after 1.6 years of treatment.[46] In the United States multicenter double-blind, placebo-controlled study of fenofibrate in 147 type IV and V hyperlipidemic patients,[58] the patients were divided into two groups: (1) triglyceride 3.95-5.63 mm/L (350-499 mg/dl) at baseline, and (2) triglyceride 5.65-16.94 mm/L (500-1500 mg/dl) at baseline. At 8 weeks, triglycerides were reduced 46% in group A and 56% in group B. Total cholesterol decreased 9% and 14%, respectively. VLDL decreased 45% and 49%, respectively, while HDL increased 20% and 23%, respectively.

Bezafibrate has been studied in Europe and in small American trials. In Europe, Olsson[59] conducted a 4.5-year study of bezafibrate in 15 type IV patients; triglycerides decreased by 28% to 39%, VLDL decreased by 38% to 52%, and total and LDL-cholesterol decreased as much as 18% and 11%, respectively. HDL increased by 10% to 19%.[59] Saku and associates[60] studied a long-acting preparation of bezafibrate and found similar results: triglycerides decreased 50% at 1 month and 54% at 4 months, with a significant increase in HDL observed.

Thus it appears there is minimal or no difference in the triglyceride-lowering ability of the various FADs in treatment of type IV disease, although there may be a slightly greater cholesterol-lowering effect with the newer agents.

Recently, a study was carried out in 44 hypertriglyceridemic subjects with mild-to-moderate cognitive impairment indicative of cerebrovascular disease.[61] One half of the group was treated with 600 mg daily of gemfibrozil and diet, while the other half was treated with diet alone. Triglyceride values dropped by 50% in the treated group but remained roughly the same in the control group. Cholesterol levels were not significantly altered in either group. HDL and LDL values were not reported. Analysis of cerebral blood flow measured by cognitive scores and the xenon[133] inhalation technique showed that gemfibrozil-treated patients had significantly higher cognitive scores and cerebral perfusion than did the untreated subjects.

In 1985, Mas reported on a patient with dementia and hyperlipidemia.[62] After treatment with diet and fenofibrate, the patient's mental status improved dramatically.

Combined Hypertriglyceridemia and Hypercholesterolemia

This section reviews only those studies where patients had elevated triglycerides and an average total cholesterol of at least 6.72 mm/L (260 mg/dl). Frequently these patients fall under the category of the type IIb phenotype. However, less clear or fluctuating lipoprotein profiles with a familial tendency toward different phenotypes are better classified under the broad category of familial combined hyperlipidemia.

The Helsinki Heart Study had 30% of the subjects who met the criteria for the type IIb classification.[6] The type IIb patients had lower mean HDL levels than the type IIa patients. Treatment effected a 4% decrease in LDL and a 12% increase in HDL. Total cholesterol and triglycerides decreased significantly, as did the incidence and number of cardiac endpoints. In fact, type IIb patients had the most significant decrease in cardiovascular morbidity and mortality compared with type IIa and IV patients.[7] This finding is logical because type IV patients appear to be at less risk for coronary heart disease than type IIb patients. Thus, gemfibrozil is most indicated in type IIb patients.

The combined results of 14 major European studies of 688 type IIb patients treated with fenofibrate found mean cholesterol decreased 23% at 1 month and 21% at 3 months; mean triglycerides decreased 44% at 3 months. LDL decreased 15% to 30% and HDL increased 0 to 22%.[46] The fenofibrate multicenter trial of 227 patients with types IIa and IIb disease found similar results. In this study, IIb was defined as cholesterol > 6.45 mm/L (> 250 mg/dl), LDL > 4.53 mm/L (> 175 mg/dl), and triglycerides > 2.82 mm/L (> 250 mg/dl). Twenty percent of the cohort was defined as IIb. Using fenofibrate treatment, type IIb patients showed a decrease in cholesterol and LDL (15.8% and 6.1%, respectively), with HDL increased by 15.3%. Mean triglycerides decreased

44% and VLDL decreased 52.7%.[15] Hunninghake and Peters reviewed 14 studies of IIb patients and concluded that patients treated with fenofibrate, bezafibrate, or ciprofibrate showed a greater reduction in total cholesterol (mean −19%, −21%, −19%, respectively), than patients treated with gemfibrozil.[25] No significant difference was noted in triglyceride reduction (48% to 37%). Although LDL-cholesterol was reduced more with fenofibrate, bezofibrate, and ciprofibrate (−20%, −17%, −21%) versus clofibrate (−4%), there was greater interpatient variability. HDL, in general, increased 10% to 20%.[25]

Vega and Grundy treated 11 predominantly hypertriglyceridemic patients with known coronary heart disease.[63] These subjects had an average pretreatment cholesterol of 6.78 mm/L (262 mg/dl), HDL-cholesterol of 0.65 mm/L (25 mg/dl) and triglyceride levels above the 95th percentage for their population. The mean LDL was 3.36 mm/L (130 mg/dl). With therapy, the average decrease in triglyceride was 63%, with an average rise in LDL of 31%. However, the synthetic rate of LDL was not increased. In fact, the production of LDL-apo B decreased. It is likely that the fractional clearance of LDL was suppressed. There was also a significant reversal in the LDL-apo B/cholesterol ratio. This ratio is abnormally high in some hypertriglyceridemic states, and this cohort was noted to have markedly increased production rates of apo B prior to therapy. In fact, close analysis reveals that gemfibrozil increases the cholesterol content of LDL far more than it increases the number of LDL particles. Finally, the LDL- cholesterol level in these patients did not rise over the 95th percentile in any of the subjects.

Manninen et al[64] conducted one of the first long-term studies using gemfibrozil in 254 type IIa and IIb patients. Regardless of the phenotype, there was a 16% decrease in total cholesterol, a 23% decrease in LDL-cholesterol, a 40% decrease in triglycerides, and a 23% rise in HDL. There was evidence for a decreased incidence of myocardial infarction, and this study set the stage for the Helsinki Heart Study.

Saku et al studied six patients with type V hyperlipoproteinemia who also had subnormal HDL levels.[20] Before therapy with gemfibrozil, the average triglyceride level was 11.06 mm/L (980 mg/dl), HDL was 0.59 mm/L (22 mg/dl), total cholesterol was 6.98 mm/L (270 mg/dl), and LDL was 2.28 mm/L (88 mg/dl). The mean reduction in triglyceride levels during therapy was 46% and in total cholesterol 80%. HDL rose by 36% and LDL cholesterol rose from subnormal levels to normal levels of approximately 2.97 mm/L (115 mg/dl). Apoprotein A-I and A-II levels, the proteins necessary for lecithin cholesterol ester transferase

(LCAT) addition and esterification of cholesterol to HDL, rose by 29% and 38%, respectively. Apoprotein B level increased by 18%.

Saku et al also studied eight patients with type V disease treated with bezafibrate SR (long-acting).[60] They found a 61% decrease in triglyceride at 2 months and a 57% decrease in triglyceride at 4 months. Total cholesterol decreased 19% and 18%, respectively, and HDL rose significantly.

Kuo et al reported the effectiveness of treatment with gemfibrozil and diet in six patients with type III disease.[65] These subjects had a mean baseline cholesterol of 15.96 mm/L (617 mg/dl), triglyceride of 12.39 mm/L (1097 mg/dl), and HDL of 1.19 mm/L (46 mg/dl). They noted a reduction in xanthomas and intermittent claudication. They also noted a reduction in mean levels of total cholesterol to 7.14 mm/L (276 mg/dl), mean triglyceride to 2.39 mm/L (212 mg/dl), and a slight increase in HDL to 1.22 mm/L (47 mg/dl).

Similar results were found in six European studies of fenofibrate treatment of type III patients.[46] Total cholesterol decreased 56% at 1 month and 48% at 6 months, from a baseline cholesterol level of 11.64 mm/L. Triglyceride levels decreased an average of 73%, from a baseline mean of 8.23 mm/L.

Hypercholesterolemia

Sixty-three percent of the subjects in the Helsinki Heart Study had type IIa lipid and lipoprotein profiles.[6] Gemfibrozil therapy resulted in an 11% decrease in LDL-cholesterol, a 9% increase in HDL, and a significant decrease in total cholesterol and triglyceride levels. The rate of new cardiovascular events was 35 per 1000 in placebo compared to 27 per 1000 in the treated group. Thus, although gemfibrozil had a beneficial effect on the lipid profile in type IIa subjects, the change in cardiovascular morbidity was less than that seen in type IIb or IV patients.[7] Interestingly, the pretherapy HDL levels in type IIb and IV patients were lower than those of type IIa patients. Therefore, the proportional rise in HDL was greater for the former two phenotypes, suggesting that the HDL-raising effect was more cardioprotective than the LDL-lowering effect.[7] Further subgroup analysis revealed that subjects with above average pretherapy HDL levels (> 1.19 mm/L [> 46 mg/dl]) had no improvement over placebo in the incidence of cardiovascular events.[57]

European studies of fenofibrate demonstrated that mean cholesterol decreased by 16% to 30% in a total of 807 type IIa patients. In general, the higher the baseline cholesterol, the greater its reduction with fenofibrate therapy. Also, VLDL decreased 26% to 31%, LDL decreased 17% to 29%, and HDL rose 0-20%.[46] In the United States multicenter trial of 172 type IIa patients treated with fenofibrate, similar results showed cholesterol decreasing 20.3%, triglycerides decreasing 37.9%, VLDL decreasing 38.4%, and HDL increasing 11.1%.

Olsson treated eight type IIa patients with bezafibrate for an average of 4.5 years and found equivalent results to fenofibrate therapy, with total cholesterol level decreasing 10% to 28%, LDL level decreasing 11% to 34%, and HDL levels rising to 12% (−2% to 12%).[59] Weisweiler conducted a comparison study of bezafibrate and gemfibrozil in the treatment of 29 patients with primary hyperlipidemia.[66] Bezafibrate caused a greater reduction in LDL-cholesterol (28% vs 18%) with a trend towards a greater reduction of total cholesterol, apo B, and triglyceride, and a trend towards greater gains in HDL. Kremer, studying 59 patients with type IIa or IIb disease,[67] similarly found a more marked reduction in total cholesterol, LDL-cholesterol, and triglyceride.

Ciprofibrate has equal efficacy compared to the other new FADs in the treatment of IIa disease. It causes an average decrease in cholesterol of 23%, a 30% decrease in triglyceride, and a 27% decrease in LDL. HDL increased by approximately 15% with the drug.[46]

Combination Drug Therapy

The principle of combination therapy, as discussed previously by our group,[68] is to combine drugs of different mechanisms to achieve an additive or synergistic effect in patients with hyperlipidemia.

East et al studied types II and IV patients to compare the combinations of gemfibrozil and colestipol with gemfibrozil and lovastatin.[69] The results are summarized in Table 1. Overall, gemfibrozil plus lovastatin proved the superior combination. Both of these combinations are theoretically sound because the mechanisms of action are all distinct. The combination of HMG-CoA reductase inhibitors and FADs is very efficacious. However, their use together is limited by an increased incidence of myositis and rhabdomyolitis. Bile-acid resins are also a good choice, however, they are known to raise triglycerides, an unwanted effect in many of the patients for whom FADs are ideal. Furthermore,

Table 1.
**Comparison of Gemfibrozil Alone and in Combination with
Colestipol or Lovastatin on the Lipid and Lipoprotein Levels of
Types IIB and IV Hyperlipoproteinemic Patients**

	Type IIB			Type IV		
	G	G + C	G + L	G	G + C	G + L
Triglyceride	−54%	−44%	−56%	−40%	−17%	−56%
VLDL-cholesterol	−64%	−54%	−69%	−33%	−32%	−65%
Total-cholesterol	−11%	−22%	−28%	7%	−17%	−24%
LDL-cholesterol	−3%	−17%	−25%	+29%	−34%	−33%
LDL Apo B	−18%	−23%	−33%	+2%	−13%	−30%
HDL-cholesterol	+26%	+10%	+26%	+26%	+16%	+35%

G = gemfibrozil; G+C = gemfibrozil + colestipol; G+L = gemfibrozil + lovastatin.

(Adapted from East, Bilheimer: Grundy[68] Annals of Internal Medicine 1988; 109: 25–32, with permission.)

there may be a slight mitigation of the HDL-raising effect with the addition of a resin compared to gemfibrozil alone.

Tuomilheto et al tested the combination of guar gum, a water-soluble fibric compound that functions like a bile-acid resin, with gemfibrozil.[70] They found that the addition of guar gum decreased total cholesterol values 13% more than gemfibrozil alone. LDL was also decreased significantly more with the combination, however, HDL levels were 5% lower with this dual therapy.

Fenofibrate has been studied in combination with colestipol for the treatment of type II disease. Sauvanet et al found that combination therapy caused an additional 10% to 15% decrease in cholesterol over fenofibrate therapy alone.[71] There was no additional triglyceride decrease with this combination. Weisweiler et al combined fenofibrate and colestipol for 8 weeks and found a significant additive effect on cholesterol, LDL-cholesterol, and apo B reduction.[72] In this study, triglycerides and HDL increased slightly (Table 2).

The combination of fenofibrate and colestipol has equal cholesterol-lowering potential when compared to simvastatin, but fenofibrate plus colestipol has greater HDL-raising potential (Table 3).[73]

When fenofibrate was combined with nicotinic acid for treatment of type IV disease, there was a greater reduction in LDL, total cholesterol, and triglycerides. However, the addition of nicotinic acid to feno-

Table 2.
Fenofibrate Versus Fenofibrate Plus Colestipol in Patients with Type II Hyperlipoproteinemia

	Fenofibrate 300mg TID	Fenofibrate 300mg TID + Colestipol 15g/d	Fenofibrate 250mg TID + Colestipol 15g/d
Cholesterol	−17%	−28%	−29%
Triglycerides	−33%	−23%	−25%
VLDL	−49%	−41%	−51%
LDL	−18%	−31%	−31%
HDL	+24%	+33%	+32%
Apo B	−10%	−19%	−19%

(Adapted from Weisweiler et al[71]*: European Journal of Clinical Pharmacology 196; 30: 191–94, with permission.)*

Table 3.
Fenofibrate Plus Colestipol Versus Simvastatin in Patients with Type II Hyperlipoproteinemia

	Fenofibrate + Colestipol	Simvastatin
LDL	−41%	−46%
HDL	+14%	+4%
Apo B	−28%	−27%
Apo A	+11%	+7%

Adapted from Weisweiler et al[72] *with permission.*

fibrate therapy caused the raised HDL measurement to return to low baseline levels.[74]

Similar results to the fenofibrate plus colestipol combination were found when bezafibrate was combined with colestipol. The addition of colestipol to bezafibrate therapy causes cholesterol to decrease an additional 9%, with triglyceride levels remaining the same.[75] Bezafibrate and colestipol has been particularly useful in the treatment of severe type IIa hypercholesterolemia inadequately treated with bezafibrate alone.[76]

Diabetes Mellitus

Noninsulin-dependent diabetes is associated with elevated triglyceride levels and low HDL levels. Todd and Ward[10] have summarized the major studies using gemfibrozil in diabetes mellitus from 1976-1982 and found that the triglyceride-lowering effect varied from 17%-57%, total cholesterol levels decreased from 1%-14%, and HDL levels rose from 6%-19%. LDL increased in some studies and decreased in others.

Garg and Grundy reported on noninsulin-dependent diabetics with hypertriglyceridemia treated with gemfibrozil.[77] Contrary to previous reports, they found that the response to therapy was the same for patients receiving oral hypoglycemics as for those receiving insulin. The patients were divided into those having marked hypertriglyceridemia (>5.65 mm/L[>500 mg/dl]) and those with moderate elevations (2.82-5.65 mm/L [250-500 mg/dl]). The average reduction in triglyceride levels in the group with marked elevation was 4.79 mm/L (425 mg/dl) or 52%, with a 55% reduction in VLDL and a 23% increase in HDL. However, LDL levels rose by 42% despite no change in LDL apo B levels. The addition of lovastatin reduced the LDL concentrations toward normal levels. Subjects with moderately increased triglyceride levels treated with gemfibrozil had a 31% decrease in triglycerides and a 36% decrease in VLDL-cholesterol. However, when compared with placebo, LDL-cholesterol rose 27%, LDL apo B rose 7%, and HDL levels did not increase compared to placebo. The results of this study suggest that gemfibrozil as monotherapy is not indicated in moderate diabetes-related hypertriglyceridemia. It may, however, be a useful adjunct to lovastatin in the diabetic patient with marked hypertriglyceridemia.

Smud et al[78] studied the effects of FADs in 64 patients with noninsulin-dependent diabetes mellitus and type II hyperlipidemia. Patients were divided into four groups: fenofibrate 300 mg daily or bezafibrate 600 mg daily, and glibenclamide 5-15 mg daily or chlorpropamide 250-500 mg daily. The results showed that both hypolipidemic agents caused a significant reduction in triglycerides, total cholesterol, LDL-cholesterol, and HDL. However, there was a significantly greater increase in HDL in the group on bezafibrate plus glibenclamide, especially in the females. In general, the groups on bezafibrate plus glibenclamide or bezafibrate plus chlorpropramide had better control over blood glucose levels than those groups on fenofibrate plus glibenclamide or fenofibrate plus chlorpropramide. Thus, this study concluded that the optimal combination for type II noninsulin-dependent diabetes mellitus patients is bezafibrate plus glibenclamide.[78] Another study by Riccardi in eight type IIb and eight type IV noninsulin-dependent diabetes mellitus patients found that the effect of bezafibrate SR had similar lipid-lowering results yet no change in blood glucose or glucose tolerance.[79] Other studies have shown bezafibrate to lower blood glucose.[80-82]

Renal Disease

Nephrotic syndrome and uremia are both known to cause hyperlipidemia. Groggel et al[83] treated 11 patients with nephrotic syndrome with gemfibrozil, achieving a 51% reduction in triglyceride levels and a 15% decrease in total cholesterol levels. LDL was decreased by 13% and HDL was increased by 18%. However, total cholesterol and LDL levels were still above normal despite reductions achieved by monotherapy with gemfibrozil. The addition of a bile-acid resin brought these values to a normal range. Bezafibrate has been studied in rats with hyperlipidemia and nephrotic syndrome. It did not significantly change cholesterol, but did significantly decrease triglycerides and significantly increase HDL.[84]

Pasternack and associates treated 18 patients with chronic renal failure with gemfibrozil, achieving a 50% reduction in triglyceride level and a 30% increase in HDL level.[85] Serum lipoprotein and hepatic lipase activity increased concurrently with the lipid alterations. This finding supports the mechanistic hypothesis that FADs enhance LPL activity. Changes in glomerular filtration rate were considered consistent with the progression of the underlying disease. There was a mean increase in serum creatinine phosphokinase (CPK) of 69% after 4 weeks of treatment; however, there was a gradual decrease after the full 24 weeks of therapy. Six patients displayed significant elevations of CPK but none were symptomatic, and all values returned to normal with the cessation of therapy. Clofibrate has been associated with myositis in patients with renal failure, and it appears from this study that CPK should be monitored carefully in the renal patient treated with gemfibrozil.

Norbeck et al[86] treated 12 patients with chronic renal failure and hyperlipidemia with bezafibrate and found triglyceride levels decreased 40%, VLDL decreased 49%, and HDL increased 17%, with each patient needing individual dosing. Individual dosing is needed because the FADs are cleared by the kidney, and fenofibrate and bezafibrate are nondialyzable. Thus, their half-life is much longer than normal in the patient with renal failure. Grutzmacher et al[17] studied 19 dialysis patients having cholesterol > 7.76 mm/L (> 300 mg/dl). With individualized bezafibrate dosing, triglycerides decreased 31%, cholesterol decreased 19%, and HDL increased. Bezafibrate has been shown to lead to muscle cramps, paresis, and elevated CPKs when dosing is not adjusted adequately for patients in renal failure.[87] Grundy does not recommend using the FADs in renal failure as the risk of myositis is significant without accurate dose adjustment.[88]

Prevention of Pancreatitis

Gemfibrozil is approved for clinical use in patients with very high elevations of serum triglycerides (types IV and V hyperlipoproteinemia) who despite dietary therapy are at risk of acute pancreatitis.[8] Patients who present with such risk usually have triglyceride levels > 22.58 mm/L (> 2000 mg/dl). Subjects with serum triglyceride levels < 11.29 mm/L (< 1000 mg/dl) usually are not at risk. Gemfibrozil can be considered for those patients with triglyceride level elevations between 11.29 and 22.58 mm/L (1000 and 2000 mg/dl) who have a history of pancreatitis, or abdominal pain suggestive of pancreatitis.

Clinical Use

It is well established that FADs are first-line therapy to reduce the risk of pancreatitis in patients with very high levels of plasma triglycerides. Results from the Helsinki Heart Study have also suggested that the hypertriglyceridemic patient with low HDL values can derive a cardioprotective effect from gemfibrozil.[6] Currently, it is not recommended to treat isolated low HDL levels with pharmacological intervention.[89]

FADs, particularly the newer generation, decrease total cholesterol and LDL levels. However, in the absence of elevated triglycerides, they should not be first-line therapy for hypercholesterolemic patients. Type IIb patients are the subset most commonly seen in clinical practice that would benefit from FAD therapy. HMG-CoA reductase inhibitors combined with FADs are excellent therapy for severe type IIb disease, however, CPK values must be closely monitored. Bile-acid resins plus gemfibrozil are also a reasonable combination for type IIb disease, however, HDL levels may drop slightly.

Gemfibrozil Dose

Gemfibrozil is approved for clinical use in the United States. The recommended dose for gemfibrozil is 600 mg before the morning meal and 600 mg before the evening meal.[8] Some patients may respond to 800 mg per day, and in most instances, the therapeutic benefit is augmented with an increase to 1200 mg daily. Some patients derive benefit from increasing the dosage of gemfibrozil to 1600 mg daily.[90]

Other FADs

Fenofibrate, bezafibrate, and ciprofibrate are not approved for clinical use in the United States. The recommended dose for fenofibrate is 300 mg daily, 100 mg with each meal, as food promotes absorption.[91] A single daily dose has been used with equivalent efficacy. The elimination half-life of fenofibrate is 20.8 hours, and 39 hours in the elderly.[23] In hepatic disease with cholestasis, the elimination half-life is increased to 44.7 hours.[23] Despite a prolonged half-life in the elderly and in hepatic disease, clearance of fenofibrate does not change due to compensatory changes in volume. However, in patients with impaired renal function, altered protein binding affects clearance and dose adjustments are needed. Fenofibrate is nondialyzable, and dose adjustment is needed for the dialysis patient.

Bezafibrate is recommended at 600 mg daily, 200 mg three times a day with meals, or as a 400 mg daily SR tablet.[17] As with fenofibrate, the dose must be adjusted in renal failure and with those on dialysis. Normally the half-life of bezafibrate is 2 hours. In patients with renal failure, the half-life is increased to 7.8 ± 3.9 hours.[92] Those patients on dialysis have half-lives as high as 17-22 hours.[17] In the elderly, it is recommended the dose adjustment be done if creatinine clearance is < 60 ml/min.[17] As discussed, bezafibrate reduces fibrinogen concentration, and has anticoagulant properties.[93] Thus, caution must be taken when combining bezafibrate with anticoagulants.

Clofibrate is available for clinical use in the United States. The recommended daily doses of 25-2000 mg, are usually divided into three daily doses.

Adverse Effects

Clofibrate, one of the earliest FADs, became unpopular because of its causative association with cholelithiasis and cholecystitis in the Coronary Drug Project.[5] The World Health Organization trial then reported a 29% increase in overall mortality in clofibrate-treated compared to placebo-treated subjects.[4] The mortality was principally due to post-cholecystectomy complications, pancreatitis, and assorted malignancies. The Helsinki Heart Study reported a decrease in cardiovascular mortality but not overall mortality in gemfibrozil-treated subjects.[6] The reason for the similarity of overall mortality rates with placebo and gemfibrozil remains a mystery at this time. Obviously, these findings have led to careful scrutiny of currently used and tested FADs.

The significant adverse effects noted with gemfibrozil in the Helsinki Heart Study included atrial fibrillation, acute appendicitis, dyspepsia, abdominal pain, and nonspecific rash.[6] The review of the European clinical trials of fenofibrate with 6.5 million patient-years shows a 2% to 15% adverse reaction rate, the most common adverse reactions being GI disturbances, dizziness and headache, muscle pains, and rash.[46] However, the only side effect significant in frequency was skin rash.[46] In the United States multicenter study of 227 patients treated with fenofibrate,[15] there was a 6% increase in side effects with fenofibrate, similar to the observations of the European studies. Three out of four of the patients who withdrew from the United States fenofibrate study had skin rashes, the fourth had fatigue and impotence.[15] Overall, the adverse experiences with bezafibrate have been similar to fenofibrate, with GI and neurological disturbances, muscle aches, and rashes most commonly seen.[15,93] After 4.5 years of treatment in 22 patients on bezafibrate, no side effects were reported by Olsson et al.[59]

In the Helsinki Heart Study, there was a 55% excess incidence of gallstones and a 64% excess incidence of cholecystectomy in the drug-treated compared to placebo-treated groups.[6] Although European studies of fenofibrate may show some increased lithogenicity of the bile, there has been no increase in the incidence of gallstone formation, either during the trials or during postmarketing surveillance.[46] Olsson et al found no increase in gallstone formation in 4.5 years of bezafibrate therapy.[59] An increased incidence of malignancy has not been observed.

The manufacturer of gemfibrozil has reported mild depressions of hemoglobin, white blood cell count, and hematocrit with the drug.[8]

The Helsinki Heart Study did not find significant alterations in these parameters.[6] Fluctuations of serum transaminase have been seen with fenofibrate therapy, as well as a decrease in alpha-gluconyl transferase and alkaline phosphatase, all without clinical significance. Also, uric acid is noted to decrease 10% to 28% on fenofibrate therapy.[46] The clinical significance of this is unknown.

There has been at least one report of an exacerbation of psoriasis in a patient treated with gemfibrozil, however, this finding was not reported by the Helsinki Heart Study.[94,95]

The combination of gemfibrozil and lovastatin has been repeatedly shown to predispose to rhabdomyolysis, and in some cases, renal failure.[96] The Helsinki Heart Study did not report any cases of myopathy in patients treated with only gemfibrozil.[6]

Bezafibrate has been shown to cause rhabdomyolysis at levels above normal in renal failure patients. Thus, caution must be taken in dosing with these patients.

Conclusions

Gemfibrozil and the new FADs can inhibit VLDL production and enhance VLDL clearance due to stimulation of lipoprotein lipase activity. The drugs lower plasma triglyceride levels while raising HDL-cholesterol levels.[97] They have variable effects on LDL levels, although the newer FADs may have greater cholesterol-lowering potential than gemfibrozil. The drugs are particularly useful in patients with very high triglycerides who are at risk of pancreatitis, and gemfibrozil specifically has been shown to reduce the risk of coronary artery disease complications in men with type IIb hyperlipoproteinemia. How these drugs protect against coronary vascular disease complications is not known, and morbidity and mortality studies with the newer FADs still need to be done.

The FADs are well tolerated, however, there is a small risk of cholelithiasis with these drugs. Combination therapy with HMG-CoA reductase inhibitors may be associated with an increased incidence of myositis and rhabdomyolitis.[98]

References

1. Thorp JM: Modification of metabolism and distribution of lipids by chlorphenoxyisobutyrate. Nature 1962; 194: 948-949.

2. Symposium on Atromide. J Atheroscler Res 1962; 3: 347-775.
3. Witiak DT, Newman HAI, Feller DR: Clofibrate and Related Analogs. New York, Marcel Dekker, 1972; pp 736-748.
4. Report from the Committee of Principal Investigators: A cooperative trial in the primary prevention of ischaemic heart disease using clofibrate. Br Heart J 1978; 40: 1069-1118.
5. Coronary Drug Project Research Group: Clofibrate and niacin in coronary artery disease. JAMA 1975; 231: 360-381.
6. Frick MH, Elo O, Haapa K, et al: Helsinki Heart Study: Primary prevention trial with gemfibrozil in middle-aged men with dyslipidemia. N Engl J Med 1987; 317: 1237-1245.
7. Manninen V, Elo O, Frick H, et al: Lipid alterations and decline in the incidence of coronary heart disease in the Helsinki Heart Study. JAMA 1988; 260: 41-51.
8. Product Insert: Parke-Davis, Division of Warner Lambert Co., AHFS Category 1988; 24: 6.
9. Smith TC: Toleration and bioavailability of gemfibrozil in healthy men. Proc Roy Soc Med 1976; 69 (Suppl 2): 24-27.
10. Todd PA, Ward A: Gemfibrozil: A review of its pharmacodynamic and pharmacokinetic properties, and therapeutic use in dyslipidaemia. Drugs 1988; 36: 314-339.
11. Okerholm RA, Keeley FJ, Peterson FE, et al: The metabolism of gemfibrozil. Proc Roy Soc Med 1976; 69 (Suppl 2): 11-14.
12. Evans JR, Forland SC, Cutler RE: The effect of renal function on the pharmacokinetics of gemfibrozil. J Clin Pharmacol 1987; 27: 994-1000.
13. Brown WV: Potential use of fenofibrate and other fibric acid derivatives in the clinic. Am J Med 1987; 83: 85-89.
14. Balfour JA, Heel RC: Fenofibrate: A review of its pharmacodynamic and pharmacokinetic properties and therapeutic use in dyslipidaemia. Drugs 1990; 40: 260-290.
15. Knopp R: Review of the effects of fenofibrate on lipoproteins, apoproteins, and bile saturability. U.S. Studies. Cardiol 1989; 76 (Suppl 1): 14-22.
16. Chapman MJ: Pharmacology of fenofibrate. Am J Med 1987; 83:21-25.
17. Grutzmacher P, Scheuermann EH, Siede W, et al: Lipid lowering treatment with bezafibrate in patients on chronic haemodyalysis: pharmacokinetics and effects. Klin Wochenschr 1986; 64: 910-916.
18. Grundy SM, Vega GL: Fibric acids: effects on lipids and lipoprotein metabolism. Am J Med 1987; 83: 9-20.
19. Nikkila EA, Yiikahri R, Huttunen JK: Gemfibrozil: effect on serum lipids, lipoproteins, post-heparin plasma lipase activities and glucose tolerance in primary hypertriglyceridemia. Proc Roy Soc Med 1976; 69 (Suppl 2): 58-63.
20. Saku K, Gartside PS, Hynd BA, et al: Mechanism of action of gemfibrozil on lipoprotein metabolism. J Clin Invest 1985; 75: 1702-1712.
21. Eckel RH: Lipoprotein lipase: a multifunctional enzyme relevant to common metabolic disease. N Engl J Med 1989; 320: 1060-1068.
22. Heller F, Harvengt C: Effect of clofibrate, bezafibrate, fenofibrate and probucol on plasma lipolytic enzymes in normolipidemic subjects. Eur J Clin Pharmacol 1983; 25: 57-63.

23. Caldwell J: The biochemical pharmacology of fenofibrate. Cardiol 1989; 76 (Suppl 1): 33-44.
24. Gavish D, Oschry Y, Fainaru M, et al: Changes in very low, low, and high density lipoproteins during lipid lowering (bezafibrate) therapy: studies in type IIA and IIB hyperlipoproteinemia. Eur J Clin Invest 1986; 16: 61-68.
25. Hunninghake DB, Peters JR: Effects of fibric acid derivatives on blood lipid and lipoprotein levels. Am J Med 1987; 83: 44-49.
26. Eisenberg S, Gavish D, Oschry Y, et al: Abnormalities in very low, low and high density lipoproteins in hypertriglyceridemia. J Clin Invest 1984; 74: 470-482.
27. Fischer WR: Heterogeneity of plasma LDL - manifestations of the physiologic phenomenon in man. Metabolism 1983; 32: 283-291.
28. Vega GL, Grundy SM: Kinetic heterogeneity of low density lipoproteins in primary hypertriglyceridemia. Arteriosclerosis 1986; 6: 395-406.
29. Ginsberg HN: Changes in lipoprotein kinetics during therapy with fenofibrate and other fibric acid derivatives. Am J Med 1987; 83: 66-70.
30. Kasaniemi YA, Grundy SM: Influence of gemfibrozil and clofibrate on metabolism of cholesterol and plasma triglycerides in man. JAMA 1984; 251: 2241-2246.
31. Shepard J, Caslake MJ, Lorimer AR, et al: Fenofibrate reduces low density catabolism in hypertriglyceridemic subjects. Arteriosclerosis 1985; 5: 162-168.
32. Packard CJ, Clegg RJ, Dominiczak MH, et al: Effect of bezafibrate on apolipoprotein B metabolism in type III hyperlipidemic subjects. J Lipid Res 1986; 27: 930-938.
33. Eisenberg S: High density lipoprotein metabolism. J Lipid Res 1984; 25: 1012-1058.
34. Schwandt P, Weisweiler P: Effect of bezafibrate on the high density lipoprotein subfractions HDL_2 and HDL_3 in primary hyperlipoproteinemia Type IV. Artery 1980; 7: 464-470.
35. Kleinman Y, Eisenberg S, Oschry Y, et al: Defective metabolism of hypertriglyceridemic lipoprotein in cultured human skin fibroblasts. Normalization with bezafibrate. J Clin Invest 1985; 75: 1796-1803.
36. Grundy SM, Ahrens EGJ, Salen G, et al: Mechanism of action of clofibrate on cholesterol metabolism in patients with hyperlipidemia. J Lipid Res 1972; 13: 531-551.
37. Shepard J, Packard CJ: An overview of the effects of p-chlorphenoxyisobutyric acid derivatives on lipoprotein metabolism. In Fears R (ed): Pharmacologic Control of Hyperlipidemia. Barcelona, Spain, Prous Sci Publishers, 1986; 135-144.
38. Hudson K, Mojumder S, Day AJ: The effect of bezafibrate and clofibrate on cholesterol ester metabolism in rabbit peritoneal macrofages stimulated with acetylated low density lipoproteins. Explor Molec Pathol 1983; 38: 77-81.
39. Schneider A, Stange EF, Ditschuneit HH, et al: Fenofibrate treatment inhibits HMG CoA reductase activity in mononuclear cells from hyperlipoproteinemic patients. Atherosclerosis 1985; 56: 257-262.

40. Blasi F, Sommariva D, Cosentini R, et al: Bezafibrate inhibits HMG CoA reductase activity in incubated blood mononuclear cells from normal subjects and patients with heterozygous familial hypercholesterolemia. Pharmacol Res 1989; 21: 247-254.
41. Berndt J, Gaumert R, Still J: Mode of action of the lipid lowering agents, clofibrate and BM 15075, on cholesterol biosynthesis in rat liver. Atherosclerosis 1978; 30: 147-152.
42. Palmer RH: Effects of fibric acid derivatives on biliary lipid composition. Am J Med 1987; 83: 37-43.
43. Bateson MC, Maclean D, Ross PE, et al: Clofibrate therapy and gallstone induction. Dig Dis 1978; 7: 623-628.
44. Angelin B, Einarsson K, Leijd B: Biliary lipid compositions during treatment with different hypolipidaemic drugs. Eur J Clin Invest 1979; 9: 185-190.
45. Kasaniemi YA, Grundy SM: Clofibrate, caloric restriction, supersaturation of bile, and cholesterol crystals. Scand J Gastroent 1983; 18: 897-902.
46. Blane GF: Review of European clinical experience with fenofibrate. Cardiology 1989; 76 (Suppl 1): 1-13.
47. Leiss O, Meyer-Krahmer K, Von Bergmann K: Biliary lipid secretion in patients with heterozygous familial hypercholesterolemia and combined hyperlipidemia. Influence of bezafibrate and fenofibrate. J Lipid Res 1986; 27: 213-223.
48. Eriksson M, Angelin B: Bezafibrate therapy and biliary lipids: effects of short-term and long-term treatment in patients with various forms of hyperlipoproteinemia. Eur J Clin Invest 1989; 17: 396-401.
49. Carvalho ACA, Colman RW, Lees RS: Platelet function in hyperlipoproteinemia. N Engl J Med 1974; 290: 434-438.$er 50 Hamsten A, Wiman B, DeFaire U, et al: Increased plasma levels of a rapid inhibitor of tissue plasminogen activator in young survivors of myocardial infarction. N Engl J Med 1985; 313: 1557-1563.
51. Torstila I, Kaukola S, Malkonen M, et al: Effect of gemfibrozil on plasma lipoproteins, apolipoproteins and the kallikrein-kinin system. Proceedings of an International Symposium: 8th Asian Pacific Congress of Cardiology 1984; 36-42.
52. Laustiola K, Lassila R, Koskinen P, et al: Gemfibrozil decreases platelet reactivity in patients with hypercholesterolemia during physical stress. Clin Pharm Ther 1988; 43: 302-307.
53. Sirtori CR, Franceschini G, Gianfranceschi G, et al: Effects of gemfibrozil on plasma lipoprotein-apolipoprotein distribution and platelet reactivity in patients with hypertriglyceridemia. J Lab Clin Med 1987; 110: 279-286.
54. Kloer HU: Structure and biochemical effects of fenofibrate. Am J Med 1987; 83: 3-8.
55. Niort G, Bulgarelli A, Cassader M, et al: Effect of short term treatment with bezafibrate on plasma fibrinogen, fibrinopeptide A, platelet activation, and blood filterability in atherosclerotic hyperfibrinogenemic patients. Arteriosclerosis 1988; 71: 113-119.
56. Leschke M, Hoffken H, Schmidtsdorff A, et al: Effect of fenofibrate on fibrinogen concentration and blood viscosity. Consequences for myocardial

microcirculation in coronary heart disease? Dtsch Med Wochenschr 1989; 114: 939-944.

57. Gotto AM: The Helsinki Heart Study Trial. Cardiol Bd Rev 1989; 6 (3 Suppl): 47-52.

58. Seidehamel RJ: Fenofibrate in Type IV and Type V hyperlipoproteinemia. Cardiology 1989; 76 (Suppl 1): 23-32.

59. Olsson AG, Lang PD, Vollmar J: Effect of bezafibrate during 4.5 years of treatment of hyperlipoproteinemia. Arterosclerosis 1985; 55: 195-203.

60. Saku K, Sasaki J, Arakawa K: Effect of slow release bezafibrate on serum lipids, lipoproteins, apolipoproteins, and post heparin lipolytic activities in patients with Type IV and Type V disease. Clin Therapy 1989; 11: 331-340.

61. Rogers RL, Meyer JS, McClintic K, et al: Reducing hypertriglyceridemia in elderly patients with cerebrovascular disease stabilizes or improves cognition and cerebral perfusion. Angiology 1989; 40: 260-269.

62. Mas JL, Bousser MG, Lacombe C, et al: Hyperlipidemic dementia. Neurology 1985; 35: 1385-1387.

63. Vega GL, Grundy SM: Gemfibrozil therapy in primary hypertriglyceridemia associated with coronary heart disease. JAMA 1985; 253: 2398-2403.

64. Manninen V, Malkonen M, Eisalo A, et al: Gemfibrozil in the treatment of dyslipidaemia. A five year follow-up study. Acta Med Scand 1982; 668 (Suppl): 82-87.

65. Kuo PT, Detwiler JG, Wilson AC: Gemfibrozil treatment of Type III hyperlipoproteinemia (familial dysbeta lipoproteinemia). (abstr.) Angiology 1986; 37: 775-776.

66. Weisweiler P: Effect of bezafibrate and gemfibrozil on serum lipoproteins in primary hypercholesterolemia. Arzneim Forsch 1988; 38: 925-927.

67. Kremer P, Marowski C, Jones C, et al: Therapeutic effects of bezafibrate and gemfibrozil in hyperlipoproteinemia Type IIA and IIB. Curr Med Res Opin 1989; 11: 292-303.

68. Frishman WH, Zimetbaum P, Nadelmann J: Lovastatin and other HMG-CoA reductase inhibitors. J Clin Pharmacol 1989; 29: 975-982.

69. East C, Bilheimer DW, Grundy SM: Combination drug therapy for familial combined hyperlipidemia. Ann Intern Med 1988; 109: 25-32.

70. Tuomilheto J, Silvasti M, Manninen V, et al: Guar gum and gemfibrozil - an effective combination in the treatment of hypercholesterolemia. Atherosclerosis 1989; 76: 71-77.

71. Sauvanet JP, Mejean L, Drouin P, et al: Treatment of long terme (24 mois) de type II par l-association colestipil et procetefene. (abstr) 42nd French Congress of Medicine, Ziege, Belgium, September 1979: 29.

72. Weisweiler P, Merk W, Jacob B, et al: Fenofibrate and colestipol: effects on serum and lipoprotein lipids and apoproteins in familial hypercholesterolemia. Eur J Clin Pharmacol 1986; 30: 191-194.

73. Weisweiler P, Schwandt P: Colestipol plus fenofibrate versus symvinolin in familial hypercholesterolaemia. Lancet 1986; ii: 1212-1213.

74. Rossner S, Olsson AG: Effects of combined procetofene - nicotinic acid therapy in treatment of hypertriglyceridemia. Atherosclerosis 1980; 35: 413-417.

75. Series JJ, Caslake MJ, Kilday C, et al: Effect of combined therapy with bezafibrate and cholestyramine on low density lipoprotein metabolism with Type IIA hypercholesterolemia. Metabolism 1989; 38: 153-158.
76. Sommariva D, Tirrito M, Bonfiglioli D, et al: Long term effect of bezafibrate and of a bezafibrate and cholestyramine combination on lipids and lipoprotein lipids in Type IIA hypercholesterolemic patients. Intl J Clin Pharmacol Res 1986; 6: 249-253.
77. Garg A, Grundy SM: Gemfibrozil alone and in combination with lovastatin for treatment of noninsulin dependent diabetes mellitus. Diabetes 1989; 38: 364-372.
78. Smud R, Sermukslis B: Bezafibrate and fenofibrate in Type II diabetics with hyperlipoproteinemia. Curr Med Res Opin 1987; 10: 612-624.
79. Riccardi G, Genovese S, Saldalmacchia G, et al: Effects of beza-fibrate on insulin secretion and peripheral insulin sensitivity in hyperlipidemic patients with and without diabetes. Atherosclerosis 1989; 75: 175-181.
80. Ruth E, Vollmar J: Improvement in diabetes control by treatment with bezafibrate. Dtsch Med Wochenschr 1982; 107: 1470-1473.
81. Bruneder H, Klein HJ: Treatment of hyperlipoproteinemia in diabetic patients. Dtsch Med Wochenschr 1981; 106: 1653-1656.
82. Wahl P, Hasslacher C, Lang PD, et al: Lipid lowering effect of bezafibrate in patients with diabetes mellitus and hyperlipidemia. Dtsch Med Wochenschr 1978; 103: 1233-1237.
83. Groggel GC, Cheung AK, Ellis-Benigni K, et al: Treatment of nephrotic hyperlipoproteinemia with gemfibrozil. Kidney Intl 1989; 36: 266-271.
84. Williams AJ, Baker FE, Walls J: The effect of bezafibrate on hyperlipidemia in experimental nephrotic syndrome rats. J Pharmacol 1985; 37: 741-743.
85. Pasternack A, Vanttinen T, Solakivi T, et al: Normalization of lipoprotein lipase and hepatic lipase by gemfibrozil results in correction of lipoprotein abnormalities in chronic renal failure. Clin Nephrol 1987; 27: 163-168.
86. Norbeck HE, Anderson P: Treatment or uremic hypertriglyceridemia with bezafibrate. Atherosclerosis 1982; 44: 125-136.
87. Rumpf KW, Barth M, Blech M, et al: Bezafibrate induced myolysis and myoglobinuria in patients with impaired renal function. Klin Wochenschr 1984; 62: 346-348.
88. Grundy SM: Management of hyperlipidemia of kidney disease (editorial review). Kidney Int'l 1990; 37: 847-853.
89. Gordon DJ, Rifkind BM: High density lipoprotein - The clinical implications of recent studies. N Engl J Med 1989; 321: 1311-1316.
90. Virtamo J, Manninen V, Malkonen M: A placebo controlled rising-dose, double-blind trial with gemfibrozil in dieting patients with primary hyperlipoproteinemia. Vasc Med 1984; 2: 22-27.
91. Bertolini S, Elicio N, Daga A, et al: Effect of a single daily dose treatment of fenofibrate on plasma lipoproteins in Type IIB patients. Eur J Clin Pharmacol 1988; 34: 25-28.
92. Anderson P, Norbeck HE: Clinical pharmacokinetics of bezafibrate in patients with impaired renal function. Eur J Clin Pharmacol 1981; 21: 209-214.

93. Monk JP, Todd PA: Bezafibrate. A review of its pharmacodynamic and pharmacokinetic properties and therapeutic use in hyperlipidemia. Drugs 1987; June: 539-576.
94. Fischer DA, Elias PM, Leboit PL: Exacerbation of psoriasis by the hypolipidemic agent, gemfibrozil. Arch Dermatol 1988; 124: 854-855 (correspondence).
95. Frick HM: Exacerbation of psoriasis. Arch Dermatol 1989; 125: 132 (correspondence).
96. Goldman JA, Fishman AB, Lee JE, et al: The role of cholesterol-lowering agents in drug-induced rhabdomyolysis and polymyositis. Arthritis Rheum 1989; 32: 358-359.
97. Manninen V, Tenkanen L, Koskinen P, et al: Joint effects of serum triglycerides and LDL cholesterol and HDL cholesterol concentrations on coronary heart disease risk in the Helsinki Heart Study: Implications for treatment. Circulation 1992; 85: 37-45.
98. Pierce LR, Wysowski DK, Gross TP: Myopathy and rhabdomyolitis associated with lovastatin-gemfibrozil combination therapy. JAMA 1990; 264: 71-75.

Chapter 6

HMG-CoA Reductase Inhibitors

William H. Frishman M.D., Peter Zimetbaum M.D.,
Melanie Derman M.D.

Increased levels of total cholesterol, LDL-cholesterol, and VLDL-cholesterol are identified as risk factors for the development of coronary artery disease (CAD).[1-5] An inverse relationship between HDL-cholesterol levels and CAD risk has also been established.[1-4]

A recent report describing 356,222 screenees of the Multiple Risk Factor Intervention Trial (MRFIT) showed that a 10% reduction in cholesterol was associated with a 11.3% reduction in the mortality rate from CAD and a 4.4% decrease from all causes.[6] The Lipid Research Clinics Program demonstrated that a reduction in total cholesterol of 13.4% and LDL-cholesterol of 20.3% led to a 19% (statistically significant) reduction in CAD death and nonfatal myocardial infarction.[7] This study also demonstrated that a small increase in HDL-cholesterol could lead to a 2% reduction in the CAD rate.[7]

The National Institutes of Health issued a consensus report based on the available data suggesting that for every 1% reduction in serum cholesterol, there is a 2% reduction in CAD morbidity and mortality over the entire distribution of cholesterol values studied.[8] They recommended that all individuals over the age of 30 years have cholesterol values 5.72 mm/L (< 200 mg/dl). For individuals with cholesterol values 6.72 mm/L (> 260 mg/dl), the panel recommended diet therapy with the addition of drug therapy, if necessary.[8]

More recently, the National Cholesterol Education Program Expert Panel suggested a cholesterol level of 6.21 mm/L (240 mg/dl) as a point for intervention (see Chapter 1).[9]

From *Medical Management of Lipid Disorders: Focus on Prevention of Coronary Artery Disease,* edited by William H. Frishman, M.D. © 1992, Futura Publishing Inc., Mount Kisco, NY.

The initial step in lowering cholesterol is a special diet that should be low in fat with substitution of saturated fatty acids with polyunsaturated fatty acids (Chapter 2). Cholesterol intake should also be reduced. Total calories should not be excessive because obesity is associated with increased production of triglycerides and VLDL-cholesterol. Since lipid levels may be reduced only minimally by special diets in certain patients,[10] drug therapy is the next step. There are several drugs that can be used.

In 1987 the Food and Drug Administration approved the marketing of lovastatin, a competitive inhibitor of 3-hydroxy-3-methylglutaryl coenzyme A reductase, the rate-limiting enzyme step in cholesterol synthesis in the body. The pharmacology and clinical efficacy of this new cholesterol-lowering drug and other drugs in this class (pravastatin and simvastatin) approved for marketing in 1991 are reviewed in this chapter.

Lovastatin

Chemistry

Lovastatin (mevinolin, MK-803, Mevacor®) is a fermentation product of the fungus *Aspergillus terreus*.[11] It is similar in structure to an earlier compound, mevastatin, a less potent inhibitor of HMG-CoA reductase, whose clinical development was limited by possible cardiogenicity in animals.[12]

The chemical structures of lovastatin and other HMG-CoA reductase inhibitors currently under investigation (simvastatin and pravastatin) are shown in Figure 1.

Pharmacology

Lovastatin, as a competitive inhibitor of HMG-CoA reductase, interferes with the formation of mevalonate, a precursor of cholesterol. Mevalonate also is a precursor of ubiquinone and dolichol, nonsterol substances essential for cell growth (Fig. 2).[13] It initially was thought that the HMG-CoA reductase inhibitors might inhibit formation of these substances, but this is not the case.[13] Nonsterol synthesis does not appear to be inhibited by HMG-CoA reductase.

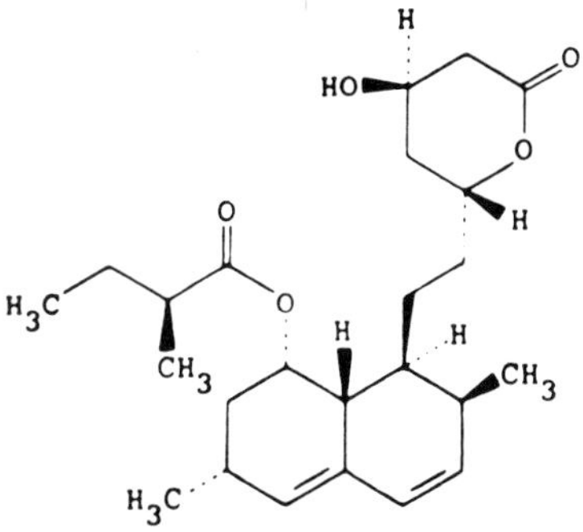

Lovastatin

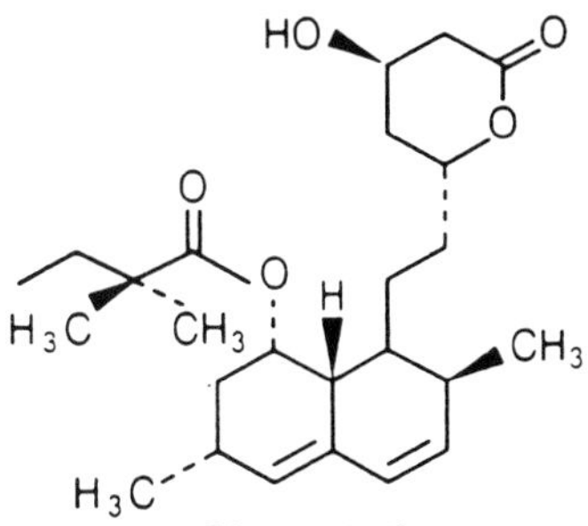

Simvastatin

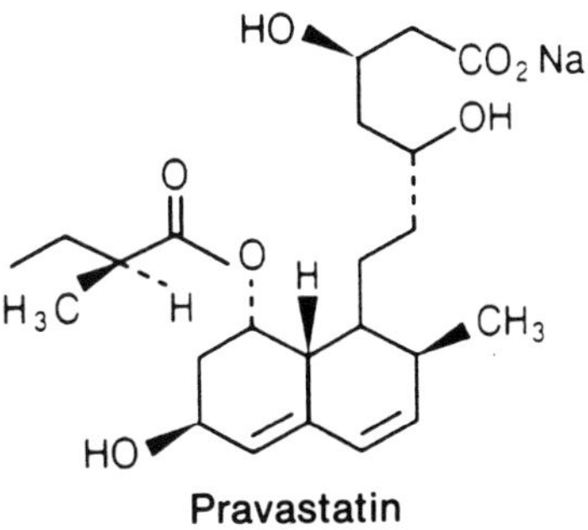

Pravastatin

Figure 1: *Structural formulas of some of the HMG-CoA reductase inhibitors.*

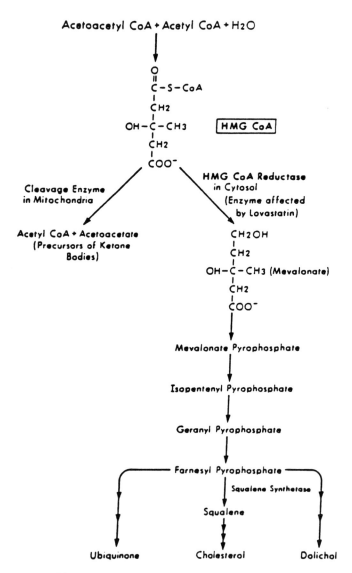

Figure 2: *Branched pathway of cholesterol synthesis.*

Pharmacokinetics

Lovastatin is an inactive lactone (prodrug) that is hydrolyzed in the liver to an active α-hydroxyacid form. The prodrug was developed rather than the active hydroxyacid form because the prodrug undergoes more efficient shunting to the liver on first pass. The potential result of this enhanced liver uptake is lower peripheral drug concentrations and fewer systemic side effects.[14] This principal metabolite is the inhibitor of the enzyme HMG-CoA reductase. The dissociation constant of the enzyme inhibitor complex (K_1) is approximately 10^{-9} M.[15,16]

An oral lovastatin dose is absorbed from the gastrointestinal tract with greater absorption at meals. The drug undergoes extensive first-pass metabolism in the liver, its primary site of action, with subsequent excretion of drug equivalents in the bile. It is estimated that only 5% of an oral dose reaches the general circulation as an active enzyme inhibitor. The drug is excreted via the bile (83%) and the urine (10%).[15,17]

Lovastatin and its β-hydroxyacid metabolite are highly bound to human plasma proteins.[17] Lovastatin crosses the blood-brain and placental barriers. The major active metabolites present in human plasma are the β-hydroxyacid of lovastatin, its 6'-hydroxy derivative, and two unidentified metabolites. Peak plasma levels of both active and total inhibitors are attained 2 to 4 hours after lovastatin ingestion. The half-life of the β-hydroxyacid is approximately 1 to 2 hours. This rapid metabolism would seem to necessitate multiple doses per day. Clinical trials, however, have indicated once or twice daily dosing is optimum. With a once daily dosing regimen, within the therapeutic range of 20-80 mg/d, steady-state plasma concentration of total inhibitors after 2 to 3 days were about 1.5 times that of a single dose.[17] Single daily doses administered in the evening are more effective than the same dose given in the morning, perhaps because cholesterol mainly is synthesized at night (12-6 a.m.).[18] A substantial clinical effect of lovastatin is noted within 2 weeks, a maximal effect at 4 to 6 weeks, and the effect completely dissipates 4 to 6 weeks after stopping the drug.

Clinical Experiences

Several investigators have demonstrated that lovastatin lowers the cholesterol levels of normal and hypercholesterolemic animals.[11,19-23] These studies demonstrate that the increased LDL receptor activity and decreased LDL synthesis are responsible for the hypocholesterolemic effect of the drug. Several studies in humans have confirmed this observation.[24-26] This increase in LDL receptor activity occurs in response to a decrement in cholesterol synthesis by HMG-CoA reductase inhibition. LDL may be reduced by either its increased clearance from the plasma or its decreased production.

Human Volunteers

Tobert and associates[27] conducted the first clinical studies with lovastatin in normal male volunteers on normal diets. The cholesterol values of the subject group ranged between (3.88 and 7.76 mm/L) (150 and 300 mg/dl). Using a placebo-control design, these investigators demonstrated that cholesterol levels were reduced significantly with active lovastatin therapy (14.6% reduction with 5 mg twice daily for 11 days, 24.5% reduction with 15 mg twice daily for 9 days, and 21.5% reduction with 50 mg used twice daily for 7 days). Serum triglycerides were not changed. In a follow-up study, doses of the drug ranging from 6.25 to 50 mg twice daily were administered for 4 weeks.[28] Clinical effects were observed by 3 days, and after 4 weeks cholesterol was reduced significantly, as well as the LDL-cholesterol and apolipoprotein B levels in plasma. No adverse effects were reported.

Heterozygous Familial Hypercholesterolemia (FH)

This autosomal dominant condition is characterized by a partial deficiency of LDL receptors, resulting in very high LDL levels, tendon xanthomas, and an increased risk of cardiovascular mortality.

Bilheimer and Grundy studied six patients with heterozygous FH using radiolabeled LDL-cholesterol and its disappearance to calculate a fractional catabolic rate (FCR) and transport rate.[24] The FCR is used to approximate LDL receptor activity[21,24,26]; the transport rate is indicative of LDL synthesis. Using 20-mg lovastatin administered twice daily, a 27% decrease in total cholesterol and a 30% reduction in LDL-cholesterol were observed, resulting from an increase in the FCR. This study suggested a direct stimulatory effect on LDL receptor activity by lovastatin, perhaps related to a stimulation of the gene for LDL receptor synthesis by the drug.[24]

Subsequent studies evaluating lovastatin's efficacy in heterozygous FM showed that lovastatin, in doses of 5 mg twice daily, produced decreases in total serum cholesterol and LDL- cholesterol.[29] Doses of 10, 20, and 40 mg twice daily were even more effective.[29-31] Patients in these studies were maintained on low cholesterol diets (≤ 300 mg/daily) and had serum cholesterol values > 7.75 mm/L (> 300 mg/dl) prior to treatment.

Despite these impressive findings, some authorities feel that lovastatin alone is often insufficient therapy for heterozygous FH.[32,33] Instead, lovastatin in combination with a bile acid sequestrant is considered a better approach.[34]

Homozygous FH

This disorder is distinguished by an absolute deficiency in LDL receptors with an exaggeration and acceleration of the processes described for heterozygous FH.

Lovastatin appears to be less effective in reducing cholesterol for this condition than for heterozygous FH and non-FH.[31,35] The drug may not be very effective in a condition where patients have few or no LDL receptors. East and colleagues[36] tested this hypothesis in a child with homozygous FH who was relatively unresponsive to lovastatin but became extremely responsive to the drug after liver transplant. The implication of these findings is that lovastatin's primary function is to increase LDL receptors, not decrease lipoprotein production.

Familial Combined Hyperlipidemia

This diagnosis is made by identifying multiple phenotypes of hyperlipidemia in a single family. Some members may have elevated LDL alone (type IIa), elevated VLDL alone (type IV), or both (type IIb). Some may have elevated chylomicrons and VLDL (type V) or elevated intermediate density lipoprotein (type III). This disorder is present in 0.5% of the population and in a large percentage of men having had a premature myocardial infarction (before age 60).[37] Lovastatin has been found to reduce cholesterol in patients with this disease.[38,39] The combination of lovastatin and gemfibrozil has been suggested as an extremely potent treatment for this condition.[37,39] However, in view of the higher risk for severe myopathy with this combination, lovastatin alone may be adequate therapy for many patients with mixed hyperlipidemia.[39]

Type 3 Hyperlipidemia (Familial Dysbeta-lipoproteinemia)

This condition is caused by an inability to remove VLDL remnants from the plasma. Case studies have suggested that lovastatin effectively lowers LDL and VLDL remnants in these patients.[40,41]

Non-FH (Polygenic)

Similar to the findings in patients with heterozygous FH, lovastatin is effective in patients with non-FH.[29,42,43] This state is characterized by an elevation of serum cholesterol > 6.21 mm/L (> 240 mg/dl) and LDL > 4.14 mm/L (> 160 mg/ dl), without other stigmata of FH (xanthomas, etc.).

Lovastatin may be more effective in normalizing cholesterol values in the non-FH patient because of lower initial levels, although the reduction in LDL-cholesterol may be greater in the FH patient.[17]

One study evaluating lovastatin in this population was the multicenter trial involving 264 patients who had primary hypercholesterolemia with an elevated LDL-cholesterol and normal triglycerides (type IIa) or mild hypertriglyceridemia (type IIb).[44] All subjects were felt to be at high risk for CAD on the basis of a variety of risk factors: all were on an American Heart Association phase I diet that was continued during the study. Patients were randomized to therapy with lovastatin (20 or 40 mg twice daily for 12 weeks) or cholestyramine (doses escalating from 4 to 8 to 12 g daily over 3 weeks and then continued at 12 mg daily for the remaining 9 weeks of the 12-week treatment period). Cholesterol fell by 27% in the 40 mg/d lovastatin group and by 34% in the 80 mg/d group, versus a 12% reduction in the cholestyramine group. In addition, LDL-cholesterol was reduced by 32% and 42%, respectively, versus 23%, and apolipoprotein B by 28% and 33% versus 21%. Both drugs produced a similar mean increase in HDL. Although cholestyramine had no significant effect on VLDL-cholesterol and apolipoprotein levels and was associated with an 11% increase in plasma triglycerides, lovastatin was associated with a reduction of VLDL-cholesterol by 34% and 31% and plasma triglycerides by 21% and 27%.

Adverse effects reported in the two groups were primarily gastrointestinal intolerance (13% in the low-dose lovastatin group, 14% in the higher dose group, and 58% in the cholestyramine group). Constipation was reported by 28% of those on cholestyramine versus 2% and 6%, respectively, on low- and high-dose lovastatin. Dyspepsia occurred in 17% on cholestyramine versus 1% on lovastatin. One patient on 40 mg lovastatin developed a myositis that reversed with discontinuation of the drug. Ophthalmological exam showed no consistent changes, and both drugs raised transaminase levels, particularly aminotransaminase levels. Increases to more than twice normal were actually more common in the cholestyramine than in the lovastatin group. The authors concluded that lovastatin is more effective and better tolerated in the short-term treatment of primary hypercholesterolemia.

The Expanded Clinical Evaluation of Lovastatin (EXCEL) study, a multicenter double-blind, diet- and placebo-controlled trial, evaluated the efficacy and safety of lovastatin in 8245 patients with moderate hypercholesterolemia (total cholesterol between 6.21 and 7.76 mm/L [240 and 300 mg/dl]).[45] Patients were randomly assigned to receive placebo or lovastatin at a dosage of 20 mg once daily, 40 mg once daily, 20 mg twice daily, or 40 mg twice daily for 48 weeks. Lovastatin produced sustained dose-related changes from baseline (for dosages of 20 to 80 mg daily), decreased LDL-cholesterol levels (24% to 40%), increased HDL-cholesterol levels (6.6% to 9.9%), decreased total cholesterol levels (17% to 29%), and decreased triglyceride levels (10% to 19%).[46] The difference between lovastatin and placebo in the incidence of clinical adverse experiences requiring discontinuation of treatment was small. Successive transaminase level elevations greater than 3 times the upper limit of normal were observed in 0.1% of patients receiving placebo and 20 mg/d, increasing to 0.9% in those receiving 40 mg daily and 1.5% in those receiving 80 mg daily. Myopathy, defined as muscle symptoms with a creatinine kinase elevation greater than 10 times the upper limit of normal, was found in only 1 patient (0.1%) receiving 40 mg once daily and 4 patients (0.2%) receiving 80 mg daily of lovastatin. The investigators concluded that lovastatin, when added after an adequate trial of a prudent diet, is highly effective and generally well tolerated in patients with moderate hypercholesterolemia.[46]

A multicenter study was undertaken to compare the effects of lovastatin (given in four different dosage regimens) and probucol in 290 patients with severe primary hypercholesterolemia.[47] Patients were all maintained on lipid-lowering diets and then randomized to receive 14 weeks of treatment with lovastatin 40 mg once daily in the morning, 40 mg once daily in the evening, 80 mg once daily in the evening, 40 mg twice daily, or probucol 500 mg twice daily. The mean reductions in total cholesterol in the five groups were 20%, 25%, 30%, 33%, and 10%, respectively. The corresponding values for LDL-cholesterol were 25%, 32%, 37%, 40%, and 8%. HDL-cholesterol increased by 9%-12% in all the lovastatin groups, but decreased by 23% in the probucol group. Triglycerides were reduced by 12%-25% in all the lovastatin groups but did not change significantly in the probucol group. The investigators concluded that lovastatin was more effective than probucol as a lipid-lowering agent.

A long-term clinical trial is now in progress where lovastatin is being used in a double-blind, placebo-controlled, primary prevention trial involving 8000 patients without clinical evidence of CAD, slight to moderate elevations of total cholesterol, and LDL-cholesterol, to establish whether treatment will decrease the rate of fatal CAD or nonfatal myocardial infarction.[48] Other studies are ongoing to evaluate the effects of lovastatin on the progression of atherosclerotic lesions of the coronary circulation using quantitative angiographic techniques. There is some recent evidence that lovastatin might reduce the incidence of restenosis following successful balloon angioplasty.[49,50] Studies in this area are also in progress.

Combination Therapy

The rationale for using lovastatin in combination with other cholesterol-lowering drugs is to cause an additive or synergistic reduction in total and LDL-cholesterol through complementary effects on LDL receptor function and other mechanisms. One interesting combination is lovastatin with bile-acid binding resins. Both drugs work to lower intracellular cholesterol and to maximize LDL receptor expression. The potential result is one of synergism without drug interaction.

In studies evaluating the efficacy of colestipol (10-20 g/daily), a bile-acid sequestrant, plus lovastatin (20-40 mg twice daily)[25,26,42] there were greater reductions in total cholesterol and LDL-cholesterol than with single drug therapy.[17] Illingworth notes that doubling the dose of lovastatin from 20-40 mg daily effects only a 5%-7% further reduction in LDL-cholesterol.[51] This is also true of the resins with their optimal dose being 16-20 mg daily. Therefore, he suggests that a combined therapy with 20 mg of lovastatin and 20 g of colestipol is superior to single dose therapy with lovastatin 40 mg twice daily.[51]

In a recent report from the Familial Atherosclerosis Treatment Study, the combination of lovastatin 40 mg daily and colestipol 30 g daily was more effective than colestipol and diet alone in reducing LDL and raising HDL in patients with CAD and elevated apoprotein B levels. There were also fewer cardiovascular events, less progression of coronary lesions, and more regression.[52]

Lovastatin (20 and 40 mg daily) when combined with nicotinic acid (3 g daily) was found to decrease LDL concentrations by 49%. Triglycerides were also reduced, making this combination particularly attractive for the treatment of type IIb hypercholesterolemia.[53] However, this duo may retard lovastatin's excretion secondary to nicotinic acid's potential impairment of hepatic metabolism.[54] This observation that nicotinic acid plus lovastatin has been associated with the development of myopathy is possibly explained by this interaction.[55]

Although the combination of lovastatin and gemfibrozil may increase the risk of myopathy, this regimen has been shown to be very effective in the treatment of severe familial combined hypercholesterolemia, as well as marked hypertriglyceridemia, in patients with noninsulin-dependent diabetes mellitus.[56]

The combination of lovastatin and probucol was found to be of little advantage compared to the use of lovastatin alone.[53]

Hoeg and coworkers[57] investigated the combination of neomycin, the aminoglycoside antibiotic that inhibits the absorption of cholesterol, with lovastatin. Lovastatin 20 mg twice daily was administered for 1 month, followed by neomycin 1 g twice daily for 2 months, then the combination for 1 month. Lovastatin alone reduced total cholesterol and LDL-cholesterol significantly, whereas the effect of neomycin alone was negligible. There was no further decrement in total cholesterol and LDL-cholesterol with combination therapy compared with lovastatin alone. In this study, combination therapy was associated with a significant reduction in HDL-cholesterol. It was concluded that there was no advantage in combining neomycin with lovastatin. Currently, investigators are examining the efficacy of triple therapy with drugs employing different mechanisms of PN action. The target of this therapy would be patients with severe and single or double drug resistance. Based on the previous findings, the most logical combination is lovastatin with nicotinic acid and a resin.[25,26,42,51,58] Studies have shown LDL reductions up to 67%, 10%-20% increases in HDL, and moderate reductions in triglycerides.[58] Triple therapy with lovastatin, colestipol, and probucol showed no advantage gained by the addition of probucol.[59]

The conclusion that may be drawn from these combination therapy trials is that hypercholesterolemia is best treated with small doses of a few synergistic but noninteractive drugs; the results being a maximal lowering of cholesterol with a minimum of side effects. Illingworth suggested an example regimen for moderate to severe hypercholesterolemia consisting of 4-8 g/d of a resin combined with 20 mg daily of lovastatin.[51]

Diabetes Mellitus

The onset of noninsulin-dependent diabetes commonly is associated with a decrease in HDL-cholesterol and increases in plasma VLDL-triglycerides and VLDL-cholesterol. In a placebo-controlled study involving 16 patients with noninsulin-dependent diabetes,[60] lovastatin 20 mg twice daily reduced total plasma cholesterol by 26%. In addition, glycemic control was maintained, and there were reductions in LDL-cholesterol of 28%, apolipoprotein B 26%, VLDL-cholesterol 42%, and triglycerides 31%. Plasma levels of HDL-cholesterol did not change with lovastatin treatment but the ratio of total to HDL-cholesterol fell by 29%.

The lipid-lowering effects of lovastatin and gemfibrozil were compared in 102 diabetic patients with primary hypercholesterolemia.[61] Two thirds of the patients were treated with oral hypoglycemic agents, and one third received diet therapy alone for their diabetes. Mean pretreatment total and LDL-cholesterol values were 7.06 and 4.99 mm/L (273 and 193 mg/dl), respectively. Patients were randomized to double-blind therapy consisting of 600 mg/d of gemfibrozil in two divided doses or lovastatin 40 mg once daily for 24 weeks of treatment. Lovastatin reduced total, LDL-, and VLDL-cholesterol by 20%, 26%, and 28%, respectively, and raised HDL-cholesterol by 14%. Gemfibrozil reduced triglycerides, VLDL-, and total cholesterol by 36%, 41%, and 9%, respectively, and raised HDL-cholesterol by 21%. Overall, lovastatin was not associated with a significant change in triglycerides, and gemfibrozil did not lower LDL cholesterol. Neither drug had a clinically important effect on fasting blood sugar or hemoglobin A1c.

Nephrotic Syndrome

The nephrotic syndrome is associated with increased levels of cholesterol and triglycerides. The elevated serum concentrations of LDL-
cholesterol, other lipids, and apoprotein B in patients with uncompli-
cated nephrotic syndrome are due to reversible increases in lipoprotein
production.[62] These lipid disorders are difficult to treat and they predispose patients to early onset of CAD. It has been suggested that the
treatment guidelines adopted by the National Cholesterol Education
Program be extended to patients with unremitting nephrotic syndrome.[63] Lovastatin has been shown to reduce plasma concentrations
of VLDL- and LDL-cholesterol in patients with nephrotic syndrome
with kinetic evidence of enhanced LDL receptor activity.[64]

Effects on Triglycerides, High Density Lipoproteins, and Other Lipoproteins

Lovastatin appears to have variable effects, with most studies
showing a reduction in triglycerides[29,31,34,43] and an increase in
HDL-cholesterol.[29,35,36,42,43,57]

There is an increasing interest in the effects of lovastatin on the
lipoprotein profile. In a thorough study of this issue, Helve and Tikkanen found that the reduction of apoprotein B is similar to that of
LDL-cholesterol. Further, a dose of 80 mg daily increased HDL_2-
cholesterol by 10%-18%. HDL_3-cholesterol levels, hepatic lipase, and
lipoprotein lipase activity, all important components of the HDL pathway, were not significantly altered.[65]

Another consideration is the effect of lovastatin on lipoprotein a
(Lp(a)), an LDL type molecule with an additional protein, apo(a), bound
to the apo B moiety (see Chapter 1). Apo(a) bears homology to plasminogen; it contains multiple copies of the kringle 4 domain of plasminogen,
as well as single copies homologous to the protease and kringle 5 do-
mains.[66] While the physiological role and metabolic pathway of Lp(a)
are not known, many feel that an elevated Lp(a) may be an independent
genetic risk factor for atherosclerotic disease.[66] Since HMG CoA reductase inhibitors are known to upregulate LDL receptors, thereby lowering
the plasma concentration of apo B particles, it is conceivable that Lp(a)
would be similarly affected. Nevertheless, reports have generated conflicting results: one study of 24 patients and another of 8 patients

demonstrate a significant increase[67,68]; yet another study of 30 patients found no change in serum Lp(a) levels.[69]

Clinical Use

Lovastatin has been shown to be effective in lowering serum cholesterol in heterozygous FH and nonFH.[19] Lovastatin doses as low as 5 mg twice daily produce significant reductions in serum cholesterol.

Patients should be placed on a standard cholesterol-lowering diet prior to drug treatment.[70] The recommended starting dose is 20 mg once daily given with the evening meal. The recommended dosing range is 20-80 mg daily in single or divided doses. Adjustments should be made at intervals of 4 weeks or more. A dose of 40 mg daily can be initiated in patients with cholesterol levels > 7.76 mm/L (> 300 mg/dl).

Twice daily dosing appears to be the most effective treatment regimen,[46] with daily evening doses being slightly less effective and daily morning doses least effective. Maximal and stable cholesterol reduction typically is achieved within 4 to 6 weeks of treatment initiation.

In patients with high cholesterol, diet and lovastatin may not reduce cholesterol to the desired level. Colestipol in combination with lovastatin may provide additional efficacy.

Studies have been done comparing lovastatin in doses of 40-80 mg daily versus cholestyramine 12 g twice daily and probucol 500 mg twice daily, with greater efficacy seen with lovastatin.[71]

Adverse Effects

Several hypercholesterolemic agents are available, each having a significant side effect profile.[72,73] Lovastatin has an acceptable rate of adverse reactions, but needs to be used with some caution.[17]

In the published trials, approximately 2% of patients were withdrawn from treatment because of adverse reactions. Gastrointestinal side effects (diarrhea, abdominal pain, constipation, flatulence) are the most commonly reported adverse side effects. Marked, persistent, but asymptomatic increases (to greater than three times the upper limit of normal) in serum transaminases have been reported in 2% of patients receiving the drug for 1 year. The increases are predominantly in SGPT and SGOT rather than alkaline phosphatase, suggesting a hepatocellular not cholestatic effect.[54] These abnormalities rapidly return to normal after the discontinuation of the drug and no permanent liver damage has been reported with the drug.[42,43] Symptomatic hepatitis in patients without underlying disease or other known hepatotoxic medications has been observed, and again, all cases resolved after stopping lovastatin. It is recommended that liver function tests be performed every 4 to 6 weeks during the first 15 months of therapy with lovastatin and periodically thereafter.

The side effect of greatest concern with lovastatin is a myopathy that appears to develop in three clinical patterns. The first, a moderate elevation in plasma creatinine kinase levels, is asymptomatic. Second, patients may develop muscle pain, primarily in the proximal muscle groups. CPK elevations may or may not be present. Finally, patients may develop a severe myopathy marked by extreme elevations in CPK, muscle pain with weakness, myoglobinuria, and, rarely, acute renal failure.[74] This finding most often occurs in the setting of concurrent immunosuppressive therapy (cyclosporine), particularly when gemfibrozil, erythromycin, or niacin was added.[75-77] Cases of myopathy have been identified as early as a few weeks and as late as two or more years after the initiation of therapy. CPK elevations appear to correlate little with the severity of the symptoms, but if CPK levels rise or muscle pain develops, it is recommended that lovastatin be reduced. If levels rise drastically (> 10 times the upper limits of normal) with muscle pain, therapy should be discontinued.

In a recent study of 11 cardiac transplant patients, all were treated with lovastatin and cyclosporine, monitored closely for 1 year, and were not treated with other hepatotoxic medications or lipid-lowering agents. None developed any evidence of hepatic, muscle, or renal toxicity, and the authors concluded that in the absence of other effective therapy, cardiac transplantation should not be a contraindication to the use of lovastatin.[78] Combinations of lovastatin with hepatotoxic agents, in the absence of cyclosporine, have been reported to be associated with myositis.[55,79,80] The FDA recently documented 12 cases of myopathy and rhabdomyolosis associated with lovastatin-gemfibrozil combination therapy, and has discouraged the use of this regimen. Although the reason that myopathy has been associated with lovastatin is not well understood, it has been postulated that drugs that impair hepatic function may alter the first-pass extraction of lovastatin and produce elevated levels, which, in turn, may be responsible for the myotoxicity. Lovastatin may disrupt the proper assembly of membrane glycoproteins, the oxidation-reduction reactions of the mitochondrial respiratory chain, or the regulation of DNA replication.[81] However, Tobert does report four cases of myositis with lovastatin monotherapy, but three of these patients had biliary stasis leading to decreased clearance of the drug.[54]

Investigators testing lovastatin have noted cataracts in dogs given at least 50 times the maximum human dosage in long-term studies.[81] Concern over cataracts dates from some 25 years ago when an unrelated antihyperlipidemic agent, citriparazel, was removed from the market after many new lens opacities were found in patients who took it.[81] Although new lens opacities were described with lovastatin, the incidence does not appear to differ from that of an untreated control population.[82] A large long-term, placebo-controlled trial assessing different doses of lovastatin has just been completed that addresses this question.[83] In this multicenter study, 8245 patients with elevated cholesterol levels were randomized to five treatment groups to receive either placebo or lovastatin in various doses (20 mg once daily, 20 mg twice daily, 40 mg once daily, or 40 mg twice daily) and followed for 48 weeks.[45,84,85] At baseline and after 24 and 48 weeks, the lens of each eye was assessed by slit-lamp examination and best-corrected visual acuity was also determined. Lens opacities were recorded with a standardized and reliable grading system of severity.[86] The frequency distribution of the opacity grades and visual-acuity assessments after 48 weeks of treatment were compared among groups after adjustment for age-group, baseline opacity, and baseline visual acuity. In patients with no lens opacities at baseline, there was no difference between placebo and lovastatin treatment in the rate of new opacity development.[84,85] Similarly, there was no difference between placebo and lovastatin treatment with regard to progression of disease in those subjects who had lens opacities at baseline.[84,85] No changes in visual acuity were observed with either treatment. The investigators concluded that there were no effects of lovastatin on the human lens after 48 weeks of treatment. However, based on this study, later effects could not be excluded.[84,85] If concern about cataract development still exists, a slit-lamp examination with dilated pupils and retro-illumination should be performed at baseline and annually for as long as lovastatin treatment continues. Any shagreen (grayish-green discoloration) in the subcapsular cortical region of the lens should be noted; vacuoles should be counted and the number recorded.[81] No changes in visual acuity have been described with the drug.

Several reports of bleeding, increase in prothrombin time, or both, have been observed in patients on concomitant warfarin anticoagulation. Although these accounts have not been attributed to lovastatin, it is recommended that prothrombin time be regulated carefully in these patients.[87]

In addition to reports of the occurrence of a rash during the clinical trials, there have been several accounts of serious hypersensitivity reactions during prescription use: anaphylaxis, arthralgia, a lupuslike syndrome, angioedema, urticaria, hemolytic anemia, leukopenia, and thrombocytopenia have all been reported. Twenty-five cases were considered serious but all recovered with discontinuation of lovastatin therapy. Since these adverse effects were never reported during the clinical trials, it is likely that the incidence is significantly less than 1/1000. Sleep disturbances characterized by insomnia or shortening of the sleep period have also been described.[88]

No effects of lovastatin on normal steroidogenesis have been described.[16] One recent report, however, does describe hypospermia in one middle-aged patient, which resolved when lovastatin was discontinued.[89] This report emphasizes the need for more long-term safety data on the HMG CoA reductase inhibitors.

Other HMG CoA Reductase Inhibitors

Simvastatin

Simvastatin (Zocor®, formerly synvinolin, MK 733), is a prodrug that is enzymatically hydrolyzed in vivo to its active form.[90] In clinical trials since 1985, simvastatin is synthesized chemically from lovastatin and differs from lovastatin by only one methyl group. Like lovastatin, it has a very high affinity for HMG CoA reductase but on a milligram-per-milligram basis, simvastatin is twice as potent.[91] Peak plasma concentrations of active inhibitor occur within 1.3 and 2.4 hours.[92]

One 12-week multicenter double-blind study comparing simvastatin to probucol found that a 20 mg and 40 mg daily dose of simvastatin lowered LDL-cholesterol by 34% and 40%, respectively. Simvastatin also reduced total cholesterol, triglycerides, and apolipoprotein B. HDL was increased.[93] As with lovastatin, interactions with warfarin and digoxin have been noted. Another multicenter study comparison with cholestyramine demonstrated that a low dose of simvastatin (10 mg) was sufficient to reduce total cholesterol by 21% and LDL by 30%, while HDL increased by 17%.[94] In comparisons of simvastatin to fibric acid derivatives, simvastatin produced greater reductions in total and LDL-cholesterol, while the latter had a greater effect on the serum triglycerides.[95-98] In a small study of patients with familial hypercholesterolemia, it was shown that 40 mg of simvastatin in combination with 12 g of cholestyramine reduced total cholesterol by 43% and LDL-cholesterol by 53%.[99]

The effects of simvastatin are achieved using a single evening dose.[100] Despite its potency, simvastatin has never been shown to disrupt adrenocortical function.[101] Side effects are predominantly headaches and dyspepsia, but asymptomatic myositis has also been noted.[93] Interestingly, some patients who experienced enzyme elevations with lovastatin and lovastatin rechallenge, tolerated simvastatin well.[102]

Simvastatin has already been explored as an agent for various hyperlipoproteinemic conditions.[103] In a recent study, 12 patients with dysbetalipoproteinemia treated with increasing doses of simvastatin (10, 20, and 40 mg twice daily) in 6-week periods had significant reductions in serum cholesterol and triglycerides.[104] As a treatment for nephrotic hyperlipidemia, simvastatin was noted to be more effective and better tolerated than cholestyramine.[105]

Simvastatin has also been evaluated for its effect on the cholesterol saturation index of gall bladder bile, a potential side effect of several hypocholesterolemic agents. A mean decline of 23% was noted in the 10 hypercholesterolemic patients studied, raising the possibility that an HMG CoA reductase inhibitor may play a future role in the treatment of gallstones.[106]

Currently, there are little available long-term data on this drug, although one study of 20 patients found that after 52 weeks on monotherapy with simvastatin, the LDL-cholesterol was still reduced by 38%, triglycerides by 17%, and HDL was increased by 19%.[107] Another 1-year study involved 20 patients aged 65 to 75 years. It also proved simvastatin effective in rapid lowering and subsequent maintenance of LDL- and total cholesterol levels. Although an initial rise in HDL was noted, the HDL levels at 52 weeks were not significantly different from baseline values, suggesting that tolerance may develop and initial elevations of HDL should be interpreted with caution.[108] Simvastatin was recently approved by the FDA for marketing in the United States.

A Scandinavian study of 4000 patients with ischemic heart disease and hypercholesterolemia will determine if simvastatin will improve total survival and reduce fatal or nonfatal myocardial infarction and sudden death for at least 3 years.[48]

Pravastatin

Pravastatin (Pravachol CS 514, SQ 3100, epstatatin) is the 6 α-hydroxy acid form of compactin.[109] The drug recently was approved for marketing by the FDA. It is the only HMG CoA reductase inhibitor administered in the active form. In vitro studies by Tsujuita et al demonstrated that pravastatin has a greater specificity for hepatic cells than lovastatin.[110] In vivo animal studies comparing pravastatin to lovastatin and simvastatin, however, found that the concentration of pravastatin in the liver was only half that of the latter two, while the concentrations in peripheral tissues was three to six times greater.[111]

In a recent study, pravastatin was found to be a specific inhibitor of hepatic HMG CoA reductase in humans.[112] Other enzymes involved in cholesterol metabolism (α-hydroxylase, which governs bile-acid synthesis and acyl-coenzyme A; cholesterol O-acetyltransferase [ACAT], which regulates cholesterol esterification) were not affected by treatment. Inhibition of hepatic HMG CoA reductase activity by pravastatin results in an increased expression of hepatic LDL receptors, which explains the lowered plasma levels of LDL-cholesterol.[112]

Multiple studies have already been conducted on humans to establish efficacy and dosage.[113-116] Despite its short plasma half-life of approximately 2 hours, a single daily dose of pravastatin has been shown to be as effective as twice daily doses.[116] As with other drugs in this class, administration of the drug in the evening rather than the morning appears to bring about greater cholesterol-lowering activity. Mabuchi et al.[117] treated patients with heterozygous FH with pravastatin 10 and 20 mg. They found a 26% and 33% decrease in LDL, respectively. HDL was significantly increased. Nakaya et al[118] also found that 5, 20, and 40 mg doses lowered the total serum cholesterol by 11.1%, 18.8%, and 25.3%, respectively in hypercholesterolemic patients. The investigators reported some mild side effects but no myositis.[118]

Pravastatin is now being compared to placebo in a double-blind, randomized, placebo-controlled trial in 3500 normocholesterolemic patients who have survived a recent myocardial infarction. Patients will be treated for up to 5 years to investigate the effects of drug therapy plus diet on subsequent coronary events in men and women.

The efficacy and safety of pravastatin compared to bile-acid binding resins in patients with heterozygous FH was assessed and compared.[119] Pravastatin reduced LDL by approximately 33% at a dose of 40 mg daily; bile resins reduced LDL by approximately 22% using an average dose of 3 to 4 packages daily; when the drugs were combined, LDL decreased by approximately 42%. CPK increased by approximately 42% with pravastatin, and the alkaline phosphatase increased by approximately 10% with the resin.

The efficacy and safety of pravastatin and gemfibrozil were compared in 385 patients with primary hypercholesterolemia in a randomized double-blind study.[120] Patients were assigned to receive either 40 mg once daily of pravastatin or 600 mg of gemfibrozil twice daily after an initial diet lead-in period. After 24 weeks, mean reductions from baseline values of plasma total and LDL-cholesterol were, respectively, 23% and 30% with pravastatin and 14% and 17% with gemfibrozil. Apolipoprotein B levels decreased 21% with pravastatin and 13% with gemfibrozil. HDL levels were raised by 5% with pravastatin compared to 13% with gemfibrozil. Triglycerides were decreased by 5% with pravastatin and by 37% with gemfibrozil. Treatment for 25 patients was discontinued during the study (8 were receiving pravastatin and 17 gemfibrozil). The incidence of clinical symptoms and laboratory alterations was low for both treatment groups. It was concluded by the investigators that both pravastatin and gemfibrozil were well tolerated, but pravastatin was more effective in reducing total and LDL-cholesterol in primary hypercholesterolemia (either familial or polygenic).[120]

Although lovastatin, simvastatin, and pravastatin have never been directly compared on a large scale, published data on similar patients suggests that over a dosage range of 20 to 80 mg daily, pravastatin and lovastatin are approximately equal in efficacy with respect to reducing LDL.[102,121,122] Furthermore, one small-scale comparison of lovastatin and pravastatin showed that these agents produced similar effects on total cholesterol, LDL-cholesterol, and apolipoprotein B, with no significant change in lipoprotein (a).[123]

Conclusions

The class of HMG-CoA reductase inhibitors have therapeutic effects similar to the bile-acid sequestrants and nicotinic acid in reducing total cholesterol and LDL-cholesterol.[16,17] Although the drugs are tolerated well, their long-term safety profile needs to be established before they can be recommended as a first-line treatment of elevated cholesterol, either alone or in combination.[121,122] More important, their effects in modifying the risk of cardiovascular morbidity and mortality also need to be established.[124]

References

1. Castelli WP, Garrison RJ, Wilson PW: Incidence of coronary heart disease and lipoprotein cholesterol levels: The Framingham Study. JAMA 1986; 256: 2835-2838.
2. Steinberg D: Lipoproteins and the pathogenesis of atherosclerosis. Circulation 1987; 76: 508-514.
3. Schaefer EJ, Levy RI: Pathogenesis and management of lipoprotein disorders. N Engl J Med 1985; 312: 1300-1310.
4. Steinberg D: Cholesterol and cardiovascular disease: current perspectives. Circulation 1987; 76: 501-503.
5. Pekkanen J, Linn S, Heiss G, et al: Ten year mortality from cardiovascular disease in relation to cholesterol level among men with and without preexisting cardiovascular disease. N Engl J Med 1990; 322: 1700-1707.
6. Stamler J, Wentworth D, Neaton JD: Is the relationship between serum cholesterol and risk of premature death from coronary heart disease continuous and graded? Findings in 356,222 primary screenees of the Multiple Risk Factor Intervention Trial. JAMA 1986; 256: 2823-2828.
7. The Lipid Research Clinics Program: The Lipid Research Clinics Coronary Primary Prevention Trial Results. I. Reduction in incidence of coronary heart disease. JAMA 1984; 251: 351-364.
8. NIH Consensus Conference: Lowering blood cholesterol to prevent heart disease. JAMA 1985; 253: 2080-2086.
9. Report of the National Cholesterol Education Program Expert Panel on Detection, Evaluation, and Treatment of High Blood Cholesterol in Adults. Arch Intern Med 1988; 148: 36-69.
10. Grundy SM: Dietary therapy for different forms of hyperlipoproteinemia. Circulation 1987; 76: 523-528.
11. Alberts AW, Chen J, Kuron G, et al: Mevinolin: a highly potent competitive inhibitor of hydroxymethylglutaryl-coenzyme A reductase and a cholesterol-lowering agent. Proc Natl Acad Sci USA 1980; 77: 3957-3961.
12. Endo A, Kuroda M, Tsijita Y: ML-236B and ML-236C, new inhibitors of cholesterogenesis produced by Penicillium citrium. J Antibiot 1976; 29: 1346-1348.
13. Brown MS, Goldstein JL: Multivalent feedback regulation of HMG-CoA reductase, a control mechanism coordinating isoprenoid synthesis and cell growth. J Lipid Res 1980; 21: 505-517.

14. Alberts AW: Discovery, biochemistry and biology of lovastatin. Am J Cardiol 1988; 62: 10J-16J.
15. Anonymous: Lovastatin for hypercholesterolemia. The Medical Letter 1987; 29: 99-101.
16. Tobert JA: New developments in lipid-lowering therapy. The role of inhibitors of hydroxymethylglutaryl coenzyme A reductase. Circulation 1987; 76: 534-538.
17. Krukemyer JJ, Talbert RL: Lovastatin: a new cholesterol- lowering agent. Pharmacotherapy 1987; 7: 198-210.
18. Parker TS, McNamara DJ, Brown C: Mevalonic acid in human plasma: relationship of concentration and circadian rhythm to cholesterol synthesis rates in man. Proc Natl Acad Sci USA 1982; 79: 3037.
19. Grundy SM: HMG-CoA reductase inhibitors for treatment of hypercholesterolemia. N Engl J Med 1988; 319: 24-33.
20. Henwood JM, Heel AC: Lovastatin. Drugs 1988; 36: 429-454.
21. Kovanen PT, Bilheimer DW, Goldstein JL, et al: Regulatory role for hepatic low density lipoprotein receptors in vivo in the dog. Proc Natl Acad Sci USA 1981; 78: 1194-1198.
22. Kritchevsky D, Tepper SA, Klurfeld DM: Influence of mevinolin on experimental atherosclerosis in rabbits. Pharmacol Res Commun 1981; 13: 921-925.
23. Kroon PA, Hand KM, Huff JW, et al: The effects of mevinolin on serum cholesterol levels of rabbits with endogenous hypercholesterolemia. Atherosclerosis 1982; 44: 41-48.
24. Bilheimer DW, Grundy SM, Brown MS, et al: Mevinolin and colestipol stimulate receptor-mediated clearance of low density lipoprotein from plasma in familial hypercholesterolemia heterozygotes. Proc Natl Acad Sci USA 1983; 80: 4124-4128.
25. Grundy SM, Vega GL, Bilheimer DW: Influence of combined therapy with mevinolin and interruption of bile-acid reabsorption on low density lipoproteins in heterozygous familial hypercholesterolemia. Ann Intern Med 1985; 103: 339-343.
26. Vega GL, Grundy SM: Treatment of primary moderate hypercholesterolemia with lovastatin (mevinolin) and colestipol. JAMA 1987; 257: 33-38.
27. Tobert JA, Hitzenberger G, Kubovetz WR, et al: Rapid and substantial lowering of human serum cholesterol by mevinolin (MK 803), an inhibitor of hydroxymethylglutaryl coenzyme A reductase. Atherosclerosis 1982; 41: 61-65.
28. Tobert JA, Bell GD, Birtwell J, et al: Cholesterol-lowering effect of mevinolin, an inhibitor of 3-hydroxy-3-methylglutaryl coenzyme A reductase, in healthy volunteers. J Clin Invest 1982; 69: 913-919.
29. Illingworth DR, Sexton GJ: Hypercholesterolemic effects of mevinolin in patients with heterozygous familial hypercholesterolemia. J Clin Invest 1984; 74: 1972-1978.
30. Illingworth DR: Comparative efficacy of once versus twice daily mevinolin in the therapy of familial hypercholesterolemia. Clin Pharmacol Ther 1986; 40: 338-343.

31. Thompson GR, Ford J, Jenkinson M, et al: Efficacy of mevinolin as adjuvant therapy for refractory familial hypercholesterolemia. QJ Med 1986; 60: 803-811.

32. Havel RJ, Hunninghaker DB, Illingworth R, et al: Lovastatin (Mevinolin) in the treatment of heterozygous familial hypercho-lesterolemia: a multicenter study. Ann Intern Med 1987; 107: 609-615.

33. Illingworth DR, Roger D, Bacon S: Treatment of familial hypercholesterolemia with lipid lowering drugs. Atherosclerosis 1989; 9 (Suppl l): 121-134.

34. Illingworth DR: Mevinolin plus colestipol in therapy for severe heterozygous familial hypercholesterolemia. Ann Intern Med 1984; 101: 598-604.

35. Luae L, Hoeg JM, Barnes K, et al: The effect of mevinolin on steroidogenesis in patients with defects in the low density lipoprotein receptor pathway. J Clin Endocrinol Metab 1987; 64: 531-535.

36. East C, Grundy SM, Bilheimer DW: Normal cholesterol levels with lovastatin (mevinolin) therapy in a child with homozygous familial hypercholesterolemia following liver transplantation. JAMA 1986; 256: 2843-2848.

37. East C, Bilheimer D, Grundy S: Combination drug therapy for familial combined hyperlipidemia. Ann Intern Med 1988; 109: 25-32.

38. Arad Y, Ramakrishnan R, Ginsberg HN: Effect of mevinolin therapy on apolipoprotein B metabolism in subjects with combined hyperlipidemia. (abstr) Clin Res 1987; 35: 496A.

39. Vega GL, Grundy SM: Management of primary mixed hyperlipidemia with lovastatin. Arch Intern Med 1990; 150: 1313-1319.

40. East CA, Grundy SM, Bilheimer DW: Preliminary report: Treatment of type 3 hyperlipoproteinemia with mevinolin. Metabolism 1986; XXXV: 97-98.

41. Grundy SA: HMG-CoA reductase inhibitors for treatment of hypercholesterolemia. N Engl J Med 1988; 319: 24-32.

42. Hoeg JM, Maher MB, Zech AL, et al: Effectiveness of mevinolin on plasma lipoprotein concentrations in type II hyperlipoproteinemia. Am J Cardiol 1986; 57: 933-939.

43. Lovastatin Study Group II: Therapeutic response to lovastatin (mevinolin) in nonfamilial hypercholesterolemia. A Multicenter Study. JAMA 1986; 256: 2829-2834.

44. Lovastatin Study Group III: Multicenter comparison of lovastatin and cholestyramine therapy for severe primary hypercholesterolemia. JAMA 1988; 260: 359-366.

45. Bradford RH, Shear CL, Chremos AN, et al: Expanded Clinical Evaluation of Lovastatin (EXCEL) Study: design and patient characteristics of a double-blind, placebo-controlled study in patients with moderate hypercholesterolemia. Am J Cardiol 1990; 66: 44B-55B.

46. Bradford RH, Shear CL, Chremos AN, et al: Expanded Clinical Evaluation of Lovastatin (EXCEL) Study. Results I: efficacy in modifying plasma lipoproteins and adverse effect profile in 8245 patients with moderate hypercholesterolemia. Arch Intern Med 1991; 151: 43-49.

47. Lovastatin Study Group IV: A multicenter comparison of lovastatin and probucol for treatment of severe primary hypercholesterolemia. Am J Cardiol 1990; 66: 22B-30B.

48. Jones PH: Lovastatin and simvastatin prevention studies. Am J Cardiol 1990; 66: 39B-43B.
49. Gellman J, Ezekowitz MD, Sarembock IJ, et al: Effect of lovastatin on intimal hyperplasia after balloon angioplasty. J Am Coll Cardiol 1991; 17: 251-259.
50. Sahni R, Maniet AR, Voci G, et al: Prevention of restenosis by lovastatin after successful coronary angioplasty. Am Heart J 1991; 121: 1600-1608.
51. Illingworth DR: New horizons in combination drug therapy for hypercholesterolemia. Cardiol 1989; 76 (Suppl 1): 83-100.
52. Brown G, Albers JJ, Fisher LD, et al: Regression of coronary artery disease as a result of intensive lipid lowering therapy in men with high levels of apolipoprotein B. N Engl J Med 1990; 323: 1289-1298.
53. Lees AM, Stein SW, Lees RW: Therapy of hypercholesterolemia with Mevinolin and other lipid lowering drugs. (abstr) Atherosclerosis 1986; 6: 544A.
54. Tobert JA: Efficacy and long-term adverse effect pattern of lovastatin. Am J Cardiol 1988; 62: 28J-35J.
55. Ayanian JZ, Fuchs CS, Stone RM: Lovastatin and rhabdomyolysin. Letter to the Editor. Ann Intern Med 1988; 109: 682.
56. Garg A, Grundy SM: Gemfibrozil alone and in combination with lovastatin for treatment of hypertriglyceridemia in noninsulin dependent diabetes mellitus. Diabetes 1989; 38: 364-372.
57. Hoeg JM, Maher MB, Bailey KR, et al: The effects of mevinolin and neomycin alone and in combination on plasma lipid and lipoprotein concentrations in type II hyperlipoproteinemia. Atherosclerosis 1986; 60: 209-214.
58. Malloy MA, Kane JP, Kunitake ST, et al: Complementarity of colestipol, niacin and lovastatin in treatment of severe familial hypercholesterolemia. Ann Intern Med 1987; 107: 616-623.
59. Witztum JL, Simmons D, Steinberg D, et al: Intensive combination drug therapy of familial hypercholesterolemia with lovastatin, probucol and colestipol hydrochloride. Circulation 1989; 79: 16-28.
60. Garg A, Grundy S: Lovastatin for lowering cholesterol values in noninsulin-dependent diabetes mellitus. N Engl J Med 1988; 318: 81-86.
61. Goldberg R, LaBelle P, Zupkis R, et al: Comparison of the effects of lovastatin and gemfibrozil on lipids and glucose control in noninsulin-dependent diabetes mellitus. Am J Cardiol 1190; 66: 16B-21B.
62. Joven J, Villabona C, Vilella E, et al: Abnormalities of lipoprotein metabolism in patients with nephrotic syndrome. N Engl J Med 1990; 323: 579-584.
63. Keane WF, Kasiske BL: Hyperlipidemia in nephrotic syndrome. N Engl J Med 1990 323: 603-604.
64. Vega GL, Grundy SM: Lovastatin therapy in nephrotic hyperlipidemia. Effects on lipoprotein metabolism. Kidney Int 1988; 33: 1160-1168.
65. Helve E, Tikkanen MJ: Comparison of lovastatin and probucol in treatment of familial and nonfamilial hypercholesterolemia: different effects on lipoprotein profiles. Atherosclerosis 1988; 72: 189-197.
66. Utermann G: The mysteries of lipoprotein(a). Science 1989: 246: 904-910.

67. Kostner GM, Gavish D, Leopold B, et al: HMG CoA reductase inhibitors lower LDL cholesterol without reducing Lp(a) levels. Circulation 1989; 80: 1313-1319.

68. Jurgens G, Ashy A, Zenker G: Raised serum lipoprotein during treatment with lovastatin (letter). Lancet April 22, 1989: 911.

69. Berg K, Leren TP: Unchanged serum lipoprotein(a) concentrations with lovastatin (letter). Lancet, September 30, 1989: 812.

70. Cobb MM, Teitelbaum HS, Breslow JL: Lovastatin efficacy in reducing low-density lipoprotein cholesterol levels on high vs low fat diets. JAMA 1991; 265: 997-1001.

71. Merck Sharp & Dohme: Mevacor package insert. West Point, Pa. August 1987.

72. Knodel LC, Talbert RL: Adverse effects of hypolipidaemic drugs. Med Toxicol 1987; 2: 10-32.

73. Anonymous: Choice of cholesterol-lowering drugs. The Medical Letter 1991; 33: 1-4.

74. Grundy SM (reply to the editor). N Engl J Med 1989; 320: 1220.

75. Norman DJ, Illingworth DR, Munson J, et al: Myolysis and acute renal failure in a heart transplant recipient receiving lovastatin (letter). N Engl J Med 1988; 318: 46-47.

76. East C, Alivizatos PA, Grundy SM, et al: Rhabdomyolysis in patients receiving lovastatin after cardiac transplantation (letter). N Engl J Med 1988; 318: 47-48.

77. Frishman WH, Zimetbaum P, Nadelmann J: Lovastatin and other HMG CoA reductase inhibitors. J Clin Pharmacol 1989; 29: 975-981.

78. Kuo PC, Kirshenbaum JM, Gordon J, et al: Lovastatin therapy for hypercholesterolemia in cardiac transplant recipients. Am J Cardiol 1989; 64: 631-635.

79. Reaven P, Witztum JL: Lovastatin, nicotinic acid, and rhab-domyolysis (letter). Ann Intern Med 1988; 109: 597-598.

80. Pierce LR, Wysowski DK, Gross T: Myopathy and rhabdomyolosis associated with lovastatin-gemfibrozil combination therapy. JAMA 1990; 264: 71-75.

81. Goldman JA, Fishman AB, Lee JE, et al: The role of cholesterol-lowering agents in drug-induced rhabdomyolysis and polymyositis. Arthritis Rheum 1989; 32: 358-359.

82. Fraunfelder F: Ocular examination before initiation of lovastatin (Mevacor) therapy. (Letter) Am J Ophthalmol 1988; 105: 91-92.

83. Hunninghake DB, Miller VT, Goldbert I, et al: Lovastatin: follow up ophthalmologic data. JAMA 1988; 259: 354-355.

84. Laties AM, Keates EU, Taylor HR, et al: The human lens after 48 weeks of treatment with lovastatin (Letter). N Engl J Med 1990; 323: 683-684.

85. Laties AM, Shear CL, Lippa EA, et al: Expanded clinical evaluation of lovastatin (EXCEL). Study Results II: assessment of the human lens after 48 weeks of treatment with lovastatin. Am J Cardiol 1991; 67: 447-453.

86. Laties A, Keates E, Lippa E, et al: Field reliability of a new lens opacity rating system using slit-lamp examination. Lens Eye Toxicol Res 1989; 6: 443-464.

87. Tobert JA, Shear CL, Cremos AN, et al: Clinical experience with lovastatin. Am J Cardiol 1990; 65: 23F-26F.
88. Tobert JA: HMG CoA reductase inhibitors for hypercholesterolemia. (Letter) N Engl J Med 1988; 319: 1222.
89. Hildebrand RD, Hepperlen TW: Lovastatin and hypospermia. (Letter) Ann Intern Med 1990; 112: 549-550.
90. Todd PA, Goa K: Simvastatin: a review of its pharmacological properties and therapeutic potential in hypercholesterolemia. Drugs 1990; 40: 583-607.
91. Stalenhoef AFH, Mol MJTM, Stuyt PMJ: Efficacy and tolerability of simvastatin (MK 733). Am J Med 1989; 87: 39S-43S.
92. Quercia RA: Focus on simvastatin: a potent HMG CoA reductase inhibitor for the treatment of hypercholesterolemia. Hosp Form 1989; 24: 559-573.
93. Pietro DA, Sidney A, Mantell G, et al: Effects of simvastatin and probucol in hypercholesterolemia (Simvastatin Multicenter Study Group II). Am J Cardiol 1989; 63: 682-686.
94. Stein E, Kreisberg R, Miller V, et al: Multicenter group 1: effects of simvastatin and cholestyramine in familial and nonfamilial hypercholesterolemia. Arch Intern Med 1990; 150: 341-345.
95. Schulzeck P, Boyanovski M, Jochim A, et al: Comparison between simvastatin and bezafibrate in effect on plasma lipoproteins and apolipoproteins in primary hypercholesterolemia. Lancet, March 19, 1988: 612-613.
96. Tikkanan XJ, Bocanegra TS, Walker JF, et al: Comparison of low-dose simvastatin and gemfibrozil in the treatment of elevated plasma cholesterol. Am J Med 1989; 87: 47S-53S.
97. Erkelens DW, Baggen MGA, Van Doormaal JJ, et al: Clinical experience with simvastatin compared with cholestyramine. Drugs 1988; 36 (Suppl 3): 87-92.
98. Deslypere JP: Comparison between low-dose simvastatin and cholestyramine in moderately severe hypercholesterolemia. Acta Cardiologica 1989; XLIV 5: 379-388.
99. Dacol PG, Cattin L, Valenti M, et al: Efficacy of simvastatin plus cholestyramine in the two-year treatment of heterozygous hypercholesterolemia. Curr Ther Res Clin Exp 1990; 48: 798-808.
100. Havel RJ: Simvastatin: a once a day treatment of hypercholesterolemia: introduction to a symposium. Am J Med 1989; 87: 1S.
101. Mol MJT, Stalenhoef AFH: Adrenocortical function in patients with simvastatin. Lancet February 17, 1990: 335.
102. Stein E: Management of hypercholesterolemia: guide to diet and drug therapy. Am J Med 1989; 87: 24S.
103. Nakandakare E, Garcia RC, Rocha JC, et al: Effects of simvastatin, bezafibrate, and gemfibrozil on the quantity of composition of plasma lipoproteins. Atherosclerosis 1990; 85: 211-217.
104. Stuyt PMJ, Mol MJTM, Stalenhoef AFH, et al: Simvastatin in the effective reduction of plasma lipoprotein levels in familial dysbetalipoproteinemia (type III hyperlipoproteinemia). Am J Med 1990; 889: 42N-45N.

105. Rabelink AJ, Henle RJ, Erkelens DW, et al: Effects of simvastatin and cholestyramine on lipoprotein profile in hyperlipidaemia of nephrotic syndrome. Lancet December 10, 1988; 1335-1338.
106. Duane WC, Hunninghake DB, Freeman ML, et al: Simvastatin, a competitive inhibitor of HMG-CoA reductase, lowers cholesterol saturation index of gallbladder bile. Hepatology 1988; 8: 1147-1150.
107. Ytre-Arne K, Nordoy K: Simvastatin and cholestyramine in the long-term treatment of hypercholesterolaemia. J Intern Med 1989; 226: 285-290.
108. Bach LA, Cooper ME, O'Brien RC, et al: The use of simvastatin, an HMG CoA reductase inhibitor, in older patients with hypercholesterolemia and atherosclerosis. J Am Geriatr Soc 1990; 38: 10-14.
109. McTavish D, Sorkin EM: Pravastatin. Drugs 1991; 42: 65-89.
110. Tsujita Y, Kuroda M, Simada Y, et al: CS 514, a competitive inhibitor of 3-hydroxy-3-methyl glutaryl coenzyme A reductase: tissue-selective inhibitor of steroid synthesis and hypolipidemic effects on various animal species. Biochem Biophys Acta 1986; 877: 50-60.
111. Germershausen JI, Hunt VM, Bostedor RG, et al: Tissue selectivity of the cholesterol-lowering agents lovastatin, simvastatin and pravastatin in rats in vivo. Biochem Biophys Res Commun 1989; 158: 667-675.
112. Reihner E, Rudling M, Stahlberg D, et al: Influence of pravastatin, a specific inhibitor of HMG CoA reductase, on hepatic metabolism of cholesterol. N Engl J Med 1990; 323: 224-228.
113. Saito Y, Goto Y, Nakaya N, et al: Dose dependent hypolipidemic effect of an inhibitor of HMG CoA reductase, pravastatin (CS 514), in hypercholesterolemic subjects: a double blind test. Atherosclerosis 1988; 72: 205-211.
114. Franceschini G, Sirtori M, Vaccarino V, et al: Plasma lipoprotein changes after treatment with pravastatin and gemfibrozil in patients with familial hypercholesterolemia. J Lab Clin Med 1989; 114: 250-259.
115. Hunninghake DB, Knopp RH, Schonfeld G, et al: Efficacy and safety of pravastatin in patients with primary hypercholesterolemia. 1. A dose-response study. Atherosclerosis 1990; 85: 81-89.
116. Hunninghake DB, Mellies MJ, Goldberg AC, et al: Efficacy and safety of pravastatin in patients with primary hypercholesterolemia. 2. Once-daily versus twice-daily dosing. Atherosclerosis 1990; 85: 219-227.
117. Mabuchi A, Kamon N, Fujita H, et al: The effects of CS 514 on serum lipoprotein, lipid and apolipoprotein levels in patients with familial hypercholesterolemia. Metabolism 1987; 36: 475-479.
118. Nakaya N, Yasuhiko H, Hiromitsu T, et al: The effect of CS 514 on serum lipids and apolipoproteins in hypercholesterolemic subjects. JAMA 1987; 257: 3088-3093.
119. Hoogerbrugge N, Mol M, Van Dormaal JJ, et al: The efficacy and safety of pravastatin, compared to and in combination with bile acid binding resins, in familial hypercholesterolemia. J Intern Med 1990; 228: 261-266.
120. Crepaldi G, Baggio G, Arca M, et al: Pravastatin versus gemfibrozil in the treatment of primary hypercholesterolemia. Arch Intern Med 1991; 151: 146-152.
121. Anonymous: Pravastatin and simvastatin for hypercholesterolemia. Medical Letter 1991; 33: 18-20.

122. Illingworth DR: Clinical implications of new drugs for lowering plasma cholesterol concentrations. Drugs 1991; 41:151-160.
123. Jacob BG, Richter WO, Schwandt P: Lovastatin, pravastatin and serum lipoprotein. (Letter) Ann Intern Med 1990; 112: 713.
124. Goldman L, Weinstein MC, Goldman P, et al: Cost-effectiveness of HMG-CoA reductase inhibition for primary and secondary prevention of coronary heart disease. JAMA 1991; 265: 1145-1151.

Chapter 7

Nicotinic Acid

William H. Frishman M.D., Jeffrey M. Drood M.D.,
Peter Zimetbaum M.D.

Nicotinic acid ([NA] pyridin-3 carboxylic acid or niacin) is a water-soluble B-complex vitamin (Fig. 1) that is used for the prophylaxis and treatment of pellagra. The substance functions in the body after conversion to either nicotinamide adenine dinucleotide (NAD) or nicotinamide adenine dinucleotide phosphase (NADP).

In 1955, Altschul and colleagues demonstrated that large doses of NA lower the concentration of plasma cholesterol in humans.[1] This property of NA is not shared by nicotinamide and appears to have nothing to do with the role of these compounds as vitamins. Subsequently, NA, in high doses, was shown to reduce triglycerides and have

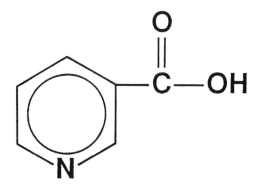

Figure 1: *Chemical structure of nicotinic acid.*

From *Medical Management of Lipid Disorders: Focus on Prevention of Coronary Artery Disease,*
edited by William H. Frishman, M.D. © 1992, Futura Publishing Inc., Mount Kisco, NY.

favorable effects in patients with various lipid and lipoprotein disorders. From the results of controlled clinical trials with NA, there is evidence that cardiovascular morbidity can be reduced with long-term therapy. In this chapter the clinical pharmacology of NA as a lipid-lowering agent is reviewed, and recommendations for its clinical use are presented.

Pharmacokinetics

NA is readily absorbed from the intestinal tract after the oral administration of pharmacological doses.[2] The level of free NA in plasma reaches a peak value between 30 and 60 minutes after ingesting a single dose of 1 g.[3] Because NA is rapidly eliminated, the doses necessary to achieve pharmacological effects (2-8 g daily)[4] are much greater than the amount needed for its physiological functions as a vitamin. When large doses of the vitamin were given to rats by intraperitoneal injection, the half-life of the compound was found to be approximately one hour in blood.[5] The half-life of NA seems to be determined primarily by the rate of renal clearance of the unchanged compound when given in high doses. At lower doses, NA is mainly excreted as its metabolites.[5]

The metabolic fate of NA is complex and varies with the dose. Under normal conditions, metabolites of NA found in the urine are mainly the products of catabolism of the pyridine nucleotides, the stored forms of the vitamin.[2] The primary route of metabolism is via methylation to N-methyl-nicotinamide, which is further oxidized to N-methyl-2- and 4-pyridone carbox-amides.[2] With pharmacological doses, the excretion of nicotinuric acid, produced by the conjugation of NA and glycine, is enhanced and seems to play a role as a detoxification product at these higher doses.[2] Once the dose is large enough to overcome the production rate of nicotinuric acid, NA is mostly excreted unchanged.[5]

Pharmacology

NA in large doses lowers total plasma cholesterol (C) and has been found to have beneficial effects on the levels of the major serum lipoproteins. Specifically, it decreases the levels of very low-density lipoprotein-triglyceride (VLDL-Tg) and low-density lipoprotein cholesterol (LDL-C) and causes an increase in the levels of high-density lipoprotein cholesterol (HDL-C).[4] This lipid-altering activity is not shared by nicotinamide and seems to be unrelated to the role of NA as a vitamin in the NAD and NADP coenzyme systems.[4] Pharmacological doses of NA result in a rapid decrease in plasma triglyceride levels, in part by lowering VLDL- Tg concentrations by 20% to over 80%.[4] The magnitude of the reduction is related to the initial VLDL levels. Within one week of initiation of therapy, concentrations of LDL-C decrease. Typically, a 10% to 15% reduction in LDL-C is observed within 3 to 5 weeks of attaining full dosage. The magnitude of the drop is also related to the dose of NA. In addition to these lipid-lowering effects, NA raises HDL-C concentrations.[4,6] Mobilization of cholesterol from peripheral tissues seems to occur after prolonged therapy, as evidenced by the regression of eruptive, tuboeruptive, tuberous, and tendon xanthomas.[4]

There are several mechanisms by which NA alters serum lipoprotein levels. NA's actions as an antilipolytic agent may be related to its effects on lowering VLDL-Tg concentration. NA has been found to decrease lipolysis in adipose tissue, resulting in decreased levels of plasma free fatty acids.[3,7-9] Carlson et al[3] found that after oral administration of 1 g of NA, a significant depression of free fatty acids as well as glycerol levels occurred in plasma, an effect that lasted 3 hours. These investigators also found reduced concentrations of triglyceride at 4 and 6 hours after drug ingestion. This single dose of NA did not alter plasma cholesterol levels. During fasting, free fatty acids released from adipose tissue serve as the major precursors for the formation of VLDL-Tg, which is synthesized mainly in the liver, and serves as the major carrier of endogenous triglyceride.[3,4] The decrease in free fatty acid release from adipose tissue that is induced by NA is thought to decrease uptake of free fatty acid by the liver and thereby reduce the hepatic synthesis of VLDL.[3]

Grundy et al[10] in an attempt to elucidate the mechanisms by which NA lowers triglyceride and cholesterol in plasma, assessed the metabolism of triglyceride and cholesterol in hyperlipidemic patients before and during treatment with the drug. Compared to baseline values, NA produced a mean reduction in total plasma triglyceride of 52% and in plasma VLDL-Tg of 36%. Furthermore, these investigators noted a reduction in transport (synthesis) of VLDL-Tg by an average of 21%. They attributed this decreased synthesis to a reduction in particle size, with less triglyceride per particle, rather than a decrease in particle number. An increased fractional catabolic rate of VLDL-Tg was also observed in most of the patients. This may be related to reports of a

NA-induced increase in the activity of lipoprotein lipase. Lipoprotein lipase is the enzyme that catalyzes the hydrolysis of triglycerides in VLDL and chylomicra to free fatty acids, which are then absorbed into adipose tissue. However, the absolute rates of triglyceride clearance from plasma were actually lower during treatment when the decreased particle size was taken into account.[10]

In the same study,[10] NA therapy resulted in a mean reduction in plasma cholesterol of 22%. Much of this decrease is attributed to a decline in the number of particles of LDL. The majority of LDL is produced by catabolism of VLDL via formation of intermediate density lipoprotein (IDL) or VLDL remnants. Therefore, one possible mechanism for the decrease in LDL seen with NA therapy is reduction in the amount of VLDL available for catabolism. However, as noted by Grundy et al[10] a reduction in LDL would not necessarily follow a decrease in the size of VLDL particles. Other possible explanations for the LDL-lowering induced by NA include increased hepatic clearance of IDL, thereby limiting the conversion of IDL to LDL, and decreased VLDL-independent synthesis of LDL.[10]

Grundy et al[10] also performed cholesterol balance studies on a number of their subjects. They found that there were no consistent changes in the fecal excretion of either neutral steroids (cholesterol) or bile acids, nor were there any detectable changes in total body synthesis of cholesterol during NA treatment. However, NA induced a slight increase in hepatic secretion of biliary cholesterol. Nevertheless, there was no significant increment in molar percent cholesterol or in percent saturation of gallbladder bile. Therefore, an increased risk of cholelithiasis should not be expected. In fact, no such increase was detected with the use of NA during the Coronary Drug Project.[11]

HDL-C comprises a class of plasma lipoproteins, the particles of which contain about one half lipid and one half protein by weight (see Chapter 1). The particles consist of a core of lipids, cholesteryl ester, triglycerides, and unesterified cholesterol. HDL, like particles of the other lipoprotein classes, act to solubilize these nonpolar constituents in the plasma by surrounding them with a surface layer of apoproteins and the polar head groups of phospholipids.[12] These surface apoproteins play important roles in regulating the enzymes involved in lipoprotein metabolism and in enabling recognition of lipoproteins by cell surface receptors.

There seem to be several sources of HDL. Apoproteins A-I and A-II, the two quantitatively major protein components of HDL, are synthesized in the liver as well as in the intestine. Apoprotein A-I is capable of attracting free cholesterol from peripheral sites by stimulating the enzyme lecithin-cholesterol acyltransferase (LCAT), which catalyzes the conversion of cholesterol to cholesteryl ester. With the incorporation of cholesteryl ester, the disc-shaped nascent HDL-C becomes the spherical HDL_3 which in turn is converted to HDL_2.[12] HDL_2, considered to be the HDL subfraction most protective against coronary artery disease, delivers excess cholesterol to the liver for excretion.

HDL is also produced through hydrolysis of the triglycerides in VLDL and chylomicra, the two triglyceride-rich lipoproteins. This hydrolysis, catalyzed by lipoprotein lipase, leaves behind an excess of surface components including cholesterol, apoproteins, and phospholipids that are transferred to HDL, thereby increasing its mass.[12] In fact, HDL concentrations associated with the HDL subfraction, are inversely related to VLDL-Tg concentrations and directly related to the activity level of lipoprotein lipase.[12-14] The other protein constituents transferred to HDL after the catabolism of chylomicra and VLDL comprise a small proportion of HDL and include the apoprotein C family of apoproteins, of which apoprotein C-I (like apoprotein A-I) acts as an activator of LCAT and apoprotein C-II acts as the specific activator of lipoprotein lipase; apoprotein D is thought to be involved in catalyzing cholesteryl ester transfer among HDL, LDL, and VLDL.[12]

As previously alluded to, there are two major subfractions of HDL: HDL_2 and HDL_3. HDL_2 is the less dense of the two, and has a higher apoprotein A-I:A-II ratio.[15] Shepherd et al[16] examined the effects of NA at pharmacological doses on the plasma levels and protein composition of HDL_2 and HDL_3. These researchers administered 3 g of NA per day to five healthy subjects over a 3-week period. As in the studies mentioned above, they found significant decreases in plasma cholesterol (15%), triglyceride (27%), and LDL-C (36%). In addition, this regimen raised HDL by 23% and increased the plasma HDL_2:HDL_3 ratio by 345%. This was associated with an absolute increase in circulating HDL_2 of 646% and a fall in HDL_3 levels of 47%. Similar results have been obtained by other investigators.[15,17] Furthermore, plasma concentrations of apoprotein A-I rose 7%, secondary to a decrease in its fractional catabolic rate, whereas concentrations of apoprotein A-II fell by 14%, mainly as a result of decreased synthesis.[16] There seemed to be a "net transfer" of apoprotein A-I from HDL_3 to HDL_2. HDL_2 and HDL_3 were associated with 6% and 94% of the circulating apoprotein A-I, respectively, prior to treatment, redistributing to 49% and 51%, respectively, during treatment.

Luria[18] studied the effects of NA at lower doses (1 g/d) on plasma HDL-C levels and total cholesterol:HDL-C ratio. This study followed a report by Alderman et al[6] that described success using a modified NA regimen that resulted in a fall in total cholesterol levels and a rise in HDL levels, the magnitude of the changes being dose dependent and significant even at less than 1 g taken twice daily. In Luria's study,[18] HDL-C levels rose 31% and the total cholesterol:HDL-C ratio dropped 27% after a mean of 6.7 months of treatment. Decreases in the total cholesterol:HDL-C ratio have been associated with slowing of the progression of coronary lesions.[19]

Flushing is a well known side effect of NA therapy. It has been observed that aspirin attenuates this bothersome effect, suggesting that the presumed vasodilation is prostaglandin mediated. Morrow et al[20] in an attempt to elucidate the substance responsible for the flush, recently measured serial metabolite levels of the vasoactive prostaglandin PGD_2 after administration of 500 mg of NA to three normal volunteers. They found that plasma levels of the PGD_2 metabolite, 9α, 11 β-PGF_2, increased by an average of 588-fold, reaching a maximum between 12 and 45 minutes after ingestion and declining to normal levels by 2 to 4 hours. These findings correlated clinically with the duration and intensity of the flushing encountered by the subjects. Urinary metabolites of two other vasoactive prostaglandins, PGI_2 and PGE_2, were also measured in one of the subjects and revealed only a modest twofold increase in dinor-6-keto PGF_1, the PGI_2 metabolite, and no increase in PGE_2 metabolite levels. However, plasma levels of these compounds were not measured. Olsson et al[21] found similar elevations in the urinary excretion of PGI_2 metabolites which they found to be significant after 2 days of NA treatment. After 28 days, these levels were not significantly different from pretreatment values. Also, in the study by Morrow et al[20] pretreatment of one of the subjects at a later date with 200 mg of indomethacin daily for 4 days prevented an increase in plasma levels of the PGD_2 metabolite. Likewise, aspirin reduces NA-induced cutaneous flushing[22] and is often used to minimize this effect in practice.

Nicotinamide does not appear to have lipid-lowering properties. Interestingly, nicotinamide also does not cause flushing and no increase in PGD2 levels is observed. One might speculate about the role, if any, that prostaglandins play in the lipid-altering effects of NA.[20] However, if levels decline with prolonged treatment as in the study by Olsson et al[21] it is then unlikely that prostaglandins play an important role in the long-term effects of NA.

Clinical Experience

As outlined above, NA has been shown to have beneficial effects on all plasma lipoprotein fractions and was identified as one of the "drugs of first choice" for the treatment of hypercholesterolemia by the Adult Treatment Panel of the National Cholesterol Education Program.[23] Studies of the clinical efficacy of NA fall into two main groups: those that examine the use of NA in patients with known coronary heart disease (CHD) and those that test its efficacy, often in combination with other lipid-lowering agents, in altering plasma lipoprotein levels in patients with various types of lipid and lipoprotein disorders.

Coronary Heart Disease

The Coronary Drug Project, a long-term, nationwide, double-blind, placebo-controlled study, looked at a number of lipid-altering regimens including NA and clofibrate in male survivors of myocardial infarction (MI).[11] In particular, the investigators assessed whether the various regimens could prevent new CHD events or prolong life in patients with clinical CHD. The subjects were men, aged 30 through 64 years with electrocardiogram-documented evidence of one or more previous MIs. Each subject was free of evidence of recent worsening of his CHD and had his last MI at least 3 months prior to entering the study. These men were randomized to either a control group that included 2789 subjects who received 3.8 g of lactose placebo daily or to one of the treatment groups. The NA group included 1119 men who received 3 g of the drug each day for 5 to $8\frac{1}{2}$ years with a mean of 6 years, 2 months. The primary endpoint for determining drug efficacy was total mortality. Other endpoints included cause-specific mortality (especially coronary mortality and sudden death) and nonfatal cardiovascular events. Subjects were also monitored for adverse effects.

Over the follow-up period, NA effected mean decreases in total serum cholesterol of 9.9% and in total triglycerides of 26.1%.[11] However, the incidence of all deaths in the follow-up period (8.5 years) was insignificantly lower than that in the placebo group (24.4% vs 25.4%).

In contrast to the findings on total mortality, the incidence of definite, nonfatal MI over the total follow-up period was 27% lower in the treatment group than in the control group (10.1% vs 13.9%). In addition, during this period the treatment group showed a 24% lower incidence of fatal or nonfatal cerebrovascular events than the placebo group. There was also a lower incidence of bypass surgery in the group receiving NA (0.9% vs 2.7%).[11]

Investigators in the Coronary Drug Project conducted a follow-up study nearly 9 years after termination of the original trial.[24] With a mean total follow up of 15 years, total mortality in the NA group was found to be 11% lower than in the placebo group (52% vs 58.2%). The men in the study had presumably stopped taking the drug after the original mean follow-up of 6.2 years. The decreased mortality is primarily due to a decrease in CHD mortality, with smaller decreases in death due to cerebrovascular causes, other cardiovascular events, cancer, and other noncardiovascular and noncancer causes.

Explanations for this observed "late benefit" of NA on mortality include the early decreases in incidence of nonfatal reinfarction and the cholesterol-lowering effects of NA on the coronary arteries.[24] It seems that patients with the largest decreases in cholesterol at 1-year follow-up had lower subsequent mortality than did subjects with increases in cholesterol. Interestingly, nearly 30% of the men in the NA group adhered poorly to the treatment regimen (took less than 60% of the amount of drug called for by the protocol); yet, there was a significant benefit in 15-year mortality.[24] This suggests that less than "optimal" doses of NA may nevertheless result in therapeutic benefits. Of course, statements regarding the efficacy of NA as a primary prevention of CHD or whether the administration of NA over longer periods of time would be beneficial or detrimental cannot be made based on the findings of this study.

In a Swedish study by Carlson et al[25] the effects of combined treatment with NA (up to 3 g daily) and clofibrate (2 g daily) were examined in 558 survivors of MI randomly assigned to one of two groups 4 months after their acute events. Both groups received advice regarding diet and the treatment group received both drugs as above. Subjects in the treatment group exhibited mean reductions in total serum cholesterol and serum triglycerides of 15% to 20% and 30%, respectively. Control group subjects showed insignificant reductions in these levels. There were no significant differences between the two groups with regard to total and CHD-related deaths. However, over a

4-year period, the number of nonfatal reinfarctions in the treatment group was reduced by 50% compared to the control group. In comparison, the Coronary Drug Project reported a 27% reduction in nonfatal reinfarctions in the NA group and insignificant reductions in the clofibrate group. Considering the more modest decreases in serum cholesterol and triglycerides (6% and 10%, respectively) found in the Coronary Drug Project as compared to those observed in this study, it has been suggested that the rate of nonfatal reinfarction may be related to the degree of serum lipid lowering.[11,25]

The Cholesterol-Lowering Atherosclerosis Study (CLAS) employed a colestipol-NA combination to test the hypothesis that aggressively lowering LDL-C and raising HDL-C will reverse or retard the progression of atherosclerotic lesions.[26] The subjects, chosen to minimize the effects of other major nonlipid risk factors for atherosclerosis, included 162 normotensive nonsmoking men aged 40 to 59 years with previous coronary bypass surgery and fasting total cholesterol levels in the range of 4.78 to 9.05 mm/L (185 to 350 mg/dl).

Subjects underwent coronary angiography and were then randomly assigned to either the treatment group or the placebo-control group. Both groups were instructed to follow a diet restricting the intake of cholesterol and saturated fat. The diets differed in that the control group followed a more lenient diet "to enhance the differential in blood cholesterol responses between the two groups'.[26] Subjects in the treatment group also took 30 g of colestipol plus 3-12 g of niacin daily. Follow-up visits included nutritional counseling and measurement of fasting blood lipids and lipoprotein levels. A repeat angiogram was performed on each subject after 2 years of treatment.

Changes in lipid values from baseline after drug treatment were as follows: decreases in total cholesterol (26%), triglycerides (22%), LDL-C (43%), and an increase in HDL-C (37%).[25] These results were all statistically significant and differed from the control group changes of −4%, −5%, −5%, and 2%, respectively.

Repeat angiography was performed on each subject at the conclusion of the study and compared to the prestudy film without knowledge of the temporal order of the films. A scoring system was employed based on a four-point scale ranging from 0 (no change) to 3 (extreme change). Signs were attached to the scores when the order of films was revealed, (−) for regression of lesion and (+) for progression. Both native arteries and bypass grafts were evaluated.[26]

The results of these readings show that the treatment group score distribution was significantly shifted toward lower scores than that of the control group, indicating less disease progression with colestipol-NA treatment. In fact, 61% of the treatment group subjects improved or remained the same, and 16.2% showed regression of atherosclerotic lesions at 2 years. This differs from the results in the placebo-control group of 39% and 2.4%, respectively. Regarding native vessels, treatment reduced the average number of lesions that progressed per subject and the percentage of subjects with new lesions.[26] Similarly, with respect to bypass grafts, the percentage of subjects either with new lesions or showing any adverse change in pre-existing lesions was significantly lower in the treatment group. Recently reported were the results of a 4-year follow-up of a subpopulation from CLAS.[27] The new data substantiate the benefit of lipid-lowering therapy on the progression and regression of coronary artery lesions.[27] These findings from CLAS suggest that following coronary artery bypass surgery patients should receive intensive interventions to beneficially alter blood lipid and lipo-protein levels.[26,27]

Recently, the results of the Familial Atherosclerosis Treatment Study (FATS) demonstrated a favorable effect of NA plus colestipol on the progression of coronary atherosclerotic disease.[28] Patients with disease, a family history of premature cardiovascular events, and elevated levels of apoprotein B 3.23 mm/L ($\geq$ 125 mg/dl) were counseled on diet and assigned to three treatment regimens: NA 4 g/d plus colestipol 30 g/d; lovastatin 40 mg/d plus colestipol; or colestipol alone (control). The combination regimens caused the greatest reductions in LDL and the greatest elevations in HDL. Bimonthly visits spanned 2.5 years between coronary angiograms. Favorable changes in clinical course and lesion severity appeared with the combination regimens. With the NA/colestipol combination, 25% of patients showed progression of coronary lesions, 39% showed regression, and only two cardiovascular events occurred. In contrast, 10 cardiovascular events occurred in the control group, 46% of patients showed region progression, and 11% regression of coronary lesions.[28]

In a smaller study, NA combined with colestipol and/or lovastatin was also shown to favor coronary lesion regression in patients with familial hypercholesterolemia.[29]

Phenotypic Hyperlipoproteinemia

Types II and IV hyperlipoproteinemia include the monogenic forms of familial hypercholesterolemia and familial hypertriglyceridemia, respectively, as well as polygenic and environmentally related forms of these conditions. Type II can be further divided into two subtypes: IIa, with elevated LDL-C only, and IIb, with elevated LDL-C and triglycerides. Elevated levels of VLDL-Tg alone are designated type IV.[30]

As described above, Shepherd et al[16] reported the effects of NA on the levels of the various lipoprotein and apolipoproteins in healthy volunteers. These investigators also studied the effects of NA (again at 3 g daily) in six type II and four type IV hyperlipoproteinemic subjects.[31] All six type II patients (three with IIa and three with IIb) met criteria for classification as having heterozygous familial hypercholesterolemia.

The results show differing effects of NA between the two groups. Type II subjects exhibited a reduction in plasma triglyceride and VLDL levels, but showed no significant changes in LDL-C or HDL-C levels or in the metabolism of apoprotein A-I and apoprotein A-II.[31] However, when the type II subjects were divided by subtype, the IIa patients also showed a marked increase in HDL-C accompanied by a 510% rise in the HDL_2:HDL_3 ratio (secondary to a 350% increase in HDL_2 and a 25% decrease in HDL_3). Apoprotein A-II synthesis also decreased. These findings are similar to those in normal subjects[16] and differ from those in the type IIb patients who demonstrated a less marked lowering of triglyceride and VLDL-C. The type IIb patients showed a slight increment in total HDL, primarily due to an increase in the HDL_3 subfraction.[31]

Changes in the lipoprotein levels in type IV subjects were similar to those in the normal subjects, including observed decreases in the functional catabolic rate of apoprotein A-I and in the synthesis of apoprotein A-II.[31] Furthermore, these investigators noted that whenever NA substantially lowers triglyceride levels (normals, IIa and IV), there are concomitant increases in HDL-C and in the HDL_2:HDL_3 ratio, as well as changes in the metabolism of apoprotein A-I and A-II. These findings may relate the action of NA as primarily a VLDL-Tg-lowering agent to its beneficial effects on HDL levels.

Hoeg et al[32] determined the effects of a combined neomycin and NA treatment on lipoprotein levels in 25 type II patients in a double-blind, randomized, placebo-controlled trial. Patients were placed on a diet restricting cholesterol and saturated fat. All patients tolerated the 2 g per day dose of neomycin, which lowered total cholesterol and LDL-C by 23% and 29%, respectively. The addition of 3 g of NA daily further lowered these values by 18% and 25%, respectively, and raised the levels of HDL-C by 32%. In addition, 92% of the subjects who tolerated the combined regimen demonstrated normalization of their plasma lipoprotein concentrations. However, 44% of the subjects were unable to tolerate the NA due to cutaneous or gastrointestinal effects.[32]

Type III hyperlipoproteinemia, less common than type II or type IV, is characterized by accumulations of circulating IDL (VLDL or VLDL-remnants), resulting in elevations of plasma cholesterol and triglycerides.[30] Three grams of NA daily in both twice a day and three times a day dosing schedules were administered to five patients with type III hyperlipoproteinemia.[33] Both regimens were effective in significantly lowering total cholesterol, total triglycerides and VLDL, as well as in elevating HDL-C levels and the HDL:LDL ratio. However, no significant changes in LDL-C were observed. The more frequent schedule resulted in higher levels of HDL-C.

Heterozygous Familial Hypercholesterolemia (FH)

Heterozygous FH is an autosomal dominant disease in which the product of the defective gene, the LDL receptor, is diminished (or absent, as in the homozygous form of the disease). Because of this deficiency, LDL cannot be removed from the circulation at a normal rate, leading to elevated levels of this lipoprotein in the blood.[4]

Most of the studies investigating the role of NA as a lipid-altering agent in patients with heterozygous FH have tested its efficacy in conjunction with other agents, most often the bile- acid binding resins. Kane et al[34] studied the effects of a colestipol-NA combination in patients who met rigorous criteria for heterozygous FH. On a diet low in cholesterol and saturated fat, colestipol alone decreased total cholesterol levels by 16%-25%. The addition of NA reduced these levels an additional 22%, resulting in a 45% decrease in total cholesterol for patients on the combined regimen, relative to diet alone. The two drugs in combination lowered LDL-C by 55% and increased HDL-C by 33%. Tendonous xanthomas, a common manifestation of heterozygous FH, were reduced significantly, indicating that cholesterol was mobilized from peripheral tissues.[34]

Similar alterations in lipid levels were found by Illingworth et al[35] and Kuo et al[36] with a colestipol-NA regimen. Furthermore, Kuo et al[36] noted that of 16 patients who completed three or more years of treatment, the 12 patients who had been "good responders" based on their lipoprotein alterations, showed neither significant progression nor development of new coronary lesions on repeated coronary arteriograms. In contrast, four "poor responders" showed varying degrees of lesion progression, that correlated well with their unstable clinical courses during the trial.[36]

Kuo et al[37] also examined the effects of combining colestipol and NA in a series of patients with FH and CHD who had demonstrated evidence of extracranial carotid artery disease. These investigators observed that, over 4.5 to 5 years of follow-up, none of the 34 patients experienced new or recurrent ophthalmological or cerebral ischemic episodes. This is consistent with stabilization of carotid artery lesions as determined by follow-up studies with intravenous digital subtraction angiography, B-scan, and ultrasonography.[37] However, it is important to note that there was no control group in this study for comparison.

In another study of treatment for heterozygous FH, researchers compared the lipid-altering ability of colestipol-NA, colestipol-lovastatin, and NA-lovastatin combinations with each other and with the triple regimen colestipol-lovastatin-NA.[38] Results indicate that the triple regimen was more effective than any of the paired combinations in lowering total cholesterol, triglyceride, and LDL-C levels. The addition of lovastatin did not significantly raise HDL-C above the levels attained by colestipol-NA. Of note, the triple regimen did not produce any adverse effects not associated with the use of the agents individually.[38]

One patient in this study with homozygous FH, aged 20 months at the onset of the trial, achieved reductions in total cholesterol and LDL-C of 59% and 58%, respectively, on the triple regimen.[38] These values are significantly lower than those achieved with any of the other combinations investigated. In addition, cutaneous xanthomas began to regress 20 months into the study, and at the time of the report, no clinical manifestations of cardiovascular disease had been noted.

Diabetes Mellitus

The most common lipoprotein abnormality seen in diabetes mellitus is an elevation of plasma VLDL-Tg, in addition to depression of

HDL-C levels and an increase in plasma LDL-C.[39] Given the beneficial effects of NA on these lipoproteins, this agent would seem to be ideal for use in these patients. Unfortunately, NA may produce hyperglyce- mia and impaired glucose tolerance even in nondiabetic patients, and a loss of diabetic control may counteract the lipid-altering effects of the drug.[4,39] However, it may be used in certain patients whose lipoprotein abnormality is unresponsive to other therapies.[39,40] The use of NA in diabetics often necessitates adjustments in dosage of hypoglycemic agents and requires close monitoring of diabetic status.

Nephrotic Syndrome

Patients with nephrotic syndrome usually have an associated hy- perlipidemia and consequently, are predisposed to early onset CHD. As reviewed by Grundy and Vega[41] this hyperlipidemia involves elevated levels of LDL-C in the early stages of the nephrotic syndrome followed by elevations in VLDL-C, and eventually, in VLDL-Tg. These increases may, in part, be related to increased hepatic production of VLDL and decreased LDL-receptor activity.[41] The use of NA in the nephrotic syn- drome has not been reported. However, one might speculate a beneficial effect in this condition given the mechanisms of hyperlipidemia postu- lated above and the decreased hepatic synthesis of VLDL-Tg associated with NA therapy.[10,42]

Lipoprotein(a) Elevations

Patients with heterozygous FH with serum cholesterol levels rang- ing from 300 to 500 mg% are markedly predisposed to premature coro- nary artery disease. However, since not all patients with FH have coro- nary artery disease, other factors must affect the atherogenicity of elevated LDL-C levels.

Lipoprotein(a) is a lipoprotein fraction that is similar to LDL and felt to be an atherogenic lipoprotein (see Chapter 1).[43] Lipoprotein (a) has an apoprotein (apoprotein a) that has a close structural relationship to plasminogen. It has been suggested that lipoprotein(a) might block the availability of true plasminogen to the blood vessel wall, thereby predisposing individuals to atherosclerosis and thrombotic events. Individuals with high lipoprotein(a) levels appear to be at increased risk for CHD.[44]

The drugs usually used to treat high LDL-C, such as the bile- acid binding resins and the HMG coenzyme A reductase inhibitors do not affect lipoprotein(a) levels. However, niacin is effective in lowering elevated lipoprotein(a) levels as is plasmapharesis.[44]

These findings have clinical significance and leave us with management questions. Should lipoprotein(a) levels be measured, and if they are elevated, should drugs such as NA be used instead of, or in addition to, other drugs used to lower LDL-C?

Clinical Use

Single Drug Therapy

NA, through its beneficial effects on VLDL-Tg, LDL-C, and HDL-C levels, is indicated in most forms of hyperlipoproteinemia and for patients with depressed HDL. This includes patients with types II, III, IV, and V hyperlipoproteinemia. It is particularly useful in patients who have elevated plasma VLDL-Tg levels as a part of their lipid profile. It is important to remember that a diet that is low in cholesterol and saturated fats is the foundation of therapy for hyperlipoproteinemia.

NA is available in 100, 125, 250, and 500 mg tablets, as well as in a time-release form. The typical dosage of NA is 3-7 g daily given in three divided doses. Therapeutic effects of the drug usually are not manifested until the patient reaches a total daily dose of at least 3 g. A greater response may be attained with periodic increases in doses up to a maximum of 7-8 g daily, although the incidence of adverse effects also increases with higher doses. In general, it is best to use the lowest dose that is necessary to achieve the desired alterations in plasma lipoprotein levels. Unfortunately, many patients cannot tolerate therapeutic doses of NA, the primary side effects being cutaneous flushing and gastrointestinal disturbance. However, certain steps can be taken to minimize these untoward effects.

NA therapy should be initiated with a low dosage regimen (100 mg daily), gradually increasing the dose every few days over a period of several weeks until the patient attains a dosage level of 3 g daily given in three divided doses. If, while increasing the dose, the patient develops any adverse effects, the dose should be cut back and then resumed at a more gradual pace. Taking the doses with meals decreases gastric irritation and cutaneous flushing.[45] Further, cutaneous flushing can be reduced or avoided by taking one aspirin tablet daily (more frequent administration is unnecessary as one tablet will inhibit cyclooxygenase for up to 2 weeks).[22,40,42] Interestingly, tachyphylaxis to the flushing phenomenon often occurs within a few days,[26] although the bothersome episodes may recur if the patient misses two or three doses.[45] Once the initial maintenance dose is reached, it is important to evaluate for therapeutic effects by measuring plasma lipoprotein values. If the therapeutic effects are unsatisfactory, the dose should be increased by 1.0 to 1.5 g per day, with periodic increases to a maximum of 7-8 g daily as needed. When doses of 4 mg daily are achieved, usually another lipid-lowering drug is added.

Regardless of the dose, it is important to make several laboratory evaluations for potential adverse effects at regular intervals. These include assessment of liver function (bilirubin, alkaline phosphatase, and transaminase levels), uric acid levels, and serum glucose levels.

NA is contraindicated in patients with active peptic ulcer disease. The drug may also impair glucose tolerance and is contraindicated in patients with diabetes that is difficult to control. NA is also associated with reversible elevations of liver enzymes and uric acid and should not be used in patients with hepatic disease or a history of symptomatic gout.[39,45]

A time-release form of NA was developed after noting that the incidence of cutaneous flushing is reduced by taking the drug with meals, suggesting that this side effect is related to the rate of gastrointestinal absorption.[46] In fact, patients taking the time-release preparation do have a lower incidence of flushing than patients with unmodified NA. However, this is outweighed by the far greater incidence of gastrointestinal and constitutional symptoms experienced by patients on the time-release form, including nausea, vomiting, diarrhea, fatigue, and decreased male sexual function.[46] In addition, the time-release preparation may be associated with more hepatotoxicity, even with low doses, including greater alkaline phosphatase and transaminase elevations.[46-48] This preparation was implicated as the cause of fulminant hepatic failure requiring liver transplant in a patient who 2 months previously began taking 6 g daily of time-release NA.[49] Prior to this time, he had taken 6 g daily of unmodified NA for 1 year without side effects.

Recently, a clinical experience was reported on describing the use of a new form of NA that employs a wax-matrix vehicle for sustained-release drug delivery.[50] Patient groups receiving 2000 and 1500 mg of NA in this formulation demonstrated significant reductions in values of LDL-C and total cholesterol when compared with diet- and placebo-treated controls. Smaller improvements were seen in HDL-C and triglycerides. A favorable side effect profile was reported with this NA formulation, perhaps related to the lower daily dose of NA used. A larger long-term clinical experience with this formulation is still needed to confirm these safety and efficacy results.

Combination Therapy

The use of combined drug therapy is beneficial in patients who are inadequately controlled on a restricted diet and NA monotherapy.[40] This is often the case in patients with heterozygous FH (type IIa) or familial combined hyperlipidemia (type IIb). One such regimen combines NA with a bile-acid binding resin, such as colestipol. This treatment takes advantage of the synergistic mechanism of action of the two agents. The resin promotes LDL catabolism and cholesterol excretion while secondarily increasing hepatic synthesis of cholesterol and VLDL, thus achieving a new steady-state with limited reduction of LDL.[35] The addition of a drug such as NA that reduces the synthesis of VLDL (and LDL) would be expected to add further therapeutic benefits to those achieved by diet and resin alone. In fact, the use of colestipol (30 g daily) in combination with NA (3-8 g daily) consistently decreases plasma levels of total cholesterol by 34% to 45% and LDL-C by 45% to 55% in patients with heterozygous FH.[34-37] In addition, this combination has been associated with the regression of atherosclerotic lesions, as well as the prevention of new lesion formation in native coronary vessels and coronary bypass grafts.[26] The addition of NA also adds the beneficial effects over diet-resin alone of increasing HDL-C levels and decreasing VLDL levels, particularly useful in familial combined hyperlipidemia.

Lovastatin is a specific competitive inhibitor of HMG-CoA reductase, the enzyme involved in the rate-limiting step of cholesterol biosynthesis. The decrease in hepatic cholesterol synthesis that occurs with lovastatin is thought to induce an increased rate of receptor-mediated uptake of LDL from the plasma as well as a decrease in LDL production, thus lowering LDL levels.[51,52] The combination of lovastatin and NA might be expected to have additive and synergistic effects given their mechanisms of action. In fact, Lees et al[53] found that when lovastatin

(20-40 mg daily) was combined with NA (3 g daily), LDL concentrations decreased by 49%, a 14% greater drop than with lovastatin alone. Triglyceride levels were also reduced, making this combination especially useful in patients with concurrent elevations in LDL-C and triglyceride (type IIb hyperlipoproteinemia). However, caution must be taken when using lovastatin and NA in combination, as NA may adversely affect liver function and thereby impair the hepatic excretion of lovastatin.[51] This interaction possibly explains the increased risk of myopathy associated with this regimen over that of monotherapy.[54]

Patients with severe heterozygous FH who inadequately respond to the use of two drugs may benefit from triple drug combinations. One such therapy with proven efficacy is NA with lovastatin and resin. This triple drug regimen decreases LDL-C levels by up to 69%, making it more effective than resin-NA, resin-lovastatin, or lovastatin-NA.[38,55,56] The triple agent combination also results in increases in HDL-C with moderate reductions in triglyceride.[38] Further, this regimen may allow for lower doses of NA and resin to achieve therapeutic changes in plasma lipoprotein levels, thus possibly reducing the incidence of adverse effects.[56]

Adverse Effects

Despite NA's efficacy in beneficially altering serum lipoprotein levels, its use is limited by a variety of troublesome and sometimes serious side effects. Some studies have experienced up to a 50% drop-out rate as a result of drug-related side effects.[18]

The Coronary Drug Project, with 1100 subjects on NA therapy, reported the common occurrences of cutaneous flushing and pruritus.[11] Other dermatological side effects include dryness of skin, rash, and acanthosis nigricans, all reversible with cessation of therapy.[57] The mechanism of the flushing is presumed to be related to the effect of NA on vasodilatory prostaglandins, and is frequently attenuated by pretreatment with aspirin.[4,20,22] This vasodilatory effect, in combination with antihypertensive therapy, may potentially result in postural hypotension.[4,57] The Coronary Drug Project also described an increased incidence of atrial fibrillation, and other transient cardiac arrhythmias were noted.[11] In addition, elevations in uric acid levels associated with an increased incidence of acute gouty arthritis were observed.

Gastrointestinal symptoms including diarrhea, nausea, vomiting, and abdominal pain were also frequent complaints encountered in the Coronary Drug Project.[11] Activation of peptic ulcer disease by NA is a potential adverse effect[4,45,57] but was not observed in this large scale study.

Liver function tests frequently are abnormal during NA therapy. Generally, there is elevation in alkaline phosphatase and hepatic transaminases. Some studies have also noted elevations in bilirubin occasionally leading to jaundice. The elevations in transaminases generally are transient and reverse with decrease in dosage or cessation of therapy, and can be minimized by increasing the dosage in gradual increments when initiating therapy.[45] Unlike the elevations in hepatic enzymes associated with HMG-CoA reductase inhibitors, the elevations that occur with the use of NA may be symptomatic. Several cases of "niacin hepatitis" progressing to fulminant hepatic failure have been described, most frequently with the time-release formulation, with biochemical, clinical, and histologic evidence of hepatocellular injury.[48,58,59] This seems to be a dose-related hepatotoxicity rather than a hypersensitivity, occurring in almost all cases at doses greater than 3 g daily. In most cases, cessation of therapy leads to eventual resolution of abnormalities, although there is one reported case of a patient on time-release NA who required liver transplantation.[49]

Hyperglycemia and impaired glucose tolerance may occur with NA therapy, and often necessitates adjustments in diet and hypoglycemic therapy in diabetic patients.[4,39,57]

The Coronary Drug Project[11] noted a statistically significant increase in CPK levels with NA therapy, and there have been reports of associated reversible myopathy.[60] The combination of lovastatin and NA has been causally implicated in at least one case of rhabdomyolysis.[61]

Conclusions

NA is a second or third choice for isolated hypercholesterolemia because of the troublesome side effects associated with the drug. However, it has a therapeutic advantage as a monotherapy in patients with severe combined hyperlipidemia when reduction of elevated concentrations of total plasma C, LDL-C, and triglyceride are needed. The drug is potentially useful for the management of all types of hyperlipoproteinemia except type I. However, untoward adverse reactions must be carefully monitored.[62] The combination of NA with a bile-acid sequestering resin, lovastatin, gemfibrozil, or probucol may allow for greater effectiveness in lowering the concentration of both LDL-C and/or triglyceride.

References

1. Altschul R, Hoffer A, Stephen JD: Influence of nicotinic acid on serum cholesterol in man. Arch Biochem 1955; 54: 558-559.
2. Fumagalli R: Pharmacokinetics of nicotinic acid and some of its derivatives. In Gey KF, Caarlson LA (eds):Metabolic Effects of Nicotinic Acid and Its Derivatives. Bern-Stuttgart-Vienna, Hans Huber Publishers, 1971; 33-49.
3. Carlson LA, Oro L, Ostman J: Effect of a single dose of nicotinic acid on plasma lipids in patients with hyperlipoproteinemia. Acta Med Scand 1968; 183: 457-465.
4. Brown MS, Goldstein JL: Drugs used in the treatment of hyperlipoproteinemias. In Goodman L, Gilman A (eds): The Pharmacologic Basis of Therapeutics, 7th ed. New York, MacMillan Publishing Co., 1985: 827-845.
5. Petrack B, Greengard P, Kalinsky H: On the relative efficacy of nicotinamide and nicotinic acid as precursors of nicotinamide adenine dinucleotide. J Biol Chem 1966; 241: 2367-2372.
6. Alderman JD, Pasternak RC, Sacks FM, et al: Effect of a modified, well-tolerated niacin regimen on serum total cholesterol, high density lipoprotein cholesterol and the cholesterol to high density lipoprotein ratio. Am J Cardiol 1989; 64: 725-729.
7. Carlson LA, Oro L: The effect of nicotinic acid on the plasma free fatty acids: Demonstration of a metabolic type of sympathicolysis. Acta Med Scand 1962; 172 :641-645.
8. Carlson LA: Studies on the effect of nicotinic acid on catecholamine stimulated lipolysis in adipose tissue in vitro. Acta Med Scand 1963; 173: 719-722.
9. Arner P, Ostman J: Effect of nicotinic acid on acylglycerol metabolism in human adipose tissue. Clin Sci 1983; 64: 235-237.
10. Grundy SM, Mok YI, Zech L, et al: Influence of nicotinic acid on metabolism of cholesterol and triglycerides in man. J Lipid Res 1981; 22: 24-36.
11. Coronary Drug Project Research Group: Clofibrate and niacin in coronary heart disease. JAMA 1975; 231: 360-381.
12. Gotto AM: High-density lipoproteins: biochemical and metabolic factors. Am J Cardiol 1983; 52: 2B-4B.
13. Castelli WP, Doyle JT, Gordon T, et al: HDL cholesterol and other lipids in coronary heart disease: the cooperative lipoprotein phenotyping study. Circulation 1977; 55: 767-772.
14. Richards EG, Grundy SM, Cooper K: Influence of plasma triglycerides on lipoprotein patterns in normal subjects and in patients with coronary artery disease. Am J Cardiol 1989; 63: 1214-1220.

15. Atmeh RF, Shepherd J, Packard CJ: Subpopulations of apolipoprotein A-I in human high-density lipoproteins: Their metabolic properties and response to drug therapy. Biochim et Biophys Acta 1983; 751: 175-188.

16. Shepherd J, Packard CJ, Patsch JR, et al: Effects of nicotinic acid therapy on plasma high-density lipoprotein subfraction distribution and composition and on apolipoprotein A metabolism. J Clin Invest 1979; 63: 858-867.

17. Walldius G, Wahlberg G: Effects of nicotinic acid and its derivatives on lipid metabolism and other metabolic factors related to atherosclerosis. Adv Exp Med Biol 1985; 183: 281-293.

18. Luria MH: Effect of low-dose niacin on high-density lipoprotein cholesterol and total cholesterol-high-density cholesterol ratio. Arch Intern Med 1988; 148: 2493-2495.

19. Arntzenius AC, Kromhout D, Barth JD, et al: Diet, lipoproteins, and the progression of coronary atherosclerosis. The Leiden Intervention Trial. N Engl J Med 1985; 312: 805-811.

20. Morrow JD, Parsons WG III, Roberts LJ II: Release of markedly increased quantities of prostaglandin D_2 in vivo in humans following the administration of nicotinic acid. Prostaglandins 1989; 38: 263-274.

21. Olsson AG, Carlson LA, Anggard E, et al: Prostacyclic production augmented in the short term by nicotinic acid. (letter) Lancet 1983; 2: 565-566.

22. Wilkin JK, Wilkin O, Kapp R, et al: Aspirin blocks nicotinic acid-induced flushing. Clin Pharmacol Ther 1982; 31: 478-482.

23. Report of the National Cholesterol Education Program. Expert panel on detection, evaluation, and treatment of high blood cholesterol in adults. Arch Intern Med 1988; 148: 36-39.

24. Canner PL, Berge KG, Wenger NK, et al: Fifteen year mortality in Coronary Drug Project patients: long term benefit with niacin. J Am Coll Cardiol 1986; 8: 1245-1255.

25. Carlson LA, Danielson M, Ekberg I, et al: Reduction of myocardial reinfarction by the combined treatment with clofibrate and nicotinic acid. Atherosclerosis 1977; 28: 81-86.

26. Blankenhorn DH, Nessim SA, Johnson RL, et al: Beneficial effects of combined colestipol-niacin therapy on coronary atherosclerosis and coronary venous bypass grafts. JAMA 1987; 257: 3233-3240.

27. Cashin-Hemphill L, Mack WEJ, Pogoda JM, et al: Beneficial effects of colestipol-niacin on coronary atherosclerosis. JAMA 1990; 264: 3013-3017.

28. Brown G, Albers JJ, Fisher LD, et al: Regression of coronary artery disease as a result of intensive lipid lowering therapy in men with high levels of apolipoprotein B. N Engl J Med 1990; 323: 1289-1298.

29. Kane JP, Malloy MJ, Ports TA, et al: Regression of coronary atherosclerosis during treatment of familial hypercholesterolemia with combined drug regimens. JAMA 1990; 264: 3007-3012.

30. Margolis S: Disorders of plasma lipids and lipoproteins. In Harvey AM, Johns RJ, McKusick VA et al (eds): The Principles and Practice of Medicine, 22nd ed. Norwalk CT, Appleton & Lange, 1988; 976-985.

31. Packard CJ, Stewart JM, Third JLHC, et al: Effects of nicotinic acid therapy on high-density lipoprotein metabolism in type II and type IV hyperlipoproteinemia. Biochim et Biophys Acta 1980; 618: 53-62.

32. Hoeg JM, Maher MB, Bon E, et al: Normalization of plasma lipoprotein concentrations in patients with type II hyperlipoproteinemia by combined use of neomycin and niacin. Circulation 1984; 70: 1004-1011.
33. Hoogwerf BJ, Bantle JP, Kuba K, et al: Treatment of type III hyperlipoproteinemia with four different treatment regimens. Atherosclerosis 1984; 51: 251-259.
34. Kane JP, Malloy MJ, Tun P, et al: Normalization of low-density lipoproteinemia levels in heterozygous familial hypercholesterolemia with a combined drug regimen. N Engl J Med 1981; 304: 251-258.
35. Illingworth DR, Phillipson BE, Rapp JH, et al: Colestipol plus nicotinic acid in treatment of heterozygous familial hypercholesterolemia. Lancet 1981; 1: 296-298.
36. Kuo PT, Kostis JB, Moreyra AE, et al: Familial type II hyperlipoproteinemia with coronary heart disease: effect of diet-colestipol-nicotinic acid treatment. Chest 1981; 79: 286-291.
37. Kuo PT, Toole JF, Schaaf JA, et al: Extracranial carotid artery disease in patients with familial hypercholesterolemia and coronary artery disease treated with colestipol and nicotinic acid. Stroke 1987; 18: 716-721.
38. Malloy MJ, Kane JP, Kunitake ST, et al: Complementarity of colestipol, niacin and lovastatin in treatment of severe familial hypercholesterolemia. Ann Intern Med 1987; 107: 616-623.
39. Dunn FL: Treatment of lipid disorders in diabetes mellitus. Med Clin N Amer 1988; 72: 1379-1398.
40. Havel RJ: Experience with individual lipid lowering drugs: nicotinic acid. Cardiovasc Rev & Rep 1990; 11: 76-77.
41. Grundy SM, Vega GL: Rationale and management of hyperlipidemia of the nephrotic syndrome. Am J Med 1989; 87: 5-3N-5-llN.
42. Grundy S: Management of hyperlipidemia of kidney disease. Kidney Intl 1990; 37: 847-853.
43. Utermann G: The mysteries of lipoprotein. Science 1989; 246: 904-910.
44. Seed M, Hoppichler F, Reaveley D, et al: Relation of serum lipoprotein concentration and apolipoprotein phenotype to coronary heart disease in patients with familial hypercholesterolemia. N Engl J Med 1990; 322: 1494-1499.
45. Witztum JL: Current approaches to drug therapy for the hypercholesterolemic patient. Circulation 1989; 80: 1101-1114.
46. Knopp RH, Ginsberg J, Albers JJ, et al: Contrasting effects of unmodified and time-release forms of niacin on lipoproteins in hyperlipidemic subjects: clues to mechanism of action of niacin. Metabolism 1985; 34: 642-650.
47. Henkin Y, Johnson KC, Segrest JP: Rechallenge with crystalline niacin after drug induced hepatitis from sustained-release niacin. JAMA 1990; 264: 241-243.
48. Etchason JA, Miller TD, Squires RW, et al: Niacin-induced hepatitis: a potential side-effect with low-dose time-release niacin. Mayo Clin Proc 1991; 66: 23-28.
49. Mullin GE, Greenson JK, Mitchell MC: Fulminant hepatic failure after ingestion of sustained-release nicotinic acid. Ann Intern Med 1989; 111: 253-255.

50. Keenan JM, Fontaine PL, Wenz JB, et al: Niacin revisited. Arch Intern Med 1991; 151: 1424-1432.
51. Illingworth DR: New horizons in combination drug therapy for hypercholesterolemia. Cardiology 1989; 76 (Suppl 1): 83-100.
52. Frishman WH, Zimetbaum P, Nadelmann J: Lovastatin and other HMG-CoA reductase inhibitors. J Clin Pharmacol 1989; 29: 975-982.
53. Lees AM, Stein SW, Lees RS: Therapy of hypercholesterolemia with mevinolin and other lipid-lowering drugs. (abstr) Arteriosclerosis 1986; 6: 544a.
54. Ayanian JZ, Fuchs CS, Stone RM: Lovastatin and rhabdomyolysis. Letter to the Editor. Ann Intern Med 1988; 109: 682.
55. Illingworth DR, Bacon SP, Larsen KK: Long-term experience with HMG-CoA reductase inhibitors in the therapy of hypercholesterolemia. Arteriosclerosis Rev 1988; 18: 161-187.
56. Stein EA, Lamkin GE, Bewley DZ, et al: Treatment of severe familial hypercholesterolemia with lovastatin, resin and niacin. (abstr) Arteriosclerosis 1987; 7: 517a.
57. Physicians Desk Reference, 46th ed. New York, Medical Economics Co., Inc., 1992: 1846.
58. Patterson DJ, Dew EW, Gyorkey F, et al: Niacin hepatitis. So Med J 1983; 76: 239-241.
59. Clementz GL, Holmes AW: Nicotinic-acid-induced fulminant hepatic failure. J Clin Gastroenterol 1987; 9: 582-584.
60. Litin SC, Anderson CF: Nicotinic-acid associated myopathy: a report of three cases. Am J Med 1989; 86: 481-483.
61. Reaven P, Witztum JL: Lovastatin, nicotinic acid, and rhabdomyolysis. Letter to the Editor. Ann Intern Med 1988; 109: 597-598.
62. Rader JI, Calvert RJ, Hathcock JN: Hepatic toxicity of unmodified and time-release preparations of niacin. Am J Med 1992; 92: 77-81.

Chapter 8

Probucol

Peter Zimetbaum M.D., William H. Frishman M.D.

Probucol was first introduced in the early 1970s and was advocated for its LDL-cholesterol-lowering properties and favorable side effect profile. However, it was soon noted that, in most instances, this drug lowered HDL-cholesterol more than it lowered LDL-cholesterol. Probucol was also challenged for its potential to prolong the ECG QT interval, which could lead to ventricular arrhythmias in nonhuman primates. Nonetheless, this agent has enjoyed fairly widespread popularity for the treatment of patients with elevated cholesterol who are unable to tolerate the side effects of the other hypocholesterolemic medications. Recently, probucol has enjoyed a resurgence in interest because of its antioxidant properties, and the potential, through this mechanism, to halt the progression of atherosclerosis despite its HDL lowering activity.

Cholesterol, LDL, and Atherogenesis

The purpose of lowering cholesterol is to decrease the formation and progression of atherosclerotic plaques and their sequelae: symptomatic and fatal vascular disease. Traditionally, it was believed that the initial event in the atherosclerotic process was injury to the arterial intima. This injury or breakdown in the subendothelial barrier was followed, in the presence of excess cholesterol, by the deposition of lipoproteins in the arterial wall and subsequent foam cell formation. Foam cells then coalesced to form fatty streaks and eventually atheroma. In this model, since the source of the injury is unknown, the only

From *Medical Management of Lipid Disorders: Focus on Prevention of Coronary Artery Disease,* edited by William H. Frishman, M.D. © 1992, Futura Publishing Inc., Mount Kisco, NY.

feasible target of therapy is elimination of the excess cholesterol. Thus, physicians strive to decrease LDL.

The above theory is fraught with one serious error. Pathological analysis shows that the fatty streak occurs before the intimal injury or loss of endothelial cells is apparent.[1] Observations by Steinberg et al have led to a new theory of atherogenesis centered on the oxidative modification of LDL.[2,3] This hypothesis is summarized as follows: in the presence of elevated plasma LDL, there is migration of LDL through the endothelium into the intima where some proportion is oxidized by endothelial cells, macrophages, and smooth muscle cells. This oxidized LDL possesses chemotactic activity causing an increased migration of monocytes into the subendothelium. These monocytes are then transformed into macrophages, and their escape is prevented by the newly modified LDL. Macrophages possess receptors for modified LDL, which then take up only the modified LDL and form foam cells.

Steinberg et al go on to suggest that oxidative modification of LDL may also lead to the formation of immune complexes in the artery that can be engulfed by macrophages,[2,3] illustrating another mechanism for the development of foam cells and thus the formation of fatty streaks.

Oxidized LDL, but not native LDL, is very cytotoxic, leading Steinberg et al to propose that perhaps its uptake by acetylated macrophages is somehow protective.[2,3] Nonetheless, eventual overload of these macrophages causes their demise and release of modified LDL. This cytotoxic lipoprotein then causes injury to and finally denudation of the overlying endothelium. Next there is platelet aggregation, growth factor release, and smooth muscle cell proliferation, leading to atheroma formation. This new theory is exciting because it not only supports the already accepted therapeutic benefit of lowering plasma cholesterol, but also proposes a role for combating LDL oxidation.

Probucol

Chemistry

The chemical name for probucol is 4-4'-([1-methyl-ethyldene] bis-[thio])bis (2,6-bis [1,1-dimethyl-ethyl]phenol) (Fig. 1). The structure is 2 butylated hydroxytoluenes connected by a sulfur-carbon-sulfur bridge. The butylated hydroxytoluene groups are potent antioxidants and the sulfur containing bis phenol is unrelated in chemical structure

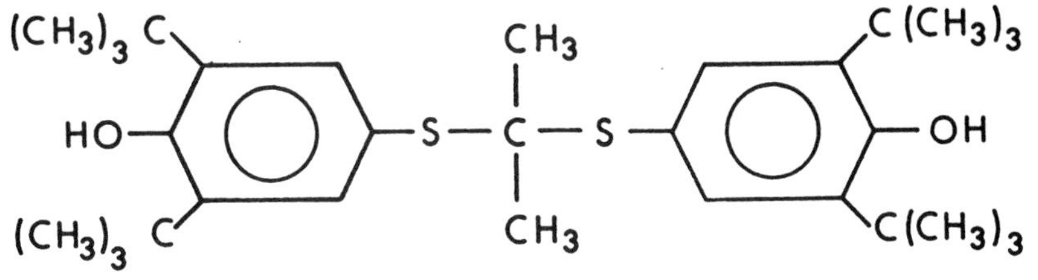

Figure 1: *Chemical structure of probucol.*

to any other cholesterol-lowering drug. Probucol is also very hydrophobic.[4]

Pharmacokinetics

Probucol is poorly absorbed from the GI tract, with only 2%-8% of the dose reaching the circulation.[5] Probucol is transported from the gut within chylomicrons and VLDL. In the plasma it is carried predominantly by LDL, VLDL, and HDL. However, Polachek et al note that there is no absolute correlation between the plasma levels of probucol and the degree of serum cholesterol-lowering.[6]

With continuous oral administration of probucol 500 mg twice daily, blood levels rise and stay relatively constant after a period of approximately 3 months.[7] Probucol accumulates in the adipose tissue, and may persist there and in the circulation for more than 6 months.[7] The major pathway of elimination is in the bile and feces. There is a small amount of renal clearance. There is no clear evidence as to whether probucol is excreted in human milk. It has been detected in animal milk, however, and is therefore contraindicated in nursing females. Probucol crosses the human placental barrier but no conclusive evidence is available regarding teratogenicity. Data in rats and rabbits show that probucol is not a teratogen but these results cannot be extrapolated to humans.[4]

Mechanisms of Action

The actions of probucol appear to be multifold, but as of yet, have not all been clearly delineated. It is felt that probucol causes an increased uptake of LDL by the liver. This increased concentration of cholesterol is then converted into bile-acids and excreted in the feces. This increased bile-acid formation leads to a depletion of hepatocyte cholesterol and an increase in cholesterol turnover. In essence, a new steady state is achieved where LDL formation is equal to LDL breakdown.[8]

Probucol has also been shown to lower cholesterol in LDL receptor deficient rabbits.[9] It is postulated that probucol enters the LDL molecule and causes an alteration in lipoprotein surface markers leading to its enhanced removal by a receptor-independent pathway.[8] The combination of these two mechanisms results in an average lowering of LDL by approximately 10%-15% when combined with diet.[10] Probucol is also known for its HDL-lowering effect, both in number and size of particles. It has been thought that probucol lowers the fractional clearance rate and turnover of HDL, thus creating a lower steady state for HDL and decreasing its absolute plasma concentrations. One would expect that this lowered HDL concentration would correlate with increased coronary artery disease. However, studies have shown this is not the case.[11]

Highly correlated with this probucol-induced lowered HDL is a regression of tendinous xanthomas, unrelated to the degree of cholesterol-lowering in patients with heterozygous familial hypercholesterolemia.[12] This finding led investigators to propose that while probucol lowers HDL levels, it also modifies this lipoprotein in a way that enhances the removal of cholesterol from peripheral tissues, i.e., augments the reverse pathway.[13]

The principle of reverse cholesterol transport, regardless of the exact mechanism, is based on the concept that HDL carries cholesterol from peripheral tissues and arterial walls. HDL is then recognized via a receptor-mediated process by the liver, where it is taken up and its cholesterol disposed of. The implications of this model suggest that a defect in this hepatic recognition process, such as lack of apoprotein E or the hepatic receptor for HDL's apoprotein E may lead to increased levels of plasma HDL despite a decreased removal of cholesterol. Conversely, a highly efficient transport system may effect such rapid uptake of HDL that plasma levels may be low despite a large efflux of peripheral cholesterol. This principle has led authorities to look beyond probucol's lowering of plasma HDL levels to its absolute effect on the reverse cholesterol pathway.[13]

Barnhardt et al[14] examined the effects of probucol on cultured rat hepatocytes. Aside from noting a lack of damage to the hepatocyte membrane by probucol, he also noted an enhanced flux of free cholesterol from HDL to liver cells. The author points out that this reduction in plasma HDL could signify an increase in reverse cholesterol transport, thus explaining Yamamoto's finding that tendon xanthoma regression increased with decreased HDL concentration.

Aburatani et al[15] found that probucol increased the levels of mRNA for apoprotein E in the spleen and brain of rabbits. As noted earlier, apoprotein E is an important factor in the recognition and uptake of HDL and chyloremnants by the liver. Thus, it is possible that although absolute concentrations of HDL seem to decrease in the presence of probucol, the functional removal of cholesterol actually is increased. There is also some evidence that probucol increases the efflux of cholesterol from the peripheral tissues.[16]

The final proposed mechanism of probucol involves its antioxidant properties, and by this action, its effect on atherosclerotic lesions. Many animal studies have shown that probucol can inhibit the progression and may cause regression of atheromas, independent of its effect on total cholesterol and despite reducing HDL levels. A similar prospective study, the Probucol Quantitative Regression Swedish Trial (PQRST,) involving humans is currently in progress.[17] This study involves a group of subjects treated with cholestyramine, diet, and either placebo or probucol, and their pre-existing femoral artery atheromas are being followed by angiography. The most current interest in probucol lies in its potential as an antioxidant to inhibit the modification of LDL and the progression of atherosclerosis. It was first demonstrated that probucol inhibited the oxidative modification of LDL by endothelial cells and the subsequent uptake by macrophages. Next, LDL receptor-deficient Watanabe rabbits were treated with either lovastatin or probucol to exclude the chance that the atherosclerotic process was inhibited by lowered cholesterol alone. The cholesterol-lowering effect was approximately equal in both groups but the probucol treated group, on autopsy, showed a significant decrease in lesions when compared with the lovastatin treated group.[18] They also found that labeled LDL that had been administered was present in greater concentrations in the atheromas of lovastatin treated rabbits compared to probucol treated rabbits.[18] The precise mechanism of probucol's antioxidant function is beyond the scope of this chapter, but it is felt that the lipophilicity of probucol and its resultant incorporation into LDL lies at the core of its effectiveness.

Clinical Experience

Monotherapy

Clinical experience with probucol as a single agent therapy is limited for reasons already outlined. In 1980, Mellies et al[19] conducted a double-blind, crossover study using probucol in a group of 19 adults with familial hyperlipidemia. All subjects were begun on a cholesterol-lowering diet and 10 received 24 weeks of placebo followed by 24 weeks of probucol. The remaining 9 subjects received 24 weeks of probucol followed by 24 weeks of placebo. It was found that all subjects on probucol lowered their cholesterol by 10.7%, with an LDL-lowering effect of 8.4% in excess of the effect of diet alone. Plasma triglyceride and VLDL levels were not significantly altered. HDL was lowered by 26% compared to the placebo group. Of note, there was excellent compliance with relatively few mild side effects.

In 1983 Yamamoto et al[20] treated eight patients with heterozygous familial hypercholesterolemia (average cholesterol 9.62 ± 1.5 mm/L [372 ± 59 mg/dl]) and nine patients with homozygous hypercholesterolemia (average cholesterol 12.39-19.5 mm/L [479-754 mg/dl]) with probucol (750-1500 mg/dl) and diet. They found that there was an initial reduction in cholesterol after 1 month of treatment but that it took 4-6 months to reach the maximal effect of a 22% reduction.

One long-term, double-blind, placebo-controlled study treating hyperlipidemic patients with cholesterol values > 6.47 mm/L (> 250 mg/dl) showed that probucol caused a 20% reduction in serum cholesterol over 9 years in 60% of subjects.[21] Over 80% of subjects had at least a 10% reduction in cholesterol from baseline values. The long duration of this study suggests that probucol maintains its efficacy over time.

Miettinen et al[22] conducted a 5-year multifactorial primary prevention trial in middle-aged men. Patients were treated with either probucol or clofibrate, with or without diuretic or beta blocker. They noted an increase over the placebo group in coronary events for those treated with a beta blocker or with clofibrate but not with probucol or diuretics. The incidence of cerebrovascular events was reduced in all groups compared to placebo. Miettinen reports that the probucol treated group had a reduction in HDL in greater proportion than the reduction in LDL. However, despite this lowered HDL, the incidence of new cardiac events was lowest in the probucol treated group.[22] There is no clear explanation for this finding in light of the understanding that HDL varies inversely with coronary heart disease. Thus, either probucol's LDL lowering effect or some other property, such as its antioxidant activity, confers protection.

Combination Therapy

Several studies have identified probucol's additive hypocholesterolemic effects when combined with other lipid-lowering drugs. Furthermore, many lipid-lowering drugs other than probucol have an HDL elevating effect that might partially counteract probucol's HDL lowering effect.

Bile Acid Resin Plus Probucol

Both Kuo[23] and Sommariva[24] in two separate studies using probucol plus colestipol and probucol plus cholestyramine, respectively, showed an additive effect with these combinations. Sommariva[24] showed that cholestyramine 16 g/d plus probucol 1 g/d lowered LDL by 32%, representing a 6% greater decrease than cholestyramine alone. There was also a substantial drop in HDL with probucol alone, but this drop was less significant when cholestyramine was combined with probucol. Kuo[23] found that colestipol 30 g/d alone lowered LDL by 33% and probucol 1 g/d alone lowered LDL by 22%. HDL-cholesterol was also lowered by 30%. However, angiography performed before and after treatment in 19 of 44 patients showed no further progression of pre-existing coronary lesions and no newly developed lesions after 4 years of therapy.[23] Together they lowered LDL by 53%. It was then found that low single dose colestipol 20 g/d effected a significant drop in LDL when added to probucol 1 g/d.[23] Furthermore, the HDL-lowering effect of probucol was counteracted by the HDL-raising effect of the resin, thus suggesting a combination that will increase compliance with the resins and decrease the potential negative effect of probucol's lowering HDL, while utilizing the strength of both drugs. However, while the combination of a bile-acid resin and probucol might alleviate the GI side effects commonly seen with either drug alone, the roughly 32% drop in HDL seen with colestipol and probucol compared to a lower HDL reduction with cholestyramine and probucol suggests that the latter combination is more favorable than the former.[25] As a result of these latter findings, it is advised to choose cholestyramine rather than colestipol for use in combination with probucol.

Lovastatin Plus Probucol

Lees et al[26] treated patients with familial hypercholesterolemia with probucol and lovastatin and found that the combination was not more effective than using lovastatin alone.

Colestipol Plus Lovastatin Plus Probucol

To date, the most comprehensive study of probucol's effect in combination with other therapies was carried out by Witztum et al.[27] This group studied patients with familial hypercholesterolemia and treated them with various combinations of probucol, lovastatin, and colestipol. Lovastatin 40 mg/d and colestipol 10 g/d lowered LDL by 56%, which was in excess of that achieved using either drug alone. Probucol 500 mg twice daily and lovastatin did not lower LDL more than lovastatin alone. Lovastatin increased HDL by 6% and probucol lowered HDL by 29%. The addition of probucol to colestipol and lovastatin had no additive effect over the combination of lovastatin and colestipol. However, tendon xanthomas were reduced significantly in the presence of probucol.

Diabetes Mellitus

Early reports from studies using probucol in the treatment of diabetes prone BB rats suggests that the antioxidant properties of the drug protect the rats from an autoimmune free radical-mediated destruction of its beta cells.[28] Studies in already diabetic rats have revealed evidence supporting the hypothesis that hyperglycemia is associated with formation of free radicals that then oxidize LDL and accelerate the atherosclerotic process in otherwise normolipidemic diabetic rats.[29] This oxidative modification is then inhibited by probucol, although no effect on hyperglycemia was seen with this intervention.

Nephrotic Syndrome

Iada et al treated 12 hyperlipidemic (279-737 mg/dl) patients with nephrotic syndrome with 500 mg/d of probucol for 12 weeks.[30] They found that probucol lowered all lipoproteins significantly without altering urinary excretion of protein.

Clinical Use

Probucol is now accepted as an excellent treatment for homozygous familial hypercholesterolemia because of its serum cholesterol-lowering effects and its ability to cause the regression of xanthomas in this population. Probucol is also a reasonable treatment for heterozygous familial hypercholesterolemia or primary moderate hypercholesterolemia, particularly because of its infrequent and generally mild side effects. Probucol's best use is probably in combination with other drugs, particularly a bile-acid resin, for the treatment of type II hyperlipidemia, whether it be of familial or polygenic origin.

There is no question that probucol consistently depresses HDL levels, in many cases to a greater degree than it lowers LDL levels. Therefore, the drug is not a good choice in a patient with low baseline levels of HDL, regardless of the LDL level.

The effectiveness and safety of probucol in children is not known, and therefore it is recommended only for adults. Tablets come in 250 mg and 500 mg dosages, with the maximum daily dose being 1000 mg. The maximum dose should be 500 mg administered with the morning meal and 500 mg with the evening meal.[4]

Adverse Effects

Side effects are few, mild, and most often GI in origin. Common side effects include diarrhea, loose stools, and flatulence. These side effects generally resolve after a few months of treatment. A major concern with probucol was raised when it was found to induce ventricular fibrillation in dogs sensitized with epinephrine. Monkeys taking probucol were then found to have a prolonged ECG QT interval which often evolved into torsades de pointes.[9] Miettinen et al conducted a 5-year prevention trial with probucol and found that there were small but significant prolongations in the QT interval with the drug.[22] However, there was no observed increase in the incidence of cardiac arrhythmias during the 5 years of the trial or during the 5 years of follow-up after completion of probucol treatment. Naukkarinen et al,[31] in a review of the above mentioned study, noted that hospital admissions secondary to arrhythmias were more frequent in the placebo group than in the probucol-treated group.

The incidence of combined biliary tract disease, defined as cholecystectomy, cholelithiasis, and cholecystitis, after 6 years of treatment with probucol was found to be 3.3%. This rate was compared to the rates observed by the Coronary Drug Project that found a 4.59% incidence for clofibrate, 3.56% for niacin, and 3.02% for placebo after 6 years of follow-up. Thus, although it is reasonable to be concerned that cholesterol-lowering drugs might have an adverse effect on the biliary system, it appears that probucol does not cause an increased risk over that of placebo.[10]

References

1. Davies PF, Reidy MA, Goode TB, et al: Scanning electron microscopy in the evaluation of endothelial integrity of the fatty lesion in atherosclerosis. Atherosclerosis 1976: 25: 125-130.
2. Steinberg D, Parthasarathy S, Carew TE, et al: Beyond cholesterol: modifications of low-density lipoprotein that increase its atherogenicity. N Engl J Med 1989; 320: 915-924.
3. Steinberg D, Witztum JL: Lipoproteins and atherogenesis. JAMA 1990; 264: 3047-3051.
4. Product Insert, Merrell Dow June 1988.
5. Marshall FN: Pharmacology and toxicology of probucol. Artery 1982; 10: 7-21.
6. Polachek AA, Katz HM, Sack J, et al: Probucol in the long-term treatment of hypercholesterolemia. Curr Med Res Opin 1970; 1: 323-330.
7. Taylor HL, Nolan RB, Tedeschi RE, et al: Combined results of the study of probucol at 1 gm/day in eight centers. Clin Pharmacol Ther 1978; 23: 131-137.
8. Beynen AC: Mode of hypocholesterolemic action of probucol in animals and man. Artery 1987; 14: 113-126.
9. Strandberg TE, VanHanen H, Miettinen TA: Probucol in long-term treatment of hypercholesterolemia. Gen Pharmacol 1988; 19: 317-320.
10. Tedeschi RE, Martz BL, Taylor HA, et al: Safety and effectiveness of probucol as a cholesterol lowering agent. Artery 1982; 10: 22-34.
11. Miettinen TA, Huttunen JK, Strandberg T, et al: Lowered HDL cholesterol and incidence of ischaemic heart disease. The Lancet August 29, 1981, p 478.
12. Yamamoto A, Hara H, Takaichi S, et al: Effect of probucol on macrophages, leading to regression of xanthomas and atheromatous vascular lesions. Am J Cardiol 1988; 62: 31B-36B.

13. Gwynne JT: Probucol, high-density lipoprotein metabolism and reverse cholesterol transport. Am J Cardiol 1988; 62: 48B-51B.

14. Barnhart JW, Li DL, Cheng WD: Probucol enhances cholesterol transport in cultured rat hepatocytes. Am J Cardiol 1988; 62: 52B-56B.

15. Aburatani H, Matsumoto A, Kodama T, et al: Increased levels of messenger ribonucleic acid for apolipoprotein E in the spleen of probucol-treated rabbits. Am J Cardiol 1988; 62: 66B-72B.

16. Goldberg RB, Mendez A: Probucol enhances cholesterol efflux from cultured human skin fibroblasts. Am J Cardiol 1988; 62: 57B-59B.

17. Walldius G, Carlson LA, Erikson U, et al: Development of femoral atherosclerosis in hypercholesterolemic patients during treatment with cholestyramine and probucol/placebo: Probucol Quantitative Regression Swedish Trial (PQRST) Status Report. Am J Cardiol 1988; 62: 37B-43B.

18. Steinberg D, Parthasarathy S, Carew TE: In vivo inhibition of foam cell development by probucol in Watanabe rabbits. Am J Cardiol 1988; 62: 6B-12B.

19. Mellies MJ, Gartside PS, Glatfetter L, et al: Effects of probucol on plasma cholesterol, high and low density lipoprotein cholesterol, and apoliprotein A1 and A2 in adults with primary familial hypercholesterolemia. Metabolism 1980; 29: 956-964.

20. Yamamoto A, Matsuzawa Y, Kishino B-I, et al: Effects of probucol on homozygous cases of familial hypercholesterolemia. Atherosclerosis 1983; 48: 157-166.

21. McCaughan D: Nine years of treatment with probucol. Artery 1982; 10: 56-70.

22. Miettinen TA, Huttunen JK, Naukkarinin V, et al: Multifactorial primary prevention of cardiovascular diseases in middle-aged men. JAMA 1985; 254: 2097-2103.

23. Kuo PT, Wilson AC, Kostis JV, et al: Effects of combined probucol colestipol treatment for familial hypercholesterolemia and coronary artery disease. Am J Cardiol 1986; 57: 43H-48H.

24. Sommariva D, Bonfiglioli D, Tirrito M: Probucol and cholestyramine combination in the treatment of severe hypercholesterolemia. Intl J Clin Pharmacol Ther Toxicol 1986; 24: 505-510.

25. Dujovne CA, Krehbrel P, Chernoff SB: Controlled studies of the efficacy and safety of combined probucol-colestipol therapy. Am J Cardiol 1986; 57: 36H-42H.

26. Lees AM, Stein SW, Lees RW: Therapy of hypercholesterolemia with mevinolin and other lipid lowering drugs. (abstr) Atherosclerosis 1986; 6: 544A.

27. Witztum JL, Simmons D, Steinberg D, et al: Intensive combination drug therapy of familial hypercholesterolemia with lovastatin, probucol and colestipol hydrochloride. Circulation 1989; 79: 16-28.

28. Drash AL, Rudert WA, Borquaye S, et al: Effect of probucol on development of diabetes mellitus in BB rats. Am J Cardiol 1988; 62: 27B-30B.

29. Chisolm GM III, Morel DW: Lipoprotein oxidation and cytotoxicity: effect of probucol on streptozotocin-treated rats. Am J Cardiol 1988; 62: 20B-26B.
30. Iida H, Izumino K, Asaka M, et al: Effect of probucol on hyperlipidemia in patients with nephrotic syndrome. Nephron 1987; 47: 280-283.
31. Naukkarinen Y, Strandberg T, Vanhanen H, et al: Probucol-induced electrocardiographic changes in a five-year primary prevention of vascular diseases. Curr Ther Res 1989; 46: 232-237.

Chapter 9

Dietary Fiber for Reducing Blood Cholesterol: Psyllium

William H. Frishman M.D., Harold Lipsky M.D.,
Mark Gloger M.D.

In recent years, there has been a growing interest in the use of dietary fiber in health maintenance and disease prevention (see Chapter 2). Some researchers have speculated that a deficiency of fiber in the Western diet might be contributing to the epidemics of diabetes mellitus, coronary artery disease, and colonic cancer.[1]

Americans have become more health conscious and aware of their diets. This awareness has probably contributed to the reported 30% decline in the death rate from coronary artery disease observed over the past 15 years.[2] In particular, fiber has been considered a possible dietary supplement for the control of systemic hypertension,[3] diabetes mellitus,[4] obesity,[5] and hyperlipidemia[6] — all known risk factors for the development of coronary artery disease.

Dietary fiber is a collective term for a variety of plant substances that are resistant to digestion by human gastrointestinal enzymes.[7,8] Fiber may be obtained either from dietary sources or from extradietary supplements. The chemical components of naturally occurring dietary fiber include cellulose, lignins, hemicelluloses, pectins, gums, and mucilages (Table 1).

Dietary fibers can be classified into two major groups based on their water-solubility.[7,8] The structural or matrix fibers (lignins, cellulose, and some hemicelluloses) are insoluble. The natural gel-forming fibers

From *Medical Management of Lipid Disorders: Focus on Prevention of Coronary Artery Disease,* edited by William H. Frishman, M.D. © 1992, Futura Publishing Inc., Mount Kisco, NY.

Table 1.
Components of Dietary Fiber

Fiber Component and Type	Biological Function	Food Source
Cellulose (insoluble)	Basic structural material of cell walls	Wheat bran, peels of apples and pears
Lignins (insoluble)	Together with cellulose form the woody cell walls of plants	Cereal grains, potatoes
Hemicelluloses (insoluble and soluble)	Surround the skeletal material of cell walls and act as the cement between them	Wheat bran, whole grains
Pectins (soluble)	Bind adjacent cell walls and hold water in interconnecting networks	Bananas, oranges, apples
Gums (soluble)	Exudates from stems or seeds that are gelatinous when moist	Oatmeal, legumes
Mucilages (soluble)	Viscous substances with water-holding properties; similar to plant gums	Seeds, seaweeds psyllium

(pectins, gums, mucilages, and the remainder of the hemicelluloses) are soluble in humans.

Both soluble and insoluble fibers cause an increased bulk of softer stool due to their increased water-retaining capabilities. In addition, soluble fibers retard gastric emptying and decrease food absorption and digestion. In various experimental studies, soluble fibers such as pectin, guar gum, oat bran, and psyllium have also been shown to reduce blood cholesterol levels.[9]

The focus of this chapter will be to examine psyllium hydrophilic mucilloid (Metamucil®), a well-known bulk laxative, as a potential cholesterol-lowering agent. Its effectiveness relates to its ability to deliver five times more soluble fiber than oat bran, and its ease of administration as a dietary supplement to patients with hypercholesterolemia.

Psyllium

Psyllium is a soluble gel-forming fiber derived from the husks of blond psyllium seeds of the genus *Plantago* plants that are grown in the

Mediterranean region and in India. The processing of psyllium involves the initial separation of the seeds from the plant husks and then grinding the husks to make the final psyllium substance. The seed husk is then enriched with mucilloid, a hydrophilic substance that forms a gelatinous mass when mixed with water. The nonutilized seed extracts are marketed as health foods or as animal feed.[9]

The chemical composition of psyllium is based on its being broken into an 85% mucilage polysaccharide and a 15% nonpolysaccharide component. The polysaccharide fraction is the active component, and is made of 63% D-xylose, 20% l-arabinose, 6% rhamrose, and 9% D-galacturonic acid as derived by acid hydrolysis and methylation analysis. Structural features of this component are those of a highly branched acidic arabinoxylan; xylan backbone with sugar 1:4 and 1:3 linkages.[10] The nonpolysaccharide component has nitrogen and other nonactive components.[10]

Clinical Trials

Several investigators have studied the activity of psyllium as a cholesterol-reducing agent. It is the universal feeling of all these investigators that psyllium is a hypocholesterolemic agent.[11-20] However, there is still debate as to the degree of cholesterol reduction with psyllium and its actual mechanism of action.

In an early clinical trial, Garvin and associates[11] demonstrated that serum cholesterol was reduced significantly by psyllium hydrophilic colloid (Metamucil®). These investigators divided their subjects (healthy male medical students) into three groups: group I maintained their normal diet and took psyllium supplements (9.6 g/d); group II ate a 'high egg' diet; group III ate the 'high egg' diet plus psyllium supplementation. Group I subjects had a 9% reduction in total cholesterol after 8 weeks of treatment. Of interest, upon stopping psyllium supplementation at week 9, a rebound increase in cholesterol (above original value) was seen. Group II subjects had an 11% increase in serum cholesterol after 8 weeks. Group III subjects had a 7% decrease in cholesterol over the 8 weeks. However, this is 18% lower than group II, the group that should be used as their comparison group. Of concern is that when psyllium supplementation was stopped in group III serum cholesterol levels rose above normal values (eggs were continued).

Psyllium Supplementation Without Modified Diet

Danielson and associates[12] studied the effects of psyllium in 26 patients with essential hyperlipidemia who continued on their previous diets. Subjects were treated for 2-29 months with psyllium, and in a retrospective analysis, assigned to four patient subgroups: group I (eight patients with increased cholesterol) showed a 16.9% reduction in serum cholesterol; group II (10 patients with increased serum triglycerides) showed a 52% reduction in serum triglycerides; group III (three patients with increased cholesterol and normal triglycerides) showed normalization of serum cholesterol levels without change in triglyceride levels; group IV (five patients with increased triglycerides and normal cholesterol) showed a marked reduction in triglycerides and no significant change in cholesterol. This study is the only trial showing psyllium to have a profound effect on triglyceride levels, and it demonstrated that psyllium affected only those lipid values that were elevated.

In 1982, Burton and Manninen[13] performed a study to measure the effectiveness of psyllium as an alternative to stimulant laxatives in the treatment of chronic constipation. They found a 20% reduction in serum cholesterol levels and no significant change in serum triglycerides. There were no changes in other metabolic parameters including serum iron, serum iron-binding capacity, and calcium. The investigators suggested that psyllium was superior to using bran alone in reducing cholesterol.

Abraham and Mehta demonstrated a relationship between the height of the pretreatment blood cholesterol level and the effectiveness of psyllium in lowering cholesterol.[15] They studied three subjects on a standard Western diet for 3 weeks followed by a psyllium-supplemented diet for the next 3 weeks. The average decrease in total cholesterol was 16%. LDL-cholesterol decreased by an average of 0.39 mm/L (15 mg/dl) and HDL-cholesterol decreased by 0.36 mm/L (14 mg/dl) (although in five of seven patients, the HDL/LDL ratio actually increased). This study was unique in that the investigators measured fecal mass and steroids. There was a doubling of fecal mass in the participants, while there was no significant change in fecal steroid, and hence, cholesterol excretion as measured in the stool. Therefore it was felt that the cholesterol-lowering effect of psyllium was independent of changes in cholesterol excretion or absorption.

One of the most convincing studies for the efficacy of psyllium as a lipid-lowering agent was performed by Anderson and associates.[16] In this double-blind, placebo-controlled study, 26 hypercholesterolemic men were treated with psyllium or placebo for 8 weeks. Subjects with types I, IV, and V hyperlipoproteinemia were excluded. The psyllium-treated group showed a 14.8% reduction in total cholesterol, a 20.2% reduction in LDL-cholesterol, and a 14.8% reduction in LDL/HDL cholesterol ratio. There were no significant changes observed in the placebo group.

Psyllium Supplementation With Modified Diet

Bell and associates[17] studied the effects of combining a Step-I diet (30% fat, 55% carbohydrate, 15% protein) with psyllium supplementation; 35 hypercholesterolemic subjects were randomized to receive placebo plus diet and 40 subjects to receive psyllium plus diet. All subjects received a Step-I diet for 12 weeks and were then treated for 8 weeks with psyllium or placebo. At 8 weeks the psyllium-treated group, when compared to placebo, showed a 4.8% decrease in total cholesterol, an 8.2% decrease in LDL-cholesterol, a 2.4% increase in HDL-cholesterol, an 8.8% reduction in apoprotein B levels, and a 10.0% decrease in the LDL/HDL ratio. They also showed a 2.7% increase in triglycerides. When the study was continued for an additional 8 weeks in 30 subjects, a diminished effect of psyllium was noted. The results of this study demonstrated a lesser effect of psyllium on cholesterol than that observed in the Anderson study.[16]

Recently, Levin and his associates[20] evaluated whether there was additional benefit of administering psyllium (5.1 g twice daily) to patients on an American Heart Association (AHA) Step-I diet to lower cholesterol levels. The effects of psyllium and a cellulose placebo on serum lipid levels were compared in 58 men and women with mild to moderate hypercholesterolemia after they had stabilized on the Step-I diet for 8 weeks. Patients were randomly assigned to receive psyllium for an additional 16 weeks of study while the diet was maintained. Little change in total cholesterol, LDL-cholesterol, or HDL-cholesterol occurred with diet alone. Psyllium was shown to lower the total and LDL cholesterol by approximately 6% and 10%, respectively, while placebo had no effect. Plasma triglyceride levels did not change substantially in either group. Curiously, the HDL-cholesterol increased by approximately 8% in the placebo group; consequently, the change in LDL/HDL ratio was similar in both groups. The effects of psyllium on LDL-cholesterol were sustained at 16 weeks. The authors concluded that psyllium as a twice daily regimen, might be a useful and safe adjunct to a prudent diet in the treatment of moderate hypercholesterolemia.

Mechanism of Action

The mechanism by which psyllium and other soluble fiber lowers serum cholesterol currently is unknown. Available information suggests that one or more of the following mechanisms may be operative. First, psyllium has been shown to bind to bile-acids in the gut and prevent their normal reabsorption.[21-23] This mechanism of action is also seen with cholestyramine and other bile-acid sequestrant drugs. Second, soluble fibers such as psyllium may interfere with micelle formation in the proximal small intestine, resulting in decreased absorption of cholesterol and fatty acids.[24,25] Finally, short-chain fatty acids are produced by bacterial fermentation of soluble fiber in the colon. These fatty acids (predominantly propionate and acetate) are rapidly absorbed into the blood stream and may inhibit hepatic cholesterol synthesis.[26] Short-chain fatty acids may also decrease hepatic cholesterol concentrations and secretions by interfering with compensatory mechanisms.[26]

Adverse Reactions and Drug Interactions

Psyllium and other soluble fibers are well tolerated by patients. In many of the clinical trials, treatment compliance was high. Bell reported 91% compliance to active treatment using 3.4 g of psyllium mixed in 240 cc of water, administered at each meal.[17] Another possible reason for the acceptability of psyllium therapy is that patients will have well-formed stools and a low incidence of side effects.

Some patients placed on psyllium report abdominal distention, excessive gas, and flatulence, but these symptoms usually subside after a few weeks. Rarely, allergic reactions to psyllium have been described.[27-29]

While there are reports indicating possible effects of psyllium and soluble fibers on reducing calcium, magnesium, zinc, copper, and iron absorption, other studies have contradicted these findings.[30,31] Animal studies have revealed the absence of teratogenic effects of psyllium.

Some studies have revealed an effect of psyllium on the binding of sodium warfarin. Any potential problem can be avoided by separating the intake of psyllium and drug ingestion by 1 to 2 hours. Finally, patients with congestive heart failure may be at risk from an excessive salt load with psyllium ingestion.

Clinical Recommendations

The current recommendation for fiber in the diet is 25-35 g/d. Fiber supplementation is widely accepted as part of achieving a healthful diet. This is in conjunction with a low-fat, low-cholesterol diet, which is considered to be 'prudent' by the American Heart Association. The Phase-I diet in the treatment of hypercholesterolemia consists of no more than 300 mg of dietary cholesterol per day, with a maximum 30% total energy as fat. This diet has been shown to decrease cholesterol by varying amounts. With the addition of fiber, the cholesterol-lowering effect of this diet can rise significantly.

The efficacy of psyllium in lowering cholesterol is consistent with many other soluble fibers.[32] Studies with 15 g of pectin added to a diet lowered cholesterol by 11%.[21] The addition of 100 g of oat bran to a diet has been shown to lower cholesterol by 19% and LDL-cholesterol by 23%.[22] However, the effectiveness of oat bran as a hypercholesterolemic intervention recently has come under question.[33,34]

The efficiency of psyllium is revealed in its ability to achieve reductions in cholesterol in studies that have used only 10.2 g of the substance daily. It is concluded that psyllium is useful as an adjunct to dietary therapy in the treatment of patients with mild-to-moderate hypercholesterolemia. Clearly, cholestyramine[35] and the new HMG-CoA reductase inhibitors[36] have greater efficacy than psyllium in reducing cholesterol. Studies combining psyllium with the other drug treatments for lowering cholesterol still need to be done.

References

1. Walker ARP: Dietary fiber and the pattern of diseases. (editorial) Ann Intern Med 1974; 80: 663-664.
2. Stamler J: Coronary heart disease: doing the 'right things.' N Engl J Med 1985; 312: 1053-1055.

3. Wright A, Burstyn PG, Gibney MJ: Dietary fiber and blood pressure. Br Med J 1979; 2: 1541-1543.
4. Anderson JW, Ward K: High-carbohydrate, high-fiber diets for insulin-treated men with diabetes mellitus. Am J Clin Nutr 1979; 32: 2312-2321.
5. Anderson JW: Dietary fiber and diabetes. In, Vahouny GV, Kritchevsky D (eds): Dietary Fiber in Health and Disease. New York, Plenum Press, 1982; 151-165.
6. Miettinen TA: Dietary fiber and lipids. Am J Clin Nutr 1987; 45 (Suppl): 1237-1242.
7. Floch M: Dietary fiber: rational recommendations. Hosp Med 1985; 21: 142-158.
8. Eastwood MA, Passmore R: Dietary fibre. Lancet 1983; 2: 202-206.
9. Chan JKC, Wypyszyk V: A forgotten natural dietary fiber: psyllium mucilloid. Cereal Foods World 1988; 33: 919-922.
10. Kennedy JF, Sandhu JS, Southgate DAT: Structural data for the carbohydrate of ispaghula husk (ex Plantago ovata Forsk). Carbohydrate Res 1979; 75: 269-274.
11. Garvin JE, Forman DT, Eiserman WR, et al: Lowering of serum cholesterol by an oral hydrophilic agent. Proc Exp Biol Med 1965; 120: 744-746.
12. Danielson A, Ek B, Nyhlin H, et al: Effect of long-term treatment with hydrophilic colloid on serum lipids. Acta Hepato Gastroenterol 1979; 26: 148-153.
13. Burton R, Manninen V: Influence of a psyllium based fiber preparation on faecal and serum parameters. Acta Med Scand 1982; 668 (Suppl): 91-94.
14. Fagerberg SE: The effect of bulk laxative (Metamucil) on fasting blood glucose, serum lipids and other variables in constipated patients with non-insulin dependent adult diabetes. Curr Ther Res 1982; 31: 166-172.
15. Abraham Z, Mehta T: Three week psyllium husk supplementation effect on plasma cholesterol concentrations, fecal steroid excretion and carbohydrate absorption in men. Am J Clin Nutr 1988; 47: 67-74.
16. Anderson JW, Zettwoch N, Feldman T, et al: Cholesterol lowering effect of psyllium hydrophilic mucilloid for hypercholesterolemic men. Arch Intern Med 1988; 148: 292-296.
17. Bell L, Hectorne K, Reynolds H, et al: Cholesterol lowering effects of psyllium hydrophilic mucilloid. JAMA 1989; 261: 3419-3423.
18. Lieberthal MM, Martens RA: Lowered serum cholesterol following the ingestion of a hydrophilic colloid. Dig Dis 1975; 20: 469-474.
19. Monari ACF, Harp JAF, Becenil M, et al: Decrease in serum lipids, glycemia, and body weight by Plantago psyllium in obese and diabetic patients. Arch Invest Med 1983; 14: 259-268.
20. Levin EG, Miller VT, Muesing RA, et al: Comparison of psyllium hydrophilic mucilloid and cellulose as adjuncts to a prudent diet in the treatment of mild to moderate hypercholesterolemia. Arch Intern Med 1990; 150: 1822-1827.
21. Kay RM, Truswell AS: Dietary fiber: effect on plasma and biliary lipids in man. In Spiller GA, Kay RM (eds): Medical Aspects of Dietary Fiber. New York, Plenum Press, 1980; 153-173.

22. Anderson JW, Story L, Seiling B, et al: Hypercholesterolemic effects of oat bran or bean intake for hypercholesterolemic men. Am J Clin Nutri 1984; 40: 1146-1155.
23. Stanley M, Paul D, Gacke D, et al: Effects of cholestyramine, Metamucil and cellulose on fecal bile salt excretion in man. Gastroenterology 1973; 65: 889-894.
24. Vahouny GV: Dietary fiber and lipid metabolism and atherosclerosis. Fed Proc 1982; 41: 2801-2806.
25. Vahouny GV, Subramaniam S, Chen I, et al: Dietary fiber and intestinal adoption: effects on lipid absorption and lymphatic transport in the rat. Am J Clin Nutr 1988; 47: 201-206.
26. Chen WL, Anderson JW, Jennings D: Propionate may mediate the hypocholesterolemic effects of certain soluble plant fiber in cholesterol fed rats. Proc Soc Exp Biol Med 1984; 175: 215-218.
27. Zaloga GP, Hierlummer VR, Engler RJ: Anaphylaxis following psyllium ingestion. J Allergy Clin Immuno 1984; 74: 79-80.
28. Maesner JE, Stephenson SH, Johnson MA: Psyllium hydrophlic mucilloid allergic reactions. Drug Intell Clin Pharm 1986; 20: 548.$er 29. Lantner RR, Espiritu BR, Zumerchik P, et al: Anaphylaxis following ingestion of a psyllium-containing cereal. JAMA 1990; 264: 2534-2536.
30. Behall KM, Scholfield DJ, Lee K, et al: Mineral balance in adult men: effect of 4 refined fibers. Am J Clin Nutr 1987; 46: 307-314.
31. Rattan J, Levin N, Graff E, et al: A high-fiber diet does not cause mineral and nutrient deficiencies. J Clin Gastroenterol 1981; 4: 389-393.
32. Anderson JW, Tietyen-Clark J: Dietary fiber, hyperlipidemia, hypertension and coronary heart disease. Am J Gastroenterol 1986; 81: 907-919.
33. Swain JF, Rouse IL, Curley CB, et al: Comparison of the effects of oat bran and low fiber wheat on serum lipoprotein levels and blood pressure. N Engl J Med 1989; 322: 147-152.
34. Connor WE: Dietary fiber - nostrum or clinical nutrient? N Engl J Med 1989; 322: 193-195.
35. Ast M, Frishman WH: Bile-acid sequestrants. J Clin Pharmacol 1990; 30: 99-106.
36. Frishman WH, Zimetbaum P, Nadelmann J: Lovastatin and other HMG-CO_A reductase inhibitors. J Clin Pharmacol 19; 29: 975-982.

Chapter 10

Other Medical Approaches for Managing Hyperlipidemia: Past, Present, and Future

William H. Frishman M.D., Melanie P. Derman M.D., Judith Mitchell M.D., Jason Lazar M.D.

In this chapter, treatment approaches for lipid disorders that were used in the past years as primary therapies will be discussed. These modalities include the use of oral neomycin and thyroxine therapy as hypocholesterolemic agents. Approaches to hyperlipidemia that are being assessed for future use will also be reviewed. These include estrogen therapy in postmenopausal women, LDL-apheresis, the use of plant sterols, and the administration in vivo of high-density lipoprotein (HDL) - very-high-density lipoprotein (VHDL).

Antibiotics

Neomycin

A hypocholesterolemic effect of neomycin was discovered with serendipity in 1958 by Samuel and Steiner.[1] During a clinical study of the effects of dietary fats on serum lipids, one patient experienced a significant drop in serum cholesterol with concomitant oral neomycin therapy for a gastrointestinal infection. This finding prompted studies

From *Medical Management of Lipid Disorders: Focus on Prevention of Coronary Artery Disease,* edited by William H. Frishman, M.D. © 1992, Futura Publishing Inc., Mount Kisco, NY.

of additional patients that confirmed neomycin's efficacy in reducing serum cholesterol.[2,3]

Chemistry (Fig. 1): Neomycin was first isolated in 1949 from Streptomyces fradiae. It is a nonabsorbable aminoglycoside antibiotic. Like other aminoglycosides of its class, neomycin has three amino sugars attached to a hexose nucleus.

Pharmacology: As an antibiotic, neomycin is bactericidal. It is known to act on the 30S unit of the bacterial ribosome, inhibiting protein synthesis and undermining the fidelity of the mRNA translation. This action, however, does not explain the lethal effect of the drug versus a broad spectrum of microorganisms including gram negatives (*Escherichia coli, Enterobacter aerogenes, Klebsiella pneumonaie*) and gram positives (*Staphylococcus aureus, S. faecalis, Mycobacterium tuberculosis*).[4]

As a hypolipidemic agent, neomycin was initially believed to act similarly to the bile-acid resins by forming insoluble complexes with the bile-acids in the intestines, thus enhancing bile-acid excretion. In vitro studies have shown that neomycin precipitates bile-acids, and clinical studies have suggested that it interferes with the integrity of the intraluminal micelles formed in the intestines.[5] Metabolic studies by other investigators, however, have demonstrated that neomycin increases fecal excretion of neutral steroids (cholesterol and metabolites) but does not change fecal bile-acid excretion.[6,7] Although the hypolipidemic effect of neomycin has also been hypothesized to be related to an alteration of the bacterial flora in the gastrointestinal tract,[8,9] this has

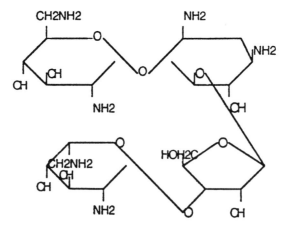

Figure 1: *Chemical structure of neomycin.*

never been confirmed. Furthermore, Samuel and Waithe examined the effects of 22 additional antibiotics and found none that decreased serum cholesterol as effectively as neomycin,[10] suggesting that a mechanism other than neomycin's bactericidal action was operative. Studies have shown that lowering of serum cholesterol in humans with neomycin is not dependent on induced steatorrhea and malabsorption. The cholesterol-lowering effects also appear to be independent of dietary fat and cholesterol.[11]

Pharmacokinetics: The hypolipidemic effect of neomycin is dependent on its presence in the intestine and it must, therefore, be administered orally. The usual dose is 2 g daily (four 500 mg tablets) which is decreased gradually to 500 mg when possible. Only 3%-6% of the antibiotic is absorbed after oral administration,[12] and this fraction is excreted in the urine. Neomycin is not altered during its transit in the alimentary canal and is eliminated quantitatively in the feces. Toxic concentrations may result from repeated administration in the setting of impaired renal function.[4]

Clinical Experience: Low-density lipoprotein (LDL) turnover studies by Kasaniemi and Grundy revealed a decline in the synthetic rate of apoprotein B with neomycin that correlated positively with the decline in the plasma level of LDL-cholesterol. Although this finding suggests that the reduction in LDL is due primarily to a decline in production following the inhibition of cholesterol absorption, the authors hypothesize that the decline may also be due to increased clearance in some patients.[13]

Hoeg et al studied the effects of neomycin in a 9-month, double-blind, randomized, crossover, placebo-controlled trial of 20 patients with type II hyperlipidemia. A 15% decline in total cholesterol was observed. Similar decline was seen for LDL, while VLDL, HDL, and triglyceride levels were not significantly altered.[14] In a crossover study of neomycin and cholestyramine in 35 patients with type II hyperlipidemia, investigators found no significant difference in the hypolipidemic effect of the two agents, but the majority of patients preferred neomycin.[15] A study by Miettinen[6] of neomycin in combination with cholestyramine demonstrated an additive hypolipidemic effect: a decline in total cholesterol of 38% and notable patient acceptance since gastrointestinal side effects are opposing and, therefore, complementary.[16] Neomycin has also been used in combination with clofibrate. An open study of 16 patients found the combined regimen to be superior to either therapy alone in one third of patients.[17] However, this finding was not confirmed in a study by Teoh where neomycin did not augment the hypocholesterolemic action of clofibrate.[18] In light of its possible toxicity and inferior efficacy compared to other available hypolipidemic agents, neomycin is considered a second-line choice in the treatment of familial hypercholesterolemia.[19]

Adverse Effects: Of the 14 patients in Hoeg's 3-month trial[14] who previously had tried cholestyramine, all preferred the neomycin regimen of two 500 mg tablets twice a day. Patients were monitored with extensive audiologic measurements and monthly blood tests; no significant renal, hepatic, or ototoxic complications were observed during the length of the study. Furthermore, none of the subjects had bacterial superinfection, and neomycin-resistant flora from stool cultures were sensitive to a variety of antibiotics.[14]

In Samuel's 20-year experience with neomycin, he found that small doses of oral neomycin produce a few side effects.[16] Approximately one third of the patients experience transient diarrhea or abdominal cramps that subside within 2 weeks. He reports that even when large daily doses were used in hepatic coma prior to bowel surgery, relatively few side effects were reported: "diarrhea, renal damage, staphylococcal enterocolitis, moniliasis, multiresistant coliform overgrowth and inhibition of digoxin absorption." Furthermore, severe hepatic or renal insufficiency or inflammatory bowel disease complicated those cases reported in the literature in which large oral doses led to deafness.

Ototoxicity by neomycin is the result of the progressive, irreversible destruction of the cochlear sensory cells in the organ of Corti. Renal toxicity appears to be secondary to renal tubular damage. This toxicity will, in turn, raise the serum concentration further and lead to ototoxicity. The parenteral route, therefore, is hazardous and, at present, there are no indications for its use via this route.

Hormonal Therapy

Thyroxine

The hormone thyroxine has been utilized as a hypercholesterolemic agent based on its effects in hypothyroid patients. Patients with clinical hypothyroidism commonly are found to have elevated concentrations of plasma cholesterol. When such patients are treated with thyroid hormone replacement, their plasma cholesterol decreases. It has been demonstrated that patients with hypothyroidism have an intrinsic and almost total defect of receptor-mediated LDL catabolism, which is reversible with hormone replacement.[20-22]

Both symptomatic and subclinical hypothyroidism may be risk factors for premature coronary artery disease.[23-27] Attempts have been made to determine whether subclinical hypothyroidism is also responsible for changes in lipoprotein fractions that could contribute to the development of premature coronary artery disease. The findings of a recent study demonstrated an increase in LDL-cholesterol and a decrease in HDL-cholesterol in patients with subclinical hypothyroidism compared to age-matched controls, while total cholesterol and triglyceride concentrations were unchanged.[28]

Clinical Experience: The hormone thyroxine has been used as a hypocholesterolemic agent in euthyroid patients. The stereoisomer dextrothyroxine (d-thyroxine) initially was chosen for clinical use because it was said to have more selective effects on metabolism when compared with levothyroxine. d-Thyroxine lowers the concentration of LDL-cholesterol by 10% to 20%, but has little effect on plasma triglycerides or on the concentration of HDL-cholesterol.[29] However, in usual therapeutic doses of 4 to 6 mg/d, d-thyroxine given to euthyroid patients can cause cardiac arrhythmias and hypermetabolic effects, such as nervousness, increased sweating, and fine tremor.[30] In the Coronary Drug Project, a higher incidence of adverse cardiovascular effects was observed in d-thyroxine-treated patients compared to placebo, requiring discontinuation of this drug treatment in the study.[31]

Arem and Patsch[32] assessed the effects of levothyroxine replacement on lipids, lipoproteins, and apolipoproteins in patients with subclinical hypothyroidism. The investigators demonstrated that after 4 months of therapy and a state of patient euthyroidism, there was a decrease in LDL-cholesterol and apoprotein B levels that was reflected in a decrease in both the ratios of cholesterol/HDL-cholesterol and LDL-cholesterol/HDL-cholesterol.

It can be concluded from the above that thyroxine replacement can alter favorably the lipid and lipoprotein levels of overt and borderline hypothyroid patients, making screening for these conditions mandatory when assessing patients with a lipid abnormality. However, the routine use of thyroxine treatment to lower LDL-cholesterol and raise HDL-cholesterol cannot be recommended in euthyroid patients because of the potential adverse effects of treatment which include cardiac toxicity.[29]

Estrogens and Progestogens

Women have an increased risk of atherosclerosis after menopause. In affluent societies, the death rate from coronary artery disease is 5-8 times greater in males than in females 25-55 years of age.[33] The difference in mortality rate narrows after menopause. These data suggest that premenopausal women have a vascular "protective factor" that is lost at menopause (natural or surgically rendered). Estrogen has been implicated as this factor or one of the factors. Estrogen may provide its protective effect through favorable actions on plasma lipids and lipoproteins.[34]

During female menopause, endogenous estrodiol levels drop and LDL-cholesterol concentration rises rapidly, with mean plasma levels eventually exceeding those of age-matched men.[35] No major change in HDL-cholesterol is seen postmenopause.[36] HDL concentrations remain lower in males than in females.[37] Thus, after menopause, levels of total cholesterol, LDL-cholesterol, and HDL-cholesterol remain higher in females than in age-matched males (Table 1).

Epidemiologic Studies: Looking at the relationships among female menopause, estrogen use, and coronary heart disease in the Framingham Study, Gordon et al reported a rise in coronary heart disease incidence after menopause.[38] They also observed that the use of exogenous estrogen after menopause was associated with a rate of coronary heart disease that was twice that observed in women not receiving estrogen therapy.[38] These observations were reconfirmed in a subsequent analysis of the Framingham population.[39]

In contrast, the majority of epidemiologic studies have shown a survival advantage in postmenopausal women with estrogen replacement therapy.[40-47]

Colditz et al[42] performed a prospective analysis of the Nurse's Health Study cohort to determine the relationship of menopause to the

Table 1.
Effects of Menopause on Plasma Lipids and Lipoproteins

Total cholesterol	↑
LDL-cholesterol	↑
HDL-cholesterol	↔
Triglycerides	↔

↑ = *increase;* ↔ = *no apparent change.*

risk of coronary heart disease. They found no increase in the rate of coronary heart disease in women receiving estrogen in the postmenopausal state compared to those not receiving treatment.

Criqui et al[43] prospectively studied the association between postmenopausal estrogen use and death from cardiovascular disease and coronary heart disease in a cohort of 1868 women, aged 59 to 79 years, residing in a retirement community. The age-adjusted death rates for cardiovascular disease and coronary heart disease were lower for those women who had never used estrogen replacement therapy. There was a greater impact of estrogen use in women who were current smokers.

Bush et al[44] followed a cohort of 2270 women, aged 40 to 69 years in a prospective manner for an average of 8.5 years. These women originally were enrolled in the Lipid Research Clinics Program. The age-adjusted relative rate of cardiovascular death in estrogen users was considerably lower compared to nonusers.

The association between low levels of HDL-cholesterol and an increased prevalence of coronary artery disease on angiography has been described,[45] with lower levels of HDL-cholesterol being associated with a greater severity of coronary artery lesions. Gruchow and colleagues[46] compared the degree of coronary artery occlusion between users and nonusers of estrogen among 933 female patients (between the ages of 50 and 75) with a diagnosis of chest pain who were referred for coronary angiography. The investigators found that estrogen users had less severe coronary occlusions than nonusers, which indicated a protective effect of postmenopausal estrogen therapy. The effect was independent of the type of menopause or other risk factors, but not independent of HDL-cholesterol levels. The investigators suggested that higher HDL levels among estrogen users may be providing a protective effect against coronary artery disease.[46]

Two recent reports have also described a benefit of estrogen replacement therapy in postmenopausal women with cardiovascular disease. Henderson and colleagues[47] conducted a prospective evaluation of 8881 postmenopausal women using a detailed health questionnaire that requested information about estrogen use: patients were followed for an average of 7.5 years. Age-adjusted, all-cause mortality in women with a history of estrogen use was 20% lower than in women who had never used estrogen. Mortality among current users was 40% lower than among those who had never used estrogen. The majority of this mortality benefit was attributable to fewer deaths from cardiovascular disease. Estrogen users also had a 20% reduction in mortality from cancer (including breast cancer); however, mortality from endometrial cancer was increased substantially among this group. The investigators proposed that favorable alterations in lipoprotein cholesterol levels contributed to the cardiovascular mortality benefit in this study.[47]

Sullivan and coworkers[48] retrospectively analyzed the relationship between postmenopausal estrogen use and survival in 2268 women undergoing coronary angiography. Patients were grouped on the basis of coronary anatomy: severe (>70% stenosis) in 1178 patients; mild (<70% stenosis) in 644; absent (0% stenosis) in 446 control patients. In the control group, 10-year survival was similar in estrogen users and nonusers. In contrast, estrogen use improved survival in women with coronary artery disease. Among patients with severe coronary artery disease, 10-year survival was 97% in estrogen users and 60% in nonusers. In the group with mild coronary artery disease, the 10-year survival was 95% and 85%, respectively. In addition, the incidence of hyperlipidemia in estrogen users was lower than that in nonusers. In a multivariate analysis, it was shown that estrogen use in postmenopausal females with coronary artery disease was an independent predictor of survival in women.[48]

Mechanism of Benefit

Effects on Lipids and Lipoproteins (Table 2): It has been observed by many investigators that various estrogen formulations used in treatment of postmenopausal females could reduce total cholesterol, VLDL-cholesterol, and LDL-cholesterol levels compared to the concentrations found in women not taking estrogens.[41,49, 50] There is some evidence that estrogens may induce the formation of hepatic LDL receptors.[34] In

Table 2.
Effects of Estrogens and Progestogens on Lipids and Lipoproteins

	Estrogen	Progestogen
Total cholesterol	↓	↑
LDL-cholesterol	↓	↑
HDL-cholesterol*	↑	↓
Triglycerides	↑	↓

↓ = *decrease;* ↑ = *increase.* *Major effect is on HDL2-cholesterol.*

a prospective analysis that compared LDL-cholesterol levels in women using estrogens to those not on therapy, the concentrations were 3.75 mm/L (145 mg/dl) versus 4.03 mm/L (156 mg/dl), respectively, a significant difference.[51]

Exogenous estrogens can also cause modest elevations in HDL-cholesterol. Bush et al[52] reported that female estrogen users had higher HDL concentrations than those women not taking the hormone (1.73 mm/L vs 1.47 mm/L [67 vs 57 mg/dl). Cauley et al[53] and Fahraeus et al[37] made a similar observation with estrogen use and also noted that the major effect of treatment was on the coronary protective HDL_2 subfraction.[37,53-55]

Estrogen replacement in postmenopausal women causes modest increases in plasma triglycerides, an effect that has been documented by several groups of investigators.[49,52-55] The clinical significance of this finding in postmenopausal females has not been determined.

Other Mechanisms (Table 3): There is mounting evidence that estrogens may have a beneficial effect on the cardiovascular system that is independent of its lipid and lipoprotein effects.[56-58] Estrogen receptors have been described in the blood vessel walls of various primates, suggesting a direct effect of estrogen in the inhibition of atheromatous plaque formation.[57] Estrogens may inhibit the formation of thromboxane, which is required for platelet adhesion to the vessel wall.[56] The inhibition of thromboxane formation also interferes with smooth muscle proliferation in the blood vessel, which could result in decreased uptake of cholesterol. Other direct effects of estrogens on the blood vessel wall include alterations in collagen and elastin, as well as changes in prostacyclin production.[56,58]

Table 3.
Possible Beneficial Effects of Estrogens in Reducing the Risk of Coronary Artery Disease in Postmenopausal Women

1. Favorable effect on LDL-cholesterol (possible increase of LDL receptors).
2. Elevation of HDL-cholesterol (HDL2); inhibition of hepatic lipase.
3. Direct effect (estrogen receptors) to prevent cholesterol deposition in vascular lesions.
4. Prevention of vasoconstrictive actions of acetylcholine on atherosclerotic vessels.
5. Interference with thromboxane effects on blood vessels.
6. Increased production of prostacyclin from blood vessels.

The effect of estrogen replacement therapy on the vasomotor responses of atherosclerotic coronary arteries was examined in ovariectomized monkeys by Williams et al.[57] The coronary arteries of monkeys treated with estrogen dilated when exposed to acetylcholine, a known endothelium-dependent dilator, whereas untreated atherosclerotic vessels constricted paradoxically. The investigators concluded that estrogen replacement could favorably modulate vasomotion of atherosclerotic coronary arteries.

Other investigators have demonstrated in animals fed an atheromatous diet that high-dose estrogens and progestins could protect against atherosclerotic disease progression in coronary arteries despite adverse changes in lipids induced by diet.[56,59]

Limited cross-sectional data suggest that estrogen use may improve carbohydrate metabolism, lowering both blood glucose and plasma insulin levels.[41] Several studies have also suggested that unopposed estrogen therapy might be associated with a lower blood pressure.[41]

Uses and Potential Risks of Estrogens

There are many therapeutic uses for exogenous estrogens in postmenopausal women. Estrogens usually are prescribed for treatment of the vasomotor, vaginal, and urinary symptoms seen in menopause.[60] They are also used for the prevention and treatment of osteoporosis.[61,62] Estrogen prevents demineralization of bone, and when progesterone is added, they can promote new bone formation.[62] Since the prevention of osteoporosis may take years, the earlier estrogen replacement is started, the greater the amount of bone mass that can be conserved.[60]

Unopposed estrogen replacement therapy is associated with an increased risk of endometrial cancer in postmenopausal women and in younger women with gonadal dysgenesis.[60,61] Although the severity grading of the cancer is usually low, estrogens can cause invasive disease.[63] To protect the endometrium, the addition of a progestogen is often required.[60] Although progestogens vary in potency, the protection is related more to the duration of progestogen exposure than to the dose.[34] With the combination of estrogen/progestogen replacement, no increase in endometrial cancer risk has been observed.[64]

Whereas the link between endometrial cancer and unopposed estrogen replacement therapy is well established, the relationship between breast cancer and estrogen replacement therapy is not clear. Some studies have shown an increased risk of breast cancer[65] with estrogen, while others show no risk or even protection.[64,66] The clarification is of utmost importance since the incidence and mortality of breast carcinoma are greater than for endometrial cancer.[61]

Dupont et al[65] recently reported on the results of a metaanalysis concerning studies of estrogen replacement therapy and breast cancer incidence. They found that women who took < 0.625 mg/d of conjugated estrogens had a risk of breast cancer that was 1.08 times that of women who did not receive this therapy. Women who took ≥ 1.25 mg/d of conjugated estrogens had a breast cancer relative risk of 2.0.[65]

The dosage and type of estrogen (i.e., with or without progestogen) may therefore affect breast cancer risk. There is also some suggestion that breast cancer risk may increase slightly with longer duration of treatment.[65,66]

Several studies have shown a protective role of progestogens against breast carcinoma when administered with estrogen in post-menopausal women.[64,67] Gambrell et al[68] found that women receiving estrogen and progestogen therapy had a lower risk of breast cancer when compared with women receiving estrogen treatment alone.

There appears to be an increased risk of cholelithiasis with estrogen replacement therapy.[60,63,64] The Boston Collaborative Drug Surveillance Program reported a 2.5 times increased risk of surgically confirmed gallbladder disease in women receiving estrogens compared to those who were not.[36]

Types of Estrogen and Estrogen/Progestogen Combination Therapy: It appears that the type of estrogen used in hormone replacement therapy can affect the responses on the cardiovascular system and on lipids and lipoproteins.[69,70] The synthetic estrogens (i.e., ethinyl estradiol and di-ethylstilbestrol) are much more potent than the natural estrogens (i.e., estradiol and estronel), and the conjugated equine estrogens (equilin and equilenin).[34]

The addition of progestogens that have markedly different androgenic potencies also have varying effects on the cardiovascular system[70] and the risks of breast[60,61] and endometrial cancers.[64] Progestogens can reduce triglycerides by increasing hepatic lipase activity, and can cause a reduction in HDL-cholesterol,[34,70,73-76] specifically HDL_2, with an attenuation or elimination of the actions of estrogens on lipids.[34,70] Newer progestogens (gestodene, desogestrel) may have a lesser metabolic effect.[77] It has been suggested that small doses of progestogens be used with estrogens to maintain the favorable effects on lipids while protecting against cancer risk.[78]

Estrogen Treatment in Males: The epidemiologic studies that have shown an increased risk of coronary artery disease in postmenopausal women compared with age-matched premenopausal women suggested a possible use for estrogen therapy in men at increased risk for myocardial infarction. The best known of these clinical trials using estrogens in men was reported by the Coronary Drug Project Research Group. In this randomized, double-blind, secondary prevention trial,[79] 8341 patients who had survived a previous myocardial infarction were randomized to receive one of four pharmacological agents that included conjugated estrogen in doses of 2.5 and 5 mg daily, or placebo. After an average follow-up of 18 months, it was observed by the Safety Monitoring Committee that an excess number of nonfatal myocardial infarctions, pulmonary emboli, cases of thrombophlebitis, and deaths were seen in the high-dose estrogen group compared with the placebo group. Those subjects receiving estrogens had an 11% incidence of new events compared to 7.5% in the placebo group. These findings led to a modification in the trial design with a discontinuation of the 5 mg/d estrogen arm of the study.[79] Three years later, the 2.5 mg/d estrogen arm of the study was stopped since the overall mortality rate was 19.9% compared to 18.8% on placebo.[80] It was concluded that estrogens were not useful and potentially harmful in men who had survived a myocardial infarction.[80]

Estrogens frequently are administered to men who have prostatic carcinoma[81-83] or who are transsexuals.[84] It is not known whether estrogen treatment will increase the risk of coronary heart disease in these individuals.

Recommendations

In the past, noncontraceptive estrogen use has been underutilized in postmenopausal females because of the fears of increasing the risk of coronary artery disease or endometrial and breast cancers. However, more recent epidemiologic studies have demonstrated that the risk of coronary heart disease is reduced in postmenopausal females who are receiving exogenous estrogens. Despite these encouraging findings, it should be pointed out that, as yet, no randomized, controlled trial of postmenopausal estrogen has evaluated multiple morbidity and mortality endpoints.[40,41,85] The Postmenopausal Estrogen/Progestin Interventions (PEPI) trial currently is underway that will evaluate cardiac risk factors in women and other issues, but not mortality. If hopes are realized, the results of the PEPI trial, coupled with other available data, will further elucidate the overall risk-benefit ratio of estrogen replacement therapy. A large multicenter controlled trial sponsored by the National Institutes of Health will soon begin that will assess prospectively the incidences of metabolic bone disease and cardiovascular morbidity and mortality in a large population of postmenopausal women. Until such data are available, however, postmenopausal women with known coronary artery disease should be evaluated carefully as candidates for estrogen replacement therapy. The use of estrogen replacement could be considered in postmenopausal women who have bothersome climacteric symptoms and are at increased risk of coronary artery disease.

If estrogen therapy is contemplated, it should be combined with doses of progestogen adequate enough to decrease the risk of endometrial cancer while small enough not to significantly affect the beneficial effects on lipids and lipoproteins seen with estrogen.

In the future, routine estrogen replacement therapy may become an important treatment modality alone or in combination with other treatments for reducing the risk of coronary artery disease in high-risk postmenopausal women.

Plasmapheresis (LDL-Apheresis)

Homozygous patients with familial hypercholesterolemia demonstrate exceedingly high plasma cholesterol and LDL-cholesterol concentrations. These individuals are at risk of developing fatal coronary artery disease and/or aortic stenosis before adulthood. Cholesterol-lowering drugs usually are ineffective by themselves in lowering cholesterol in these patients, and other therapies have been proposed including liver transplantation, biliary diversion, portacaval shunt, hyperalimentation, and plasmapheresis.[86-90] Plasma exchange for the treatment of homozygous patients was first used in 1975.[91] A more refined technique, LDL-apheresis, has now become an accepted life-time therapy for these patients. It enables one to remove LDL from patients without needing to replace other plasma constituents.[86] The procedure is rarely used in heterozygous patients with familial hypercholesterolemia.

Several methods have been developed for selective removal of atherogenic lipoproteins.[86] Selective removal of LDL (LDL-apheresis) relies on the principle of affinity-chromatography and the various methodologies used have been described.[86] Numerous studies have demonstrated immediate changes in lipoproteins and plasma components with LDL-apheresis including marked reductions in plasma cholesterol, LDL-cholesterol,[92-94] and lipoprotein(a),[95] while plasma HDL-cholesterol and Apo A-1 were shown to increase, decrease, or remain the same.[92-94,96,97]

It has been suggested that LDL-apheresis might cause an increase in the turnover rate of Apo E-containing HDL, with possible increments in cholesterol removal from peripheral tissues.[86,96,97]

Drug therapy has been combined with LDL-apheresis with greater benefit on cholesterol reduction than with either therapy alone.[93,98,99] There is some early suggestion that LDL-apheresis can cause regression or stabilization of coronary atherosclerotic lesions in patients with familial hypercholesterolemia as assessed by angiographic techniques.[93,100,101] However, much larger numbers of patients and a longer period of treatment will be needed to establish whether LDL-apheresis can, in fact, cause significant regression of atherosclerotic lesions.

Newer Pharmacological Approaches

β-Sitosterol (Plant Sterols)

β-Sitosterol is a plant sterol with a structure similar to that of cholesterol except for the substitution of an ethyl group at C24 of its side chain. Despite this structural relation to cholesterol, it is poorly absorbed from the intestine. β-Sitosterol is known to compete with cholesterol for incorporation into mixed micelles, thereby reducing intestinal cholesterol absorption.[102,103] The importance of dietary intake of plant sterols on cholesterol absorption and serum cholesterol has been demonstrated in human beings—dietary intake of plant sterols is negatively related to fractional cholesterol absorption and overall cholesterol synthesis.[104-108] β-Sitosterol may also inhibit 7-α-hydroxylase.[109,110]

β-Sitosterol is used for treatment of hypercholesterolemia in Europe. It is quite effective in reducing cholesterol by 5%-15%.[107] It is a very safe substance, although a high dose is required (6 g), taken before meals and at bedtime. Another plant sterol, β-Sitostanol, has been shown to reduce serum cholesterol more effectively than sitosterol at a lower dose.[111]

The plant sterols are indicated only for the treatment of excess LDL in patients with polygenic hypercholesterolemia who appear to be extremely sensitive to small amounts of dietary cholesterol.

Acyl Coenzyme A Transferase (ACAT) Inhibitors

The inhibitors of ACAT catalyzed cholesterol esterification are thought to be potent inhibitors of intestinal cholesterol absorption. A novel ACAT inhibitor, CC 277,082, was shown to reduce elevations in both liver and serum cholesterol in cholesterol-fed rats.[112] Fecal analysis in this study revealed an 80% increase in neutral sterol excretion in the first 24 hours after an oral dose of labeled-14C cholesterol. These agents may have use as hypercholesterolemic drugs in human beings.

HDL Infusion

Several large epidemiologic studies have shown the inverse relationship between the incidence of coronary heart disease and HDL-cholesterol levels.[113,114] Recently, a study was completed where HDL-VHDL was infused in rabbits to determine the in vivo effects on the development of atherosclerosis.[115] The experimental animals (n=31) all received a 0.5% cholesterol-rich diet for 8 weeks. During this period, 50 mg/week of homologous HDL-VHDL protein was intravenously administered to the treatment group; the control group received a matching volume of normal saline. During the study, plasma lipid values were similar in both groups. At the completion of the study, the animals were sacrificed, and atherosclerotic lesions of the intimal aortic surface were less prevalent in the treated group. The values of total and free cholesterol, esterified cholesterol, and phospholipids deposited within the vessel wall were significantly lower in the HDL-treated animals. Cholesterol accumulation in the liver was also significantly less in the treated group.

The investigators concluded that the administration of homologous HDL-VLDL lipoprotein fraction to cholesterol-fed rabbits reduced the extent of aortic fatty streaks and reduced lipid deposition in the arterial wall and liver without modification of the plasma lipid levels. It was suggested that HDL-VHDL infusions could play a role in enhancing reverse cholesterol transport, thus inhibiting the development and/or progression of atherosclerosis.

Inhibitors of CETP, Enhancers of 7-α-Hydroxylase, and Lipoprotein Lipase Activity

With advances in molecular biology and an increased knowledge of cholesterol homeostasis, newer approaches to the treatment of lipid disorders are being conceived.

Cholesteryl ester transfer protein (CETP) is involved in the regulation of plasma cholesterol identification and the transfer of cholesteryl esters between lipoprotein particles.[116-119] Families with human CETP deficiency have relatively high HDL-cholesterol levels and a relatively low risk of having coronary artery disease.[117] Drugs that inhibit the action of CETP could be extremely useful in modifying the lipoproteins of individuals at risk for developing premature atherosclerotic vascular disease.

The enzyme 7-α-hydroxylase is the regulatory substance in the conversion of cholesterol to bile salts.[120] Bile-acid biosynthesis represents the major route of catabolism and removal of cholesterol in the body. The cloning of the regulatory enzyme recently has been reported.[121] This is a significant finding since the regulation of this important enzyme can be studied on the molecular level. An understanding of the molecular mechanisms that regulate this enzyme might make a clinical impact if an enzyme-enhancing drug could be developed. This drug would potentially reduce plasma cholesterol levels while having a preventive influence on gallstone production.

Lipoprotein lipase has also been cloned and its regulation is being studied on the molecular level.[122-126] The enzyme catalyzes the hydrolysis of glycerides and phospholipids of various lipoproteins. An enhancement of lipoprotein lipase activity could favorably influence the levels of triglyceride and various lipoproteins in the plasma.

References

1. Samuel P, Steiner A: Effect of neomycin on serum cholesterol level of man. Proc Soc Exp Biol Med 1959; 100: 193-195.

2. Samuel P, Holtzman CM, Meilman E, et al: Effect of neomycin on exchangeable pools of cholesterol in the steady state. J Clin Invest 1968; 47: 1806-1818.
3. Samuel P, Holtzman CM, Goldstein J: Long-term reduction of serum cholesterol levels of patients with atherosclerosis by small doses of neomycin. Circulation 1967; XXXV: 938-945.
4. Sande MA, Mandell GL: Antimicrobial agents. In Gilman AG, Rall TW, Niles AS, et al (eds): Goodman and Gilman's The Pharmacological Basis of Therapeutics, 8th ed. New York, Macmillan Publishing Co., 1990; 1098-1106.
5. Thompson GR, Barrowmann J, Gutierrez L, et al: Action of neomycin on absorption, synthesis and/or flux of cholesterol in man. J Clin Invest 1971; 50: 319-323.
6. Miettinen TA: Effects of neomycin alone and in combination with cholestyramine on serum cholesterol and fecal steroids in hypercholesterolemic subjects. J Clin Invest 1979; 64: 1485-1493.
7. Sedaghat A, Samuel P, Crouse JR, et al: Effects of neomycin on absorption, synthesis and/or flux of cholesterol in man. J Clin Invest 1975; 55: 12-21.
8. Samuel P, Holtzman CM, Meilman E, et al: Effect of neomycin and other antibiotics on serum cholesterol levels and on 7α-dehydroxylation of bile-acids by the fecal bacterial flora in man. Circ Res 1973; XXXIII: 393-402.
9. Samuel P, Schussheim A, Lieberman S, et al: Relation of serum cholesterol to in vitro 7α-dehydroxylation of primary bile- acids by fecal bacteria in infants and children. Pediatrics 1974; 54: 222-228.
10. Samuel P, Waithe WI: Reduction of serum cholesterol concentrations by neomycin, para-aminosalicylic acid, and other antibacterial drugs in man. Circulation 1961; XXIV: 578-591.
11. Samuel P, Meilman E, Siil TE: Dietary lipids and reduction of serum cholesterol levels by neomycin in man. J Lab & Clin Med 1967; 70: 471-479.
12. Breen KJ, Bryant EE, Levinson JD, et al: Neomycin absorption in man. Ann Intern Med 1972; 76: 211-218.
13. Kesaniemi YA, Grundy SM: Turnover of low density lipoproteins during inhibition of cholesterol absorption by neomycin. Arteriosclerosis 1984; 4: 41-48.
14. Hoeg JM, Schaefer EJ, Romano CA, et al: Neomycin and plasma lipoproteins in Type II hyperlipoproteinemia. Clin Pharmacol Ther 1984; 36: 555-565.
15. Schade RWB, van't Laar A, Majoor CLH, et al: A comparative study of the effects of cholestyramine and neomycin in the treatment of Type II hyperlipoproteinaemia. Acta Med Scand 1976; 199: 175-180.
16. Samuel P: Treatment of hypercholesterolemia with neomycin - a time for reappraisal. N Engl J Med 1979; 30: 595-597.
17. Samuel P, Holtzman CM, Meilman E, et al: Reduction of serum cholesterol and triglyceride levels by the combined administration of neomycin and clofibrate. Circulation 1970; XLI: 109-114.

18. Teoh PC: Effect of combined administration of clofibrate and neomycin on serum cholesterol levels in familial Type II hyperlipoproteinaemia. Curr Med Res Opin 1973; l: 535-539.
19. Illingworth DR, Bacon S: Treatment of familial hypercholesterolemia with lipid-lowering drugs. Arteriosclerosis 1989; 9: I121-134.
20. Thompson GR, Soutar AK, Spengel FA, et al: Defects of receptor-mediated low density lipoprotein catabolism in homozygous familial hypercholesterolemia and hypothyroidism. Proc Natl Acad Sci USA 1981; 78: 2591-2595.
21. Chait A, Bierman EL, Albers JJ: Regulatory role of triiodothyronine in the degradation of low density lipoprotein by cultured human skin fibroblasts. J Clin Endocrinol Metab 1979; 48: 887-889.
22. Thompson GR, Soutar AV, Spengel FA: Defects of receptor mediated low density lipoprotein catabolism in homozygous familial hypercholesterolemia and hypothyroidism in vivo. Proceedings of the National Academy of Sciences 1981; 768: 2591-2595.
23. Bastenie PA, Vanhaelst L, Bonnyns L, et al: Preclinical hypothyroidism: a risk factor for coronary heart disease. Lancet 1971; 1: 203-204.
24. Fowler PBS, Swale J, Andrews H: Hypercholesterolaemia in borderline hypothyroidism: stage of premyxoedema. Lancet 1970; 2: 488-491.
25. Bastenie PA, Vanhaelst L, Neve P: Coronary artery disease in hypothyroidism: observations in preclinical myxoedema. Lancet 1967: 2: 122l-1222.
26. Dean JW, Fowler PBS: Exaggerated responsiveness to thyrotrophic releasing hormone: a risk factor in women with coronary artery disease. Br Med J 1985; 290: 1555-1561.
27. Heller RF, Miller NE, Lewis B, et al: Associations between sex hormones, thyroid hormones and lipoproteins. Clin Sci 1981; 61: 649-651.
28. Althaus BU, Staub JJ, Ryff-De Leche A, et al: LDL/HDL changes in subclinical hypothyroidism: possible risk factors for coronary heart disease. Clin Endocrinol 1988; 28: 157-163.
29. Burman KD: Is long-term levothyroxine therapy safe? Arch Intern Med 1990; 150: 2010-2012.
30. Illingworth DR: Lipid-lowering drugs. Drugs 1987; 33: 259-279.
31. Coronary Drug Project: Findings leading to further modifications of its protocol with respect to d. thyroxine. JAMA 1972; 220: 996-1002.
32. Arem R, Patsch W: Lipoprotein and apolipoprotein levels in subclinical hypothyroidism. Arch Intern Med 1990; 150: 2097-2100.
33. Ryan KJ: Estrogens and atherosclerosis. Clin Obstet Gynecol 1976; 19: 805-815.
34. Lobo RA: Cardiovascular implications of estrogen replacement therapy. Obstet Gynecol 1990; 7S: 18S-25S.
35. Fahraeus L: The effects of estradiol on blood lipids and lipoproteins in postmenopausal women. Obstet Gynecol 1988; 72 (S Suppl): 18S-22S.
36. Boston Collaborative Drug Surveillance Program: Surgically confirmed gallbladder disease, venous thromboembolism and breast tumors in relation to post menopausal estrogen therapy. N Engl J Med 1974; 15: 290.

37. Fahraeus L, Wallentin L: High-density lipoprotein subfractions during oral and cutaneous administration of 17 β-estradiol to menopausal women. J Clin Endocrinol Metab 1983; 56: 797-801.

38. Gordon T, Kannel WB, Hjortland MC, et al: Menopause and coronary artery disease. Ann Intern Med 1978; 89: 157-161.

39. Wilson PWF, Garrison RJ, Castelli WP: Post-menopausal estrogen use, cigarette smoking, and cardiovascular morbidity in women over 50. The Framingham Study. N Engl J Med 1985; 313: 1038-1043.

40. Stampfer MJ, Colditz GA: Estrogen replacement therapy and coronary heart disease: a quantitative assessment of the epidemiologic evidence. Prevent Med 1991; 20: 47-63.

41. Barrett-Connor E, Bush TL: Estrogen and coronary heart disease in women. JAMA 1991; 265: 1861-1867.

42. Colditz GA, Willett WC, Stampfer MJ, et al: Menopause and the risk of coronary heart disease in women. N Engl J Med 1987; 316: 1105-1110.

43. Criqui MH, Suarez L, Barrett-Connor E, et al: Postmenopausal estrogen use and mortality: results from a prospective study in a defined, homogeneous community. Am J Epidemiol 1988; 128: 606-614.

44. Bush TL, Barrett-Connor E, Cowan LD, et al: Cardiovascular mortality and noncontraceptive use of estrogen in women: results from the Lipid Research Clinics Program Follow-up Study. Circulation 1987; 75: 1102-1109.

45. Pearson TA, Bulkley BH, Achuff SC, et al: The association of low levels of HDL-cholesterol and arteriographically defined CAD. Am J Epidemiol 1979; 109: 285-295.

46. Gruchow HW, Anderson AJ, Barboriak JJ, et al: Postmenopausal use of estrogen and occlusion of coronary arteries. Am Heart J 1988; 115: 954-963.

47. Henderson BE, Paganini-Hill A, Ross RK: Decreased mortality in users of estrogen replacement therapy. Arch Intern Med 1991; 151: 75-78.

48. Sullivan JM, Vander Zwaag R, Hughes JP, et al: Estrogen replacement and coronary artery disease. Arch Intern Med 1990; 150: 2557-2562.

49. Lagrelius A, Johnson P, Lunell NO, et al: Treatment with oral estrone-sulphate in the female climacteric. 1. Influence on lipids. Acta Obstet Gynecol Scand 1981; 60: 27-31.

50. Campos H, Wilson PW, Jimenez D, et al: Differences in apolipoproteins and low-density lipoprotein subfractions in postmenopausal women on and off estrogen therapy: results from the Framingham Offspring Study. Metabolism 1990; 39: 1033-1038.

51. The Lipid Research Clinics Program: The Lipid Research Clinics Coronary Primary Prevention Trial Results. 1. Reduction in incidence of coronary heart disease. JAMA 1984; 251: 351-364.

52. Bush T, Cown LD, Barrett-Connor E, et al: Estrogen use and all cause mortality: preliminary results from the Lipid Research Clinics Program Follow-up Study. JAMA 1983; 249: 903-906.

53. Cauley JA, LaPorte RE, Kuller LH, et al: Menopausal estrogen use, high-density lipoprotein cholesterol sub-fractions and liver function. Atherosclerosis 1983; 49: 31-39.

54. Krauss RM, Perlman JA, Ray R, et al: Effects of estrogen dose and smoking on lipid and lipoprotein levels in postmenopausal women. Am J Obstet Gynecol 1988; 158: 1606-1611.

55. Wahl PW, Warnick GR, Albers JJ, et al: Distribution of lipoproteins, triglyceride and lipoprotein cholesterol in an adult population by age, sex and hormone use - the Pacific Northwest Bell Telephone Company Health Survey. Atherosclerosis 1981; 39: 111-124.

56. Adams MR, Clarkson TB, Koritnik DR, et al: Contraceptive steroids and coronary artery atherosclerosis in cynomolgus macaques. Fertil Steril 1987; 47: 1010-1018.

57. Williams JK, Adams MR, Klopfenstein S: Estrogen modulates responses of atherosclerotic coronary arteries. Circulation 1990; 81: 1680-1687.

58. Sternleitner A, Stanczyk FZ, Levin JH, et al: Decreased in vitro production of 6-keto-prostaglandin F/d by uterine arteries from postmenopausal women. Am J Obstet Gynecol 1989; 161: 1677-1681.

59. Hough JL, Zilversmit DB: Effect of 17 β-estradiol on aortic cholesterol content and metabolism in cholesterol-fed rabbits. Arteriosclerosis 1986; 6: 57-63.

60. Huppert LC: Hormonal replacement therapy: benefits, risks, doses. Med Clin North Am 1987; 71: 23-39.

61. Gambrell RD: The menopause: benefits and risks of estrogen- progestogen replacement therapy. Modern Trends 1982; 37: 457-474.

62. Ettinger B, Genant HK, Cann CE: Long-term estrogen replacement therapy prevents bone loss and fractures. Ann Intern Med 1985; 102: 319-324.

63. Stampfer MJ, Willett WC, Colditz GA, et al: A prospective study of post-menopausal estrogen therapy and coronary artery disease. N Engl J Med 1985; 313: 1044-1049.

64. Nachtigall LE, Nachtigall RH, Nachtigall RD, et al: Estrogen replacement therapy. II. A prospective study in the relationship to carcinoma and cardiovascular and metabolic problems. Obstet & Gynecol 1979; 54: 74-79.

65. Dupont WD, Page DL: Menopausal estrogen replacement therapy and breast cancer. Arch Intern Med 1991; 151: 67-72.

66. Steinberg J, Thacker SB, Smith J, et al: A meta-analysis of the effects of estrogen replacement therapy on the risk of breast cancer. JAMA 1991; 265: 1985-1990.

67. Gambrell Jr. RD: Role of progestogens in the prevention of breast cancer. Maturitas 1986; 8: 169-176.

68. Gambrell RD, Maier RC, Sanders BI: Decreased incidence of breast cancer in postmenopausal estrogen-progestogen users. Obstet Gynecol 1983; 62: 435-443.

69. Knopp RH, Walden CE, Wahl PW, et al: Effects of oral contraceptives on lipoprotein triglyceride and cholesterol: relationships to estrogen and progestin potency. Am J Obstet Gynecol 1982; 142: 725-731.

70. Fotherby K: Oral contraceptives and lipids. (editorial) Br Med J 1989; 289: 1049-1050.

71. Knopp RH: Effects of sex steroid hormones on lipoprotein levels in pre- and post-menopausal women. Can J Cardiol 1990; 6 (Suppl B): 31B-35B.

72. Sonnendecker EW, Polakow ES, Benade AJ, et al: Serum lipoprotein effects of conjugated estrogen and a sequential conjugated estrogen-medrogestone regimen in hysterectomized post-menopausal women. Am J Obstet Gynecol 1989; 160: 1128-1134.

73. Mattsson LA, Cullberg G, Samsioe G: A continuous estrogen-progestogen regimen for climacteric complaints. Effects on lipid and lipoprotein metabolism. Acta Obstet Gynecol Scand 1984; 63: 673-677.

74. Mattsson LA, Samsioe G: Estrogen-progestogen replacement in climacteric women, particularly as regards a new type of continuous regimen. Acta Obstet Gynecol Scand 1985; 130: 53-58.

75. Rossner S, Frankman O, Marsk L: Effects of ethinylestradiol/D-norgestrel combinations on serum lipoproteins. Acta Obstet Gynecol Scand 1980; 59: 255-258.

76. Bradley DD, Wingerd J, Petitti DB, et al: Serum high-density lipoprotein cholesterol in women using oral contraceptives, estrogens and progestins. N Engl J Med 1978; 299: 17-20.

77. Harvengt C, Desager JP, Gaspard U, et al: Changes in lipoprotein composition in women receiving two low-dose oral contraceptives containing ethinylestradiol and gonane progestins. Contraception 1988; 37: 565-575.

78. Wolfe BM, Huff W: Effects of combined estrogen and progestin administration on plasma lipoprotein metabolism in postmenopausal women. J Clin Invest 1989; 83: 40-45.

79. The Coronary Drug Project Research Group. The Coronary Drug Project: Initial findings leading to modifications of its research protocol. JAMA 1970; 214: 1303-1313.

80. The Coronary Drug Project. Findings leading to discontinuation of the 2.5 mg/d estrogen group. JAMA 1973; 226: 652-657.

81. Wallentin L, Varenhorst E: Plasma lipoproteins during anti-androgen treatment by estrogens or orchidectomy in men with prostatic carcinoma. Horm Metab Res 1981; 13: 293-297.

82. Wallentin L, Varenhorst E: Changes of plasma lipid metabolism in males during estrogen treatment for prostatic carcinoma. J Clin Endocrinol Metab 1978; 47: 596-599.

83. Moorjani S, Dupont A, Cabrie F, et al: Changes in plasma lipoproteins during various androgen suppression therapies in men with prostatic carcinoma: effects of orchiectomy, estrogen, and combination treatment with luteinizing hormone-releasing hormone agonist flutamide. J Clin Endocrinol Metab 1988; 66: 314-322.

84. Damewood MD, Bellantoni JJ, Bachorik PS, et al: Exogenous estrogen effect on lipid/lipoprotein cholesterol in transsexual males. J Endocrinol Invest 1989; 12: 449-454.

85. Vandenbrocke JP: Postmenopausal oestrogen and cardioprotection. Lancet 1991; 337: 833-834.

86. Mabuchi H: Use of LDL-apheresis in the management of familial hypercholesterolemia. Curr Opin Lipidol 1990; 1: 43-47.

87. Starzl TE, Bahnson HT, Hardesty RL, et al: Heart-liver transplantation in a patient with familial hypercholesterolemia. Lancet 1984; 1: 1382-1383.

88. Deckelbaum RJ, Lees RS, Small DM, et al: Failure of complete bile diversion and oral bile-acid therapy in the treatment of homozygous familial hypercholesterolemia. N Engl J Med 1977; 296: 465-470.

89. Starzl TE, Putnam CW, Chase HP, et al: Portacaval shunt in hyperlipoproteinaemia. Lancet 1973; ii: 940-944.

90. Torvik H, Fischer JE, Feldman HA, et al: Effects of intravenous hyperalimentation on plasma lipoproteins in severe familial hypercholesterolaemia. Lancet 1975; i: 601-604.

91. Thompson GR: Plasma exchange for hypercholesterolemia. Lancet 1981; 1; 1246-1248.

92. Stoffel W, Borberg H, Greve V: Application of specific extracorporeal removal of low density lipoprotein in familial hypercholesterolemia. Lancet 1981; ii: 1005-1007.

93. Thompson GR, Barber M, Okabayashi K, et al: Plasmapheresis in familial hypercholesterolemia. Arteriosclerosis 1989; 9 (Suppl 1): 152-157.

94. Parker TS, Gordon BR, Saael SD, et al: Plasma high density lipoprotein is increased in man when low density lipoprotein (LDL) is lowered by LDL-pheresis. Proc Natl Acad Sci USA 1986; 83: 777-781.

95. Schenck I, Keller CH, Hailer S, et al: Reduction of Lp(a) by different methods of plasma exchange. Klin Wochenschr 1988; 66: 1197-1201.

96. Franceschini G, Apebe P, Calabresi I, et al: Alterations in the HDL system after rapid plasma cholesterol reduction by LDL-apheresis. Metabolism 1988; 37: 752-757.

97. Koizumi J, Inazu A, Fujita H, et al: Removal of apolipoprotein E-enriched high density lipoprotein by LDL-apheresis in familial hypercholesterolemia: a possible activation of the reverse cholesterol transport system. Atherosclerosis 1988; 74: 1-8.

98. Mabuchi H, Fujita H, Michishita I, et al: Effects of CS 514 (eptastatin), an inhibitor of 3-hydroxy-3-methylglutaryl coenzyme a (HMG-CoA) reductase, on serum lipid and apolipoprotein levels in heterozygous familial hypercholesterolemic patients treated by low density lipoprotein (LDL) apheresis. Atherosclerosis 1988; 72: 183-188.

99. Riesen WF, Descoeudres C, Mordasini R, et al: Selective elimination of atherogenic lipoproteins by dextran sulfate cellulose. Schweiz Med Wochenschr 1989; 119: 55-58.

100. Keller CH, Spengel FA: Changes of atherosclerosis of the carotid arteries due to severe familial hypercholesterolemia following long-term plasmapheresis, assessed by duplex scan. Klin Wochenschr 1988; 66: 149-152.

101. Mabuchi H, Koizumi J, Michishita I, et al: Effects on coronary atherosclerosis of long-term treatment of familial hypercholesterolemia by LDL-apheresis. Contrib Infus Ther 1988; 23: 87-96.

102. Ikeda I, Tanaka K, Sugano M, et al: Inhibition of cholesterol absorption in rats by plant sterols. J Lipid Res 1988; 29: 1573-1582.

103. Ikeda I, Tanaka K, Sugano M, et al: Discrimination between cholesterol and sitosterol for absorption in rats. J Lipid Res 1988; 29: 1583-1592.

104. Tilvis RS, Miettinen TA: Serum plant sterols and their relation to cholesterol absorption. Am J Clin Nutri 1986; 43: 92-97.

105. Kesaniemi YA, Miettinen TA: Cholesterol absorption efficiency regulates plasma cholesterol level in the Finnish population. Eur J Clin Invest 1987; 17: 391-395.
106. Miettinen TA, Kesaniemi YA: Cholesterol absorption: regulation of cholesterol synthesis and elimination and within-population variations of serum cholesterol levels. Am J Clin Nutri 1989; 49: 629-635.
107. von Bergmann K: Lipid-lowering drugs working in the intestine. Curr Opin Lipid 1990; 1: 48-50.
108. Gylling H, Miettinen TA: Serum noncholesterol sterols related to cholesterol metabolism in familial hypercholesterolemia. Clin Chim Acta 1988; 178: 41-49.
109. Boberg KM, Akerlund J-E, Bjorkhem I: Effects of sitosterol on the rate-limiting enzymes in cholesterol synthesis and degradation. Lipids 1989; 24: 9-12.
110. Shefer S, Salen G, Nguyen L, et al: Competitive inhibition of bile-acid synthesis by endogenous cholestanol and sitosterol in sitosterolemia with xanthomatosis. Effect of cholesterol 7-alpha-hydroxylase. J Clin Invest 1988; 82: 1833-1839.
111. Heinemann T, Pietruck B, Kullak-Ublick G, et al: Comparison of sitosterol and sitostanol on inhibition of intestinal cholesterol absorption. Agents Actions 1988 (Suppl 26): 117-122.
112. Largis EE, Wang CH, DeVries VG, et al: CL-277,082: a novel inhibition of ACAT-catalyzed cholesterol esterification and cholesterol absorption. J Lipid Res 1989; 30: 681-690.
113. Miller NE, Forde OM, Thelle DS: The Tromso Heart Study: high density lipoproteins and coronary heart disease. A prospective case-control study. Lancet 1977; 1: 965-968.
114. Gordon T, Castelli WP, Hjortland MC, et al: High density lipoprotein as a protective factor against coronary heart disease: The Framingham Study. Am J Med 1977; 62: 707-714.
115. Badimon JJ, Badimon L, Galvez A, et al: High density lipoprotein plasma fractions inhibit aortic fatty streaks in cholesterol-fed rabbits. Lab Invest 1989; 60: 455-461.
116. Brown ML, Hesler C, Tall AR: Plasma enzymes and transfer proteins in cholesterol metabolism. Curr Opin Lipidol 1990; 1: 122-127.
117. Brown ML, Inazu A, Hesler CB, et al: Molecular basis of lipid transfer protein deficiency in a family with decreased high-density lipoproteins. Nature 1989; 342: 448-451.
118. Agellon LB, Quinet EM, Gillette TG, et al: Organization of the human cholesteryl ester transfer protein gene. Biochem 1990; 29: 1373-1376.
119. Kondo I, Berg K, Drayna D, et al: DNA polymerization at the locus for human cholesteryl ester transfer protein (CETP) is associated with high density lipoprotein cholesterol and apolipoprotein levels. Clin Genet 1989; 35: 49-56.
120. Edwards PA, Fogelman AM: Cellular enzymes of cholesterol metabolism. Curr Opin Lipidol 1990; 1: 136-139.

121. Noshiro N, Nishimoto M, Morohashi K, et al: Molecular cloning of cDNA for cholesterol 7α hydroxylase from rat liver microsomes. Nucleotide sequence and expression. FEBS Letts 1989; 257: 97-100.
122. Olivecrona T, Bengtsson-Olivecrona G: Lipases involved in lipoprotein metabolism. Curr Opin Lipidol 1990; 1: 116-12l.
123. Persson B, Bengtsson-Olivecrona G, Enerback S, et al: Structural features of lipoprotein lipase. Lipase family relationships, binding interactions, non-equivalence of lipase cofactors, vitellogenin similarities and functional subdivision of lipoprotein lipase. Eur J Biochem 1989; 179: 39-45.
124. Deeb SS, Peng R: Structure of the human lipoprotein lipase gene. Biochem 1989; 28: 4131-4134.
125. Enerback S, Bjursell G: Genomic organization of the coding region of the guinea pig lipoprotein lipase gene; evidence for exon fusion and unconventional splicing. Gene 1989; 84: 391-397.
126. Kirchgessner TG, Heinzeman C, Antonarakis SE, et al: Human lipoprotein lipase gene: structure, genetics and evolution. Arteriosclerosis 1989; 9: 691a.

Part IV
Special Articles

Chapter 11

The Effects of Cardiovascular Drugs on Plasma Lipids and Lipoproteins

William H. Frishman M.D., Brian F. Johnson M.D.,
George Pulos M.D., Margaret A. Danylchuk Pharm D.,
Marcia Brown, M.D., Eliot J. Lazar M.D.*

The past 10 to 20 years have witnessed a substantial improvement in the outlook of a variety of cardiovascular disorders, with a corresponding improvement in life expectancy. To a major extent, this reflects the availability of new medications and improved knowledge about how to use drug therapy in managing cardiovascular disease. Many agents have multiple uses. Diuretics and angiotensin-converting enzyme (ACE) inhibitors are recommended for both hypertension and congestive heart failure, for example, and many β-blockers and calcium channel blockers are valuable in ischemic heart disease and hypertension.

Despite the very favorable impact of these drugs on cardiovascular diseases, there are concerns about the potentially detrimental effect of some agents on plasma lipids and lipoprotein profiles.[1-8] Such concerns probably apply equally in heart failure and ischemic heart disease, but the agents have been studied mainly in patients with hypertension.

It is well established that control of severe hypertension is associated with increased life expectancy, with clear benefit to the risk of

Portions of this chapter were adapted from an earlier work by Johnson BF, Danylchuk MA: Med Clin N Amer 1989; 73: 449-473, with permission.

*Dr. Lazar contributed to this chapter prior to his appointment as a consultant to the Department of Health and Human Services. No official support or endorsement by HHS is intended or should be inferred.

From *Medical Management of Lipid Disorders: Focus on Prevention of Coronary Artery Disease,* edited by William H. Frishman, M.D. © 1992, Futura Publishing Inc., Mount Kisco, NY.

cerebrovascular accident and cardiac and renal failure.[9,10] However, the effects of antihypertensive treatment on the development of atherosclerosis and particularly coronary artery disease are less well defined.[8] Whereas some studies of mild hypertension have provided evidence of some reduction in the risk of coronary heart disease (CHD),[11] many others have failed to show any reduced frequency of CHD manifestations with treatment.[10] Recently, in a very large placebo-controlled study in the United Kingdom[12] neither a thiazide nor propranolol produced significant reduction in manifestations of CHD. This is of particular importance because CHD is the most frequent cause of death in patients with hypertension.

It seems clear that control of hypertension usually is feasible using one or more of the available therapeutic agents.[10] The major challenge for the future is to reduce the high incidence of CHD in hypertension.[8] At this time, it seems reasonable to examine the hypothesis that agents that are equally effective in lowering blood pressure have equally beneficial effects on life expectancy. Because the available agents have been shown to have different effects on plasma lipids and lipoproteins, it should be considered that they also may have different effects on the development of coronary artery disease.[3,7] This chapter provides a review of the reported data on the effects of cardiovascular medications on plasma lipids and lipoproteins, and provides some inferences about how these effects impact the drug selection process for individual patients.

Diuretics

Diuretics have long been a first-line antihypertensive therapy and are known to have metabolic consequences. The propensity of thiazides to reversibly induce hyperglycemia and glycosuria and worsen established diabetes mellitus has been known for many decades. Although it is very difficult to study the impact of many years of treatment, the Medical Research Council Trial[13] demonstrated persistent hyperglycemia in the thiazide-treated group over an average period of 5 years, and in a small group of subjects followed for 14 years, Murphy and coworkers[14] demonstrated persistent and worsening glucose intolerance. Bloomgarden and colleagues[15] showed 18% higher mean glycosylated hemoglobin levels in 89 insulin-dependent diabetic subjects on long-term hydrochlorothiazide (HCTZ) therapy, compared with 255 diabetics not taking diuretics. It commonly is stated that the hyperglycemia results from impaired pancreatic secretion of insulin, secondary to diuretic-induced hypokalemia. Profound potassium deficiency induced in animals causes hyperglycemia secondary to reduced insulin secretion.

In studies by Basabe et al of daily doses of 100 mg of HCTZ,[16] it was found that the hyperglycemic effect was not inhibited by preventing hypokalemia with concurrent spironolactone, and was associated with increased circulating levels of insulin. Similarly, chlorothiazide was reported to increase plasma insulin levels.[17]

The observation of a thiazide-induced state that resembled obesity and noninsulin-dependent diabetes suggested the possibility that thiazides also might be associated with increased hepatic synthesis of triglycerides.[18] The results of a follow-up study were presented by Johnson et al at the Medical Research Society in London,[19] demonstrating a 28% increase in mean triglyceride levels in a group of 14 hypertensive patients treated with 100 mg of HCTZ daily for 4 weeks. In that study, a small and nonsignificant increase in total serum cholesterol was observed. Ames and Hill, however, were the first to demonstrate significant increases in both triglycerides and cholesterol.[20]

These basic conclusions have been confirmed in many other studies (Table 1).[21-48] All tables in this chapter list only reports of single drug usage in which more than 10 patients were studied. In addition, a primary objective of the study was the assessment of drug-induced changes in plasma lipoprotein fractions. The studies listed in Table 1 mainly were relatively short-term, with high dosing of a thiazide diuretic, but with variations in treatment duration and in the laboratory methods used to determine the plasma lipids. Despite these differences, there is reasonable consistency in the overall conclusions. Thiazide diuretics increase triglycerides to a substantial but variable extent, with a corresponding increase in very low-density lipoprotein (VLDL), the predominant transport system for triglycerides. It also is apparent, however, that low-density lipoprotein (LDL) cholesterol levels are increased, so total cholesterol levels rise. The main area of controversy relates to changes in high-density lipoprotein (HDL) cholesterol where there is much more variability. Most investigators have found no significant effect, although two studies did detect increases[35,39] and two studies indicated decreases.[41,47]

The consistency of patient response to the thiazides also is debated.[49] Ames and Hill[30] demonstrated obvious variability in response, but this was not reported by Grimm and coworkers.[28] Only one investi-

Table 1.
Thiazide Diuretics and Chlorthalidone (% Change from Baseline)

Reference	# Pts.	Drug	Duration (weeks)	TC	TG	LDL-C	VLDL-C	HDL-C	HDL-C/ TC-C	LDL-C/ HDL-C	APO A-I	APO A-II	APO B
Rosenthal et al.[21] 1980	21	Chlor	12	8*	16*	9*	9	-12					
van Brummelen et al.[22] 1979	10	HCTZ	36	7*	1			8					
Gluck et al.[23] 1980 (males)	19	Chlor	6	8	4	18*	5	-6*			0	-3	0
(females)	10		6	1	8	4	6	11			-1	2	5
Goldman et al.[24] (1980)	302†	Chlor	52	5*	8*	10*		0					
Crisp et al.[25] 1980	13	Cyclop	8	3.5	14	12		-7					
Mordasini et al.[26]	12	Chlor	6	11	11	15*	-5	-6					
Joos et al.[27] 1980		HCTZ	3	8*	25*	10*	38*	1					
Grimm et al.[28] 1981	39	Chlor	6	7*	18*	6	13*	7					
	39	HCTZ	6	9*	13*	10*	7*	5					
Bauer et al.[29] 1981	13	HCTZ	4	5.4	13	6	7	1					
Ames & Hill[30] 1981	40	Chlor	52	7*	33*			2					
	47	HCTZ		5*	28*			-2					
Boehringer et al.[31] 1982	22††	Chlor	6	1	4	3	35	2			-5*	-2	0
	18**	Chlor	6	13*	-7	21*	-20	20			-5	-7	16*
Grimm et al.[32] 1982	14	HCTZ		5*	19*	5	24*	0					
	16	Chlor		5*	26*	8	24*	3					
Meier et al.[33] 1982	18	Chlor	6		5	28*		-7					

Study	n	Drug	Duration									
Schiffl et al.[34] 1982	17	Clop	4	7	13	13*	40	8			10*	9*
Valimaki et al.[35] 1983	24	HCTZ	12	10*	12	12*	21*	7			6*	3*
Fagar et al.[36] 1983	11	HCTZ	12	5	26*	1	43*	4			16*	9
Johnson et al.[37] 1984	20	Poly	4	4*	14*	3	8	8				
Holtzman et al.[38] 1984	21	Chlor	12	8*	16*	9*	9	-10				
Johnson et al.[39] 1986	16	HCTZ	24	10.5*	27*	7*	26*	12*				
Middeke et al.[40] 1987	14	HCTZ	3 yrs	11*	12*	13*		8			0	2
Trost et al.[41] 1987	16	HCTZ	24	9.8	26*			-8.4*	-19.4*			
Hjortdahl et al.[42] 1987	39	HCTZ	24	1.2	7.6			-13.1	-10.2			
Yoshino et al.[43] 1987	15	Trich	24	2.8	12	NS		0.9	NS	NS		
Holtzman et al.[44] 1987	21	Chlor	12	8.1*	16*	17*		5	-17*	22.5*		
Lehtonen et al.[46] 1987	13	HCTZ	24	2	29	-0.2	28	0.7	-0.5	1		
Lasser et a.[45]	28	HCTZ	28	11*	15	13.2*		1.4		12.7		
Frithz[47] 1989	42	HCTZ	12	8.8*	6*	17.4*		-11*	-19*	39*		
Pollare et al.[48] 1989	50	HCTZ	32	5	15*	5.6*		0.7	-5			

TC = total cholesterol; TG = triglyceride; LDL-C = low-density lipoprotein cholesterol; VLDL-C = very low-density lipoprotein cholesterol; HDL-C = high-density lipoprotein cholesterol; APO = apoprotein; Chlor = chlorthalidone; HCTZ = hydrochlorothiazide; Cyclop = cyclopenthiazide; Clop = clopamide; Poly = polythiazide; Trich = trichlorome; * = $p < 0.05$; † = HDL and LDL-C determined in 89 pts.; †† = premenopausal; ** = postmenopausal.

gator[31] has suggested that thiazide diuretics have a different effect on plasma lipids in pre- and postmenopausal women. These differences of opinion hardly seem surprising in view of the small numbers of subjects in most studies. As also would be expected, observed changes more often were statistically significant in the larger studies reported.

There is insufficient information about the effects of thiazide diuretics on apolipoproteins to determine whether, for example, there are increased concentrations of LDL particles or whether thiazides increase the cholesterol content of LDL particles, which otherwise remain unchanged. There also is inadequate information about the relation of drug dose to altered lipid profile. No major difference between daily chlorthalidone doses of 50 and 100 mg were reported by either Goldman's[24] or Grimm's[50] groups. Although only 9 postmenopausal black women were studied, McKenney and coworkers[51] demonstrated an equal and approximately 20% increase in LDL-cholesterol with daily doses of either 12.5 or 112.5 mg of HCTZ. Frishman et al found no significant effects on plasma lipids when using 6.25 mg of HCTZ.[52]

The questions of the sustained hyperlipidemic effect of continued thiazide treatment remains controversial.[49] In the studies of Johnson et al,[39] the effects of short-term treatment were dissipated within 2 to 4 weeks of discontinuing HCTZ. With continued treatment, however, there was no evidence of any change in the hyperlipidemic effects after 6 months. In 25 renal hypertensive subjects, 6 years of treatment with a HCTZ-amiloride combination produced a 20% increase in mean plasma cholesterol.[53] In their study in diabetics, Bloomgarden and associates[15] found lesser diabetic control associated with a 13% higher mean LDL cholesterol level in patients on long-term HCTZ.

There obviously are major difficulties in conducting studies of longer term diuretic treatment. Regardless of attempts to maintain behavioral stability in a study sample, patients frequently change their diet or level of exercise. Long-term studies that have included thiazide diuretics as a major component of therapy have not been designed to look specifically at changes in lipids, and therefore would not be expected to detect moderate changes accurately. In such trials, moreover, the control groups often have shown evidence of decline in lipid levels over the course of the study. Assuming that these changes represent alterations in diet and exercise in the entire study sample, they could obscure the continuing effect of treatment in the group of patients receiving thiazides.[13,54] In the Multiple Risk Factor Intervention Trial,[54] for example, all subjects received intensive dietary advice aimed at lowering cholesterol levels, but mean cholesterol levels declined less in patients receiving thiazide diuretics than in other patients. It has been shown that dietary modification can prevent the hyperlipidemic effects of thiazides.[28] It has been pointed out[55] that for several years a consistent decline in mean levels of serum cholesterol has been occurring in the general population.

It must be concluded that long-term studies would need to be designed to take these features into account to allow any chance of demonstrating the effect of continued diuretic treatment.

At present, the only reasonably large, long-term study that has shown significant effects of diuretics is that conducted by the Veterans Administration-NHLBI Cooperative Trial Group.[24] In 302 patients treated with chlorthalidone for 1 year, significant increases of 8% in triglycerides and 5% in total cholesterol were seen.

In general, it would be expected that diuretics that have a relatively similar chemical structure would have thiazidelike effects on plasma lipids. As shown in Table 2, however, studies of such agents (for example, furosemide) have been relatively rare.[27,30] Indapamide is an interesting drug that has less structural similarity to the thiazides than the already mentioned agents. It has diuretic activity but also has independent vasodilator properties at the recommended dose levels of 2.5 to 5 mg daily. The few available reports strongly suggest that these dose levels are not associated with changes in plasma lipids.[56-59] Again, relatively little attention has been paid to diuretic drugs that are unrelated chemically to the thiazides. Little can be concluded about these agents, especially in view of the inconsistency in reported changes with agents such as spironolactone.[32,60,61]

Possible Mechanisms for the Hyperlipidemic Effect

Diuretic therapy with thiazides appears to enhance VLDL and triglyceride synthesis in the liver. Plasma insulin levels are higher with diuretic therapy,[35,62] perhaps due to increments in growth hormone,[1,56] and insulin is known to stimulate triglyceride synthesis.[63] If lipoprotein lipase remains intact, then the excess hepatic VLDL synthesized in the liver could be secreted and metabolized to LDL-cholesterol, thereby also raising the total cholesterol level. The observation that certain diuretics produce significant changes in serum lipid levels while others do not may be related to their effects on serum insulin levels. Diuretics

Table 2.
Nonthiazide Diuretics

Reference	# Pts.	Drug	Duration (weeks)	TC	TG	LDL	VLDL	HDL-C	APO A-I	APO A-II	APO B
Joos et al.[27] 1980	12	Furosemide	3	5*	37*	4	56*	−3			
Ames & Hill[30] 1982	14	Furosemide	52	0	17			−15			
Valimaki et al.[35] 1983	24	Piretanide	12	15*	28*	15*	538	−3	11*		28*
Meyer-Sabellek et al.[57] 1985	20	Indapamide	26	3	−5	−3	−10	16			
Gerber et al.[58] 1985	69	Indapamide	6–8	2	4	2	0	2	0	2	5*
Yoshino et al.[43] 1987	8	Indapamide	48	3*	10			5*			
Leonetti et al.[59] 1990	248	Indapamide	48	0.4	−0.1			2.4			

TC = total cholesterol; TG = triglyceride; LDL = low-density lipoprotein; VLDL = very low-density lipoprotein; HDL-C = high-density lipoprotein-cholesterol; APO = apoprotein; * = p < 0.05.

can also raise catecholamines, thereby inhibiting phosphodiesterase and increasing cAMP activity.[5] This action would stimulate lipolysis and an increase in serum triglycerides. However, there is no known pathway that could provide a direct link between this effect and the observed increments in LDL cholesterol levels.[5] It has been suggested that diuretics might independently increase apoprotein B levels with a parallel increase in LDL-cholesterol.[5,31]

Beta-Adrenergic Blockers

Because of the intense competition between manufacturers of the various β-adrenergic blockers, these drugs have had extensive evaluation. As shown in Table 3, the nonselective agent propranolol has been studied in doses of 30 to 480 mg daily for periods of 3 days to 96 weeks.[29,45,64-88] Reported changes in total and LDL-cholesterol levels have been small, inconsistent, and usually not significant. By contrast, about half of the studies have shown significant increases in triglyceride levels, with the majority of studies reporting mean increases of > 15%. As would be expected, a similar trend is apparent in the smaller number of reports of VLDL-cholesterol levels. The greatest interest, however, has been directed to the mean reductions in HDL-cholesterol levels seen in all but three of the studies and reported as statistically significant in more than half. From Table 3, it appears that a median reduction of HDL-cholesterol of about 10% is produced by usual clinical doses of propranolol. These changes are convincing. There is a growing body of information showing reductions in both the HDL_2 and HDL_3 subfractions, and reductions in apoproteins I (A-I) and apoproteins II (A-II) (Table 3), although the information is not strong enough to draw definite conclusions. There is insufficient information about the relative effects of propranolol on patients with initially normal or elevated plasma lipids, although Dujovne and colleagues[71] suggest that the percentage changes are similar.

The limited information about other nonselective β-blockers is illustrated in Table 4. The trend for these agents to increase triglycerides and decrease HDL-cholesterol, again, is variable, but generally similar to that seen with other β-blockers without ISA.[88-94] Only one study[91] has suggested that lipid changes may worsen with increasing duration of β-blocker therapy.

Table 3.
β-Adrenergic Blockade (Propranolol) (% Change from Baseline)

Reference	# Pts.	Dose (mg)	Duration (weeks)	TC	TG	LDL	VLDL	HDL	HDL₂	HDL₃	LDL/HDL	HDL/TC	APO A-I	APO A-II	APO B
Streja & Mymin[64] 1978	16	40–240	2	−5.5	−0.4	−2.6		−12*							
Leren et al.[65] 1980	23	40–160	8	−1	24			−13*							
Ruhling et al.[66] 1980	10	75	4	−2*	9			−5*							
Schauer et al.[67] 1980	25	120	8	−2*	16*			−9*							
Bauer et al.[29] 1981	10	80–230	4	−5.7	16	0	15.5	−22							
Day et al.[68] 1984	53	160	12	−1.4	34*	−6	42*	−17*							
Birnbaum et al.[69] 1983	20	90–240	8	−5.6*	20.3	−9*		−7							
Ponti et al.[70] 1983	11	160	6	8.4*	20*			−7.6							
Dujovne et al.[71] 1984	8N 9H	40–360	24	0.1 1	27* 23*	−5 0	30.5 14.5	−4 −4							
Leon et al.[72] 1984	18	80–320	12	0.5	28.3*			10.4*							
Weber et al.[73] 1984	15	80–320	4	6	5.3			2.4							
Durrington et al.[74] 1985	11	160	2	2.2	8.3	3.1	25	−6.4	−12.7	2.9					1.4
Flamenbaum et al.[75] 1985	46	80–240	52	3.6	21			−11							
Harter et al.[76] 1986	10	40–120	12	0	17		21	−19	−22	−18					
Johnson et al.[77] 1986	19	40–160	3	−1	13*	−2		−8*							

Velasco et al.[78] 1986	10	40–240	8	4	14.4	-5.5	20*	-8	-49*	2				
Harvengt et al.[79] 1987	10	120	0.5	-0.4	24.8*	2.3		-14.7*				1.4	-2.5	7*
Malini et al.[80] 1987	19	80–240	6	1	18.6*	2.2		-4.2				-21.4		-8.6
Northcote et al.[81] 1987	21	40–80	52	1.5	5	-3.8	27.9*	-10.7	15*	-9.2*		1	-5.3	5.7
Miller et al.[82] 1987	7	80–160	48	-5	28*	-2.9	23	-23.6*	8.6		25.6			
Lijnen et al.[83] 1987	50	40–80	12	.27	3.9		3.5				-7.1			
Magarian et al.[84] 1987	45	40	96	4.23*	44.5*	6.3*	20.6*	-9.4*			-17.3*			
Fogari et al.[85] 1989	17	160	96	0.9	35*	-1.98		-37.2*			57.3			
Leon et al.[86] 1989	13	120–240	16	1.48	32*	-1.45	37.9*	-15.6	-3.75	15	-13	-6.15	-4.31	8.3*
Alderman[87] 1989	38	120–240	48	1	7.15	4.5	.84	13.57		-1.2	3.6			
Sirtori et al.[88]	10N	40–120	16	-7.87	30.2	-13.4	46.4†	-7.8			-6.1	-10.13		-7.3†
	8H	40–120	16	-3.62	39.6	-10.3	15.2†	-41.2*			-2.35	-12.94		12.94†
Lasser et al.[45] 1989	27	40–480	28	4.81	20.6*	8.2	14.2*				24.15*			

TC = total cholesterol; TG = triglyceride; LDL = low-density lipoprotein; VLDL = very low-density lipoprotein; HDL-C = high-density lipoprotein-cholesterol; APO = apoprotein; * = $p < 0.05$; † = after 5th week; N = normolipidemic; H = hyperlipidemic.

Table 4.
Other Nonselective β-Blockers (% Change from Baseline)

Reference	# Pts.	Drug/ Dose (mg)	Duration (weeks)	TC	TG	LDL	VLDL	HDL	HDL$_2$	HDL$_3$	LDL/ HDL	HDL/ TC	APO A-I	APO A-II	APO B
Harvengt et al.[79] 1987	10	Nadolol/ 160	0.5	-0.5	16.8	-0.5		-7.8*					-0.3	2.3	11.3
Waal-Manning[89] 1981	13	Nadolol/ 50–200	10	1.5	-14.5	-2	29	-3							
Northcote et al.[90] 1987	10	Sotalol/ 360	24	1.2	25*	1.9	20.5	-10.3					2.5	-0.4	2.9
Lehtonen et al.[91] 1979	12	Sotalol/ 160–640	4	-3.6	4.2		0.5	-14.8*							
			12	4	24.5	*LDL + VLDL*	11*	-19*							
			24	7.8*	32		16.8*	-24*							
			52	13.8	39.7		24*	-26*							
Richard et al.[92] 1986	10N	Teratolol/5	12	10*	20*	11	13.5	8					2.3		
	10H	5	12	-9	22*	-7	19	4					13.6		
Gundersen et al.[93] 1985	20	Timolol/20	52	3.3	27*			-4.5*							
Leren et al.[94] 1988	63	Timolol/10	24	3.2*	34.5*	7.6*		-11.3*			17.1*				

TC = total cholesterol; TG = triglyceride; LDL = low-density lipoprotein; VLDL = very low-density lipoprotein; HDL-C = high-density lipoprotein-cholesterol; APO = apoprotein; * = p < 0.05.

It has been claimed that β_1 selective blockers have relatively less effect on plasma lipids than propranolol. For the most extensively studied agents, such as metoprolol[68,93,97-106] and atenolol[74,79,85,107-119] (Table 5), however, the range of observed changes appears to overlap those reported for propranolol. The possibility that β_1 selective agents have less impact on plasma lipids seems dubious because there have been few direct comparisons of selective and nonselective agents in the same laboratories. Limited information suggests that the main effect of atenolol upon apolipoproteins is to reduce the level of A-I.

There is more convincing evidence for a unique effect on plasma lipids of β-blockers with intrinsic sympathomimetic activity (ISA).[134] As illustrated in Table 6, many have been reported to have no adverse effect or to possess a potentially beneficial effect by increasing HDL-cholesterol. Unfortunately, not all drugs with ISA have shown consistent effects, possibly reflecting their differing degrees of ISA potency. At present, there is insufficient evidence to make generalizations about this subgroup of β-blockers, although it does seem likely that pindolol, the agent with the most ISA, does not increase triglyceride or lower HDL-cholesterol, as commonly seen with other β-blockers.

Although the predominant effects of labetalol are those of β-blockade, its additional α_1-blocking-properties are of great interest. It might be anticipated that the drug would demonstrate a combination of the effects of nonselective β-blockers, such as propranolol, with those of drugs such as prazosin. As shown in Table 7, few studies have shown significant effects on plasma lipids. It is not clear whether the considerable variability in different reports represents experimental variability or perhaps differing degrees of expression of the relative α_1 and β-blocking properties of the drug in different patient samples. Although inconclusive, it seems that labetalol is less likely to cause potentially adverse effects on plasma lipids than most β-blockers.

As with the thiazide diuretics, there is relatively little information about the continuation of these effects with sustained β-blocker treatment. Some of the studies listed in Tables 3 to 7, however, involved 96 weeks of treatment. These studies show results compatible with those reported following short periods of treatment. In addition, the Veterans Administration Cooperative Study Group[135] reported a 25% increase in triglyceride values in 118 patients who received propranolol for 1 year.

Table 5.
β-Adrenergic Blockers (β₁-Selectivity)

Reference	# Pts.	Dose (mg)	Duration (weeks)	TC	TG	LDL	VLDL	HDL	HDL₂	HDL₃	LDL/HDL	HDL/TC	APO A-I	APO A-II	APO B
Acebutolol															
Birnbaum et al.[69] 1983	20	600–1800	8	-7.5	-2	-11.6*		-2.4							
Giuntoli et al.[95] 1984	16	400	52	5.8	24.7	-0.7		16.7							
Lehtonen[96] 1984	18	400–800	24	-4	2.3	-4.8	2.2	-6.8							
Miller et al.[82] 1987	8	400	48	-7	1.18	-7.48	-5.47	-1.7	9	-31.3*	-4.27				
Atenolol															
England et al.[97] 1980	34	100	12	-0.8	6.1			-10*					-9.8*		5.3
Eliasson et al.[107] 1981	15	100–200	32	6.9	20.5*	3.6	22.9*	0.7							
Rossner et al.[98] 1983	20	50	12	-0.3	6	-1.5	3.4	-2.1							
Day et al.[68] 1984	53	100	12	3	19.4*	-5	32.5*	-7*							
Lehtonen & Marniemi[108] 1984	18	100	24	8*	27*			-12*	-29*	-3.8					
Rouffy & Jaillard[109] 1984	26	100–200	12	2.9*	18*	5.6*	20*	-10.1*	-6.1*				-6.4*		2.9*
Durrington et al.[74] 1985	11	50	2	-2.5	11.7	0.3	3.4	-7.8	-11.3	1.5					-8.6
Lithell et al.[100] 1986	21	50	24	-2	2.3	-2.9	2	-5	-2	-5.5			-9*	-3.4	0.7
		100	24	-4.5	13	-7.5	17*	-6.6*	0	-12.3			-10*	-6.9	0
Neusy & Lowenstein[110] 1986	19	50–100	52	-1.9	17.5*	-4.2		-4.4	-20	0					
Pasotti et al.[99] 1986	15	100	12	1	20	3		1							
Rouffy & Jaillard[111] 1986	30	100–200	24	3*	22*	7*		-8*	-4				-9*		5*
Valimaki et al.[112] 1986	21	100	24	0	-2.9	-1.9		2.3	1.9	4					
Frick et al.[113] 1987	50	50–100	52	0.6	32.4*		-5.6*								-8.6
Harvengt et al.[79] 1987	10	100	0.5	-2	7.5	8.9		-19*					-4.3	-6.2	6.7
Nash et al.[114] 1987	40	50–100	10	-2.5	9.4			-6.2							

Study	n	Dose	Weeks	TC	LDL	HDL-C	TG	VLDL					
Ott et al.[115] 1987	56	50–100	20	0.7	6.1		−9						
Mazzola & Guerrasio[116] 1987	20	50–100	8	2.4	6.45*		−4				−5.26		12.3
Herpin et al.[117] 1988	10	50–100	8	−9.5	8.8	0.59	0.87			−0.72	−6.58		
Takashi et al.[118] 1989	6	50–100	12	−0.56	13.6		4.4						
Fogari et al.[85] 1989	25	100	96	−0.33	24.8*	−0.9	−18.6*		28.6*				
Superko et al.[119] 1989	14	50–100	48	2.7	20.3	1.3	−2.1		20.9		−5		
Lithell[101] 1989	60	50–100	32	0	18.3	−5.4*	−7.8*	22.6*		3.4			
Linden et al.[101] 1990	20	100	4	1.54	−3.37	3.17	−1.22						3.95
Bisoprolol													
Frithz & Weiner[120] 1986	41	2.5–40	54	4	20.5	0	0						
Lithell et al.[100] 1986	24	10	24	−1.7	17*	−2.9	−12.4*	22*	25.8	−1.5	−12	−6.5	4.5
	21	20	24	−3.8	13.8	−5.7	−14.7*	19.7*	33.9*	−1.5	−12	−7.6	1.5
Frithz & Weiner[121] 1987	43	2.5–40	12	3	5	0.3	0.7						
Fogari et al.[85] 1989	20	10	96	0.46	19*	0.24	−0.53			−0.45			
Metoprolol													
England et al.[97] 1980	34	200–400	12	−1	10*		−13*					−9.1*	−2.3
Pasotti et al.[102] 1982	16	100–200	12	6.2	0.5	5.6	0.7						
Frishman et al.[103] 1983	38	100–400	12	−6.6*	10.1	−6.6*	−6.2						
Rossner & Weiner[98] 1983	20	200	12	2.5	26.4	−3.3	−7.7	22.5*					
Day et al.[68] 1984	53	200	12	−1.4	12.5*	−4.4	−13*	26.3*					
Ferrara et al.[106] 1986	30	200	10	1	14*		−16.2*						−2.6
Pasotti et al.[99] 1986	15	200	12	6	10.6	3	−21						
Holtzman et al.[44] 1987	21	200–400	12	−2.38	22*	0	−7.5	−8*		−1.0			
Maternson et al.[104] 1989	138	100–400	48	1.8	24.5*	−0.7	2.85			4.3*			
Lithell[100] 1989	60	40–480	32	4.8	20.6*	−1.36	−5.8*	32.8*					6.74
Linden[101] 1990	20	100	4	−0.6	−8	1.3	−2.5						
Foss & Jensen[105] 1990	53	50–200	24	−2	10.3*	−1.1	−5.6*			−9.36*			

TC = total cholesterol; TG = triglyceride; LDL = low-density lipoprotein; VLDL = very low-density lipoprotein; HDL-C = high-density lipoprotein-cholesterol; APO = apoprotein; * = p < 0.05.

Table 6.
β-Adrenergic Blockers (Intrinsic Sympathomimetic Activity (% Change from Baseline))

Reference	# Pts.	Dose (mg)	Duration (weeks)	TC	TG	LDL	VLDL	HDL	HDL$_2$	HDL$_3$	LDL/HDL	HDL/TC	APO A-I	APO A-II	APO B
Alprenolol															
Jurgensen et al.[122] 1982	33	400	52	1.5	0	4.4	-16.7	12							
Bopindolol															
van Brummelen et al.[123] 1986	24	1-4	12	-2	24	-12		0							
Celiprolol†															
Herrmann et al.[124] 1988	15	200	12	-5.25	-23.4*	-8.1		29.6*			28.2*				
Fogari et al.[85] 1989	18	400	96	-5	-13.8	-4.2		11.2			-13.9				
Sirtori et al.[88] 1989	9N	200-600	16	-5.17	-18.12	-6.8	-19.4††	6.4			-11.36		-7.68		-14.95
	9H	200-600	16	-5.64	3.53	-10.5	21.8††	1.96			-8.6		6.84		3.5
Dilevalol†															
Frishman et al.[125] 1988	42	100-800	48	0	22	-1*		15			-0.29				
Materson et al.[104] 1989	311	200-1600	48	.45	12.7	-1.7		9.1			-5.86				
Mepindolol															
Pasotti et al.[99] 1986	15	10	12	-2	23	-10		4							
Fogari et al.[85] 1989	18	10	96	-2.2	-14	-1.66		4.48			-6.3				
Oxprenolol															
Simons et al.[126] 1982	12	160-320	32	6.6	25	6.8	33	10.3							
Day et al.[68] 1984	53	160	12	-1.3	21*	-3.9	35*	-11.5*							
Penbutolol															
Valimaki[112] 1986	21	40	24	6	22.6	6	35	-12*	-11	-13.8					
Pindolol															
Miettinen et al.[127] 1982	12	10	5 yr	8.7	31			0.8							

Study	n	Dose (mg)	Duration (wk)	TC	TG	LDL	VLDL	HDL					
Pasotti et al.[102] 1982	16	7.5–15	12	0.3	1.8	4		16.6*					
Karmakosk et al.[128] 1983	13	5–15	16	4.3	−20.4	10.9		−3.9					
Lehtonen & Marniemi[108] 1984	20	10–20	52	1.1	6.6	−2.7	6.3	10.2			5.3	−0.4	
Durrington et al.[74] 1985	11	10	2	−1.2	24*	−6.7	42.6	−2.8	−12.7	8			−4.3
Lehtonen[129] 1985	11	10–20	24	−3.9	3.4	−5.3	3.3	3.3					
Carlson et al.[130] 1987	47	5–15	24	−1.2	19*	−3.9*	13.3*	−1.5		−2.4			
Harvengt et al.[79] 1987	10	15	0.5	−2.2	1.7	0		−7.6*			0.2	0	−12.6
Northcote & Ballantyne[90] 1987	19	2.5–5	52	−3.1	0	−2.4	−6	−3	15.9	−5.5	4.3	−1.2	9.3
Roman et al.[131] 1987	17	10–20	24	.47	−20.9*	.5		−17.9*		−16.3*			
Herpin et al.[117] 1988	11	15	8	−5.7	20.3	12.9	1.7			10.1	−4.9		2.67

TC = total cholesterol; TG = triglyceride; LDL = low-density lipoprotein; VLDL = very low-density lipoprotein; HDL = high-density lipoprotein; APO = apoprotein; * = p < .05; † = after 5th week; † = celiprolol and dilevalol have partial β2-agonist activity.

Table 7.
α-β-Adrenergic Blockade (Labetalol) (% Change from Baseline)

Reference	# Pts.	Dose (mg)	Duration (weeks)	TC	TG	LDL	VLDL	HDL
Frishman et al.[103] 1983	38	200–1200	12	0	0.7	0.7		−0.8
Ponti et al.[70] 1983	11	400	6	6.2	1.2			−7.4
Weber et al.[73] 1984	25	400–1200	4	0.4	11.7			23
Flamenbaum et al.[75] 1985	59	200–1200	52	2	2			4
Ohman et al.[132] 1985	25	400–800	6	0	25			−12.5*
Farry et al.[133] 1989	20	200–400	16	.85		2.35		

TC = total cholesterol; TG = triglyceride; LDL = low-density lipoprotein; VLDL = very low-density lipoprotein; HDL = high-density lipoprotein; * = $p < 0.05$.

Mechanisms of Lipid Modifying Effect

Different mechanisms have been proposed to explain the lipid modifying effects of β-adrenergic blockers.[1,5] The most likely one appears to relate to the effects of these drugs on lipoprotein lipase (LPL)[136-138] that is seen with nonselective β-blockade (propranolol). Since unopposed α-adrenergic stimulation inhibits LPL activity,[139] a reduction in LPL would retard VLDL and triglyceride catabolism, resulting in higher triglyceride concentrations. Subsequently, HDL-cholesterol, a product of VLDL catabolism, would decrease. Some β-blockers, especially those having ISA or combined α-β-blockade, appear to have less influence on triglyceride and HDL levels.[134] These observations suggest that these drugs do not inhibit LPL activity to the same degree as propranolol. Propranolol has also been shown to inhibit insulin release,[140-143] which can further impair LPL activity and decrease the removal of triglycerides from the circulation.

Some β-adrenergic blockers (propranolol, metoprolol) have been shown to decrease lecithin cholesterol acyltransferase (LCAT) activity and by this mechanism suppress HDL cholesterol levels.[144] A-I is specifically decreased with some β-blockers.[145,146] Pindolol, a β-blocker with ISA, has been shown to increase LCAT activity, A-I levels, and HDL cholesterol.[147]

Since β-blockers decrease free fatty acid levels in the blood, it is unlikely that increased triglyceride synthesis could explain the changes in serum lipid levels.[68,148]

Alpha$_1$-Adrenergic Blocking Agents

In strong contrast to the potentially detrimental effects of thiazide diuretics and β-blocking agents on lipids and lipoproteins, many studies have suggested that the α_1-blocking agents may produce desirable changes in lipid profiles. Early studies by Kirkendall and associates[149] and by Leren's group[65] showed that customary clinical doses of prazosin for 8-week periods produced small but significant reductions in total cholesterol levels. In contrast with patients given propranolol, Leren's group showed that those receiving up to 4 mg daily of prazosin showed no reduction in HDL-cholesterol but a significant drop in non-HDL-cholesterol levels.[65] The two drugs also had opposite effects on serum triglycerides.[65] As illustrated in Table 8, most subsequent studies have reported similar trends. Although not always significant, almost all studies have shown some degree of reduction in total cholesterol and triglyceride levels. There also is reasonably consistent reporting that total cholesterol levels fall because of reduction in non-HDL-cholesterol levels. It is of particular interest that HDL-cholesterol levels are preserved and, often, significantly increased by about 5%. As a result, the relative proportions of HDL- to non-HDL-cholesterol levels may be improved more dramatically.

It would be anticipated that other α_1-blocking agents would have effects similar to those of prazosin, and the information currently available (Tables 9 and 10) tends to support this view.

There is an obvious need for studies of the long-term effects of this group of agents on plasma lipids. Few studies have followed more than 10 patients for a period of at least a year, but these studies show changes similar to those of shorter term administration. In view of the potential importance of the reported observations with the α_1-blockers, there is a clear need for additional studies to validate the long-term efficacy of these agents in increasing the ratio of HDL- to non-HDL-cholesterol levels.

Mechanisms of Action

α_1-Adrenergic inhibitors appear to have a favorable effect on lipoprotein metabolism.[175] The drugs on average reduce triglycerides by 7.5%, total cholesterol by 4.5%, and raise HDL-cholesterol by 8%. Consequently, the ratio between HDL-cholesterol and total cholesterol is augmented.[5]

There are multiple explanations for the benefit of α_1 blockade.[1] First, LPL activity has been shown to increase with prazosin and doxazosin,[176] and this action could increase catabolism of VLDL and decrease triglyceride levels.[65] Increased catabolism of VLDL could explain the increase in HDL observed with these drugs. A-I is increased with prazosin.[111] High-dose doxazosin in vitro has been shown to increase LDL receptor activity, and this effect could lower LDL- cholesterol and total cholesterol levels.[177] Finally, prazosin can inhibit phosphodiesterase activity, and concurrent increments in 3' 5'-adenosine monophosphate could modulate cholesterol metabolism and fatty acid synthesis in the liver.[178]

Table 8.
α₁-Adrenergic Blockade (Prazosin) (% Change from Baseline)

Reference	# Pts.	Dose (mg)	Duration (weeks)	TC	TG	LDL	VLDL	HDL	HDL_2	HDL_3	LDL/HDL	HDL/TC	APO A-I	APO A-II	APO B
Leren et al.[65] 1980	23	0.5-4	8	-8.9*	-16.2*	LDL + VLDL -10.1*		-4.1							
Harvard et al.[150] 1982	17	3-18	12	-3.8*	3.9			2.8							
Kokubu[151] 1982	14	1.5-12	12	-0.7	0.9	-4.5		12.5*							
Kather et al.[152] 1984	15	1-15	12	2.9	6.4			8.6*							
Rouffy & Jaillard[109] 1984	26	0.5-15	12	-7.9*	-9.9*	-13.4*	-18.8*	13.1*	14.6*				10.5*	-7.5*	
Takabatake et al.[153] 1984	15	1.5-15	52	2	-7.3			17*							
Cambien & Plouin[155] 1985	15	0.5-3	5	-3.1	-1.1			-3.3							-3.6
Deger[154] 1986	32	1-20	4	-3.7	-4	-6.4*		6.1							
Ferrara et al.[106] 1986	30	4	10	-6.9*	2.9			12.5*							4.7
Harter et al.[76] 1986	10	2-12	12	0	-8*		-6*	16*	4	19*					
Neusy & Lowenstein[110] 1986	11	2-20	52	-12*	-3.4	-16.9*		-6	-13	0					
Rouffy & Jaillard[111] 1986	29	2-15	24	-9*	-9*	-14*		13*	10				16*		-8*
Torvik & Madsbu[156] 1986	49	1-20	16	-6.4	-10.1			2							
Velasco et al.[78] 1986	10	1-8	8	-11*	-13.9	-7.7	-23	-15.8	-5	-4.5					
Magarian et al.[84] 1987	16	Var	16-24	-2	15	0	-3	-6							

Table 8.—Continued
α_1-Adrenergic Blockade (Prazosin) (% Change from Baseline)

Reference	# Pts.	Dose (mg)	Duration (weeks)	TC	TG	LDL	VLDL	HDL	HDL2	HDL3	LDL/ HDL	HDL/ TC	APO A-I	APO A-II	APO B
Nakamura[157] 1987	16	1-3	8	-12	-20			0					1		-8
Pool[158] 1987	49	1-20	18-24	-6.4	-10.3			2							
Stamler et al.[159] 1988	49	1-10	96	-5.6*	12.5*	.01		0.1				0.2			
Lasser et al.[45] 1989	29	2-20	28	0.6	1.3	-2.6		12.1			-11.5				
Rockhold et al.[160] 1987	193	1-10	12-20	-2	17.1*	-5.67*	-20.4			-2.94					
Alderman[87] 1989	34	2-20	48	-4.56	0.1	-5.9		6.28	10.45	3.77	11.44				
Farry et al.[133] 1989	20	1-10	8	-1.62	0.1	-16.55		-7.8			-9.57				
Swislocki et al.[161] 1989	12	1-10	10	-3.6*	-7.7*	-3.85*	-28.9*	21.05*			-21*				

TC = total cholesterol; TG = triglyceride; LDL = low-density lipoprotein; VLDL = very low-density lipoprotein; HDL = high-density lipoprotein; APO = apoprotein; * = $p < 0.05$.

Table 9.
α₁-Adrenergic Blockade (Doxazosin) (% Change from Baseline)

Reference	# Pts.	Dose (mg)	Duration (weeks)	TC	TG	LDL	VLDL	HDL	HDL₂	HDL₃	LDL/HDL	HDL/TC	APO A-I	APO A-II	APO B
Lehtonen et al.[162] 1986	18	1–16	20	−8.9*	−4.7*	−16.9*	−3.3	8*	19.4	0					
Frick et al.[163] 1986	39	1–16	20–52	−1.7	−5*			3.9*							
Torvik & Madsbu[164] 1986	46	1–16	16	−3.9	−12.6*			6.3							
Frick et al.[113] 1987	46	1–16	52	−1.6	−5.9*			7.2*				8.7			
Hjortdahl et al.[42] 1987	40	1–16	24	−3.9	−7.2			−0.7							
Nash et al.[114] 1987	38	1–16	10	−2.9	−11			2				5.2			
Ott et al.[115] 1987	51	1–16	20	−0.8	−1.7			0.7				6.9			
Pool[158] 1987	142	1–16	10–24	−1.2	−9.1*			7.6							
	46	1–16	18–24	−3.9	−12.6			6.3							
	25	1–16	18–24	−5.6	−14.6*			3.5*							
	39	1–16	52	−1.7	−5*			3.9*							
Torvik & Madsbu[156] 1987	52	1–16	52	−3.6	−1.17			5				8.9			
1987															
Trost et al.[41] 1987	19	2–20	24	−6.1	−17.4			13				19.7*			
Mazzola & Guerrasio[116] 1987	20	1–16	8	−7.1*	−8.1*			11*				9.75*			
Cubeddu et al.[165] 1988	49	1–16	15	−4.7	−4.8	−9.0*		0.3				3.0			
Giorgi et al.[166] 1988	20	1–10	8	−3	−7.8*			6.0*				9.45*			
Talseth et al.[167] 1988	110	1–16	52	−1.1	−4.7			−3.1*				4.4*			

Table 9.—Continued
α₁-Adrenergic Blockade (Doxazosin) (% Change from Baseline)

Reference	# Pts.	Dose (mg)	Duration (weeks)	TC	TG	LDL	VLDL	HDL	HDL₂	HDL₃	LDL/HDL	HDL/TC	APO A-I	APO A-II	APO B
Nechwatal et al.[168] 1988	36	1–16	10	.54	6.15			16.3				2.7			
Taylor et al.[169] 1988	31	1–16	18	−1.92	−0.68			0.66				2.63			
Ames & Kiyasu[170] 1989	15	1–16	10	0	−1.49	−2.8		9.4	8.57				−11.1*	−5.68	.1

TC = total cholesterol; TG = triglyceride; LDL = low-density lipoprotein; VLDL = very low-density lipoprotein; HDL = high-density lipoprotein; APO = apoprotein; * = p < 0.05.

Table 10.
Other α_1-Adrenergic Blockade (% Change from Baseline)

Reference	# Pts.	Dose (mg)	Duration (weeks)	TC	TG	LDL	VLDL	HDL	HDL$_2$	HDL$_3$	LDL/ HDL	HDL/ TC	APO A-I	APO A-II	APO B
Trimazosin															
Singleton & Taylor[171] 1983	48	100–800	52	−3.8*	5.4		2								
Taylor et al.[172] 1983	42	100–300	52	−4.8	−5.4		2								
Lehtonen[129] 1985	11	100–400	24	5.4	−13.4	10.5	−13.6	10.5	−13.6	2.2					
Terazosin															
Ferrier et al.[173] 1986	15	2–20	8	−5.5	−3.5	−5.4	3.6	0							
Deger[148] 1986	128	5–20	4	−2.5*	−8	−3.6* (LDL + VLDL)		−1.6							
	38	5–20	4	−3.1	−1.6	−5* (LDL + VLDL)		4.2							
Indoramin															
Martinez[174] 1986	29		12	−4.7	−13.37	−8.8*		0.5			−17.65*	37.15*			10.91*

TC = total cholesterol; TG = triglyceride; LDL = low-density lipoprotein; VLDL = very low-density lipoprotein; HDL = high-density lipoprotein; APO = apoprotein; * = $p < 0.05$.

Centrally Acting Agents (α_2-Agonists)

It has been suggested that clonidine and methyldopa can suppress cholesterol synthesis in extrahepatic and hepatic cells through inhibitory effects on both β_2- and α_2 adrenoreceptors. Surprisingly, there have been few studies that have assessed α_2-agonists and the changes in lipid profiles.

Following the early report by Kirkendall et al of a mean 8% decrease in total cholesterol in hypertensive patients receiving clonidine,[149] subsequent studies have confirmed this slight reduction (Table 11).[179-181] Kaplan[182] reported that guanabenz produced a 10% reduction in total cholesterol and a 14% reduction in LDL-cholesterol in 39 patients after 4 weeks of treatment. In a retrospective analysis of 87 diabetic patients who were receiving guanabenz for an average of 7 months for the treatment of coexisting hypertension, total cholesterol was noted to decrease by a mean of 6%.[183] McCarron[184] also found a 7% reduction in total cholesterol after both 4 weeks and 6 months of guanabenz treatment of hypertensives. Similarly, Hauger-Klevene et al[185,186] showed that 2 years of treatment with guanfacine in 30 patients was associated with significant reductions of 14% in total cholesterol and 15% in triglyceride levels. Finally, Fillingim's group[187] demonstrated no significant difference between guanfacine and placebo in 21 patients followed for 8 weeks. Taken together, these studies strongly suggest that α_2 stimulants have no detrimental effects and probably reduce total cholesterol levels. A more detailed study assessing the effects of these agents on lipoproteins and apoproteins is indicated.

Although there have been only a few studies of methyldopa, two small studies both showed significant reductions in HDL-cholesterol levels. In one study,[30] 17 patients followed for 1 year showed no change in total cholesterol or triglyceride levels, but a 15% reduction in HDL-cholesterol. In 14 patients followed for 12 weeks, Leon and associates[72] demonstrated tendencies for reduction in both total cholesterol and triglycerides, but the only significant change was an 11% reduction in HDL-cholesterol level. In contrast, Velasco and coworkers[188] reported a mean 10% increase in HDL-cholesterol levels when methyldopa was given to patients already taking HCTZ.

Adrenergic Neuron Blockers

In this category, only debrisoquine has been studied, with Weidmann and coworkers,[189] reporting that 4 weeks of treatment in 20 pa-

Table 11.
Centrally Acting Agents and Direct Vasodilators (% Change from Baseline)

Reference	# Pts.	Dose (mg)	Duration (weeks)	TC	TG	LDL	VLDL	HDL	LDL/HDL	HDL/TC
Clonidine										
Kirkendall et al.[149] 1978	16	0.1–1.2	12	−8.2*						
Karlberg et al.[179] 1985	23	.045–0.2	26	−5.5	12.1	2.34	1.49	−0.65	−2.97	−5.3
Nilson-Ehle et al.[180] 1987	20	.075–0.3	12	−1.92	−0.59	1.03		5.88	−0.5	
Guanabenz										
Kaplan[182] 1984	39	−16	96	9.84*	12.12	14.3*		−3.07	−11.5	7.42
Pinacidil										
Rockhold et al.[160] 1987	36	12.5–75	12–20	−9.8*	−21.6*	−8.1*		3.6*	−0.5*	

TC = total cholesterol; TG = triglyceride; LDL = low-density lipoprotein; VLDL = very low-density lipoprotein; HDL-C = high-density lipoprotein-cholesterol;
* = $p < 0.05$.

tients produced significant reductions in total cholesterol and apoprotein B levels. Tendencies for general reductions in mean lipid levels were noted, about 2% in HDL, 6% in LDL, 8% in total cholesterol, 14% in triglycerides, and 29% in VLDL-cholesterol.

The complex effects of reserpine include actions in both the central nervous system and adrenergic neurons. Its effect on lipids has been studied only by Ames and Hill[30] who reported no significant effect of treatment for up to 1 year.

Direct Vasodilators

Deming and coworkers[190] demonstrated a 12% reduction in total cholesterol in seven patients receiving high doses of hydralazine for 16 weeks. However, no significant effect was seen with doses that would be more usual today. Gerber and colleagues[191] have reported a significant 24% increase in HDL-cholesterol and 17% in apoprotein B levels in 12 patients receiving carprazidil for a period of 16 weeks. Another new vasodilator, endralazine, produced no significant effect on lipid profiles.[192]

Of course, vasodilator drugs normally are given as add-on therapy to patients insufficiently controlled by one or more other agents. In 11 patients who were controlled inadequately by nadolol and chlorthalidone, a mean dose of 7 mg of minoxidil was reported by Johnson and colleagues[193] to produce a 20% improvement in the ratio of HDL- to total cholesterol. Compared with measurements made while the patients were receiving nadolol and chlorthalidone, a significant increase in mean HDL-cholesterol level and decrease in mean LDL-cholesterol level were noted. Although very limited, these studies suggest that the more powerful vasodilators tend to improve plasma lipid profiles.

Pinacidil is a vasodilator with a novel mechanism of action, which involves opening of potassium channels in vascular smooth muscle. In a recent study [160] the drug was also shown to improve the lipid profile of hypertensive patients (Table 11).

Angiotensin-Converting Enzyme Inhibitors

In contrast to HCTZ and propranolol therapy, the ACE inhibitors do not affect blood glucose and may favorably influence plasma lipids and lipoproteins.

The initial report of Ohman's group was that captopril, administered to 20 patients for 2 years, produced no significant effect on triglyceride or total cholesterol levels.[194] Reporting on two multicenter trials, Weinberger[195] confirmed the lack of an effect on mean total cholesterol levels with daily doses of 75 to 100 mg of captopril. In parallel groups of approximately 80 patients, HCTZ (40-50 mg daily) produced significant increases in total cholesterol over 6 weeks, whereas patients receiving both HCTZ and captopril showed smaller, nonsignificant tendencies for total cholesterol to rise. More recently it has been suggested that captopril and enalapril, longer-acting nonsulfhydrl ACE inhibitors, actually may cause a modest reduction in triglycerides and total cholesterol, while causing a modest rise in total and HDL-cholesterol and the HDL_2 subfraction (Table 12). These findings need to be confirmed in larger studies. The drugs certainly can blunt some of the lipid changes seen with thiazide diuretics.[1] Many other ACE inhibitors are in clinical trials. It is assumed that their effects on serum lipids will be similar to those of captopril and enalapril.

Calcium Channel Blockers

The metabolic effects of the calcium channel blockers were reviewed in a recent article by Schoen et al.[203] In experimental studies, verapamil and nifedipine were shown to increase LDL receptor activity.[4] It is also known that nifedipine can stimulate neutral cholesterol ester hydrolase activity, which results in an increased intracellular free cholesterol concentration. Increased cellular cholesterol may induce HDL binding activity at the cell surface and enhance efflux of cholesterol, leading to an increase of HDL in plasma.[4]

Reports of the metabolic effects of this group of drugs have also been discussed by Trost and Weidmann in an extensive review of clinical studies carried out between 1972-1987.[204] Of 43 studies, five were conducted in noninsulin-dependent diabetic subjects. The drugs studied were diltiazem in nine reports, verapamil in nine studies, nifedipine in 22 studies, and another dihydropyridine (usually nitrendipine) in 12 reports. In general, the better quality studies were those of short duration, including five double-blind, placebo-controlled trials in which no evidence of any effect on plasma lipoproteins was observed. In almost all of the studies, in which the duration of treatment varied from a few weeks to 5 years, no change was observed in total cholesterol,

Table 12.
Angiotensin-Converting Enzyme Inhibitors (% Change from Baseline)

Reference	# Pts.	Dose (mg)	Duration (weeks)	TC	TG	LDL	VLDL	HDL	HDL$_2$	HDL$_3$	LDL/HDL	HDL/TC	APO A-I	APO A-II	APO B
Captopril															
Ohman et al.[194] 1984	20	25–150	96	1.52											
Saltvedt et al.[196] 1986	23	25–100	24	5.55			19.6*								
Ghirlanda et al.[197] 1986	17	25–100	24	−13.66*	−15.33	−15.78		−1.93				13.1*			
Costa et al.[199] 1988	24	25–50	24	−18.0*	−25*			21.95*				47.55*			
Pollare et al.[48] 1989	48	25–50	32	−1.0	−1.4	7.4		−3.0				−2.18			
Sasaki & Arakoua[100] 1989	17	25–50	12	0.46	5.8	−7.97	5.62	3.77	25.5*	−18.21*	−11.72		6.71*	1.32	4.85
Foss & Jensen[105] 1990	51	25–100	24	0.6	−10.6*	0.9		6.2			−6.64	5.4			
Enalapril															
Perani et al.[198] 1987	12	20–40	16	1.0	26.0*	−3.0		23.0*	42.0*	−14.0*		22.0*	11.0*		
Taylor et al.[169] 1988	31	10–40	18	−2.81	−1.35			1.45				4.46			
Leren et al.[94] 1988	57	10–20	24	1.5	−9.0	2.1		0.7			−0.7				
Sasaki & Arakowa[201] 1989	21	2.5–10	12	1.33	−15.73	4.38	−9.76		−6.5	−7.93	2.63				
Zofenopril															
LaCourciere & Gagne[202] 1989	18	5–10	12	2.53	1.08	−4.57		−0.1	−5.0	5.63	−1.2	6.52			2.75

TC = total cholesterol; TG = triglyceride; LDL = low-density lipoprotein; VLDL = very low-density lipoprotein; HDL-C = high-density lipoprotein-cholesterol; APO = apoprotein; * = p < 0.05.

triglyceride, or HDL-cholesterol levels. Even within the few studies in which significant changes were reported, no consistent trend was apparent. In 38 studies reporting on HDL-cholesterol levels, for example, three showed a significant increase, two showed a decrease, and the rest showed no change. Similarly, almost all of the studies in diabetic subjects showed no influence of any of the calcium channel blockers on either glucose homeostasis or plasma lipids. It appears reasonable to conclude that none of the currently available calcium channel blockers has any clear effect upon plasma lipids. More recent studies (Table 13) have suggested the same conclusion.

Combination Regimens

Often, combinations of antihypertensive drugs are used to manage patients with high blood pressure. Several studies have examined combination antihypertensive therapies and their influence on lipoprotein metabolism. This experience has been reviewed by Lardinois and Neuman.[1] Most studies in this review combined a thiazide diuretic with a nondiuretic agent. Results from studies where nondiuretic combinations were used have also been reported.

The overall conclusions that were reached by Lardinois and Neuman[1] were that combination regimens that include a thiazide diuretic plus a β-adrenergic blocker devoid of ISA, reserpine, or methyldopa have the greatest adverse effects on serum lipid values—often worse than with thiazides alone.[1] Combination regimens that include a thiazide diuretic plus either an α_1-adrenergic blocker, a β-blocker with ISA, or an ACE inhibitor have a more favorable lipid profile. The adverse effects of thiazides on lipids can be neutralized by the addition of another drug having a more favorable lipid profile. Finally, it appears that nondiuretic antihypertensive combinations that include agents that are lipid neutral would also be beneficial.[1]

Conclusions

For many of the agents frequently prescribed in the treatment of cardiovascular disease, there appears to be ample evidence that specific changes in the levels of plasma lipids and lipoproteins occur. The extent of these changes for drugs for which there are reports sufficient to

Table 13.
Calcium Channel Blockers (% Changes from Baseline)

Reference	# Pts.	Dose (mg)	Duration (weeks)	TC	TG	LDL	VLDL	HDL	HDL₂	HDL₃	LDL/HDL	HDL/TC	APO A-I	APO A-II	APO B
Amlodipine														
Osterloch[210] 1989	847		48	2.2	-1.9										
Diltiazem														
Schulte et al.[205] 1986	19	240–360	8	-2.55	-0.7	-7.8*	26.1	3.2			-10.7	5.7			
Pool et al.[208] 1988	50	240–360	8	0.46	3.55	3.9		2.0							
Pollare et al.[209] 1989	26	180–360	24	-3.8	-13.4	-1.0	-12.5	1.7					-2.9		
Nifedipine														
Schulte et al.[205] 1986	18	40–60	8	-3.6	-27.9	6.56	-33.3*	-7.5			-15.1	-3.9			
Nisoldipine														
Perani et al.[206] 1987	15	5–20	6	5.0	6.0	1.0		14.0*	16.0	13.0*	-9.24	7.94	12.0*		3.0
Takahashi et al.[118] 1989	7	2.5–5.0	12	-13.83*	-12.7			7.41				-7.9			
Nitrendipine														
Nechwatal et al.[168] 1988	36	10–20	18	-3.36	16.67			2.96				-0.38			
Verapamil														
Lehtonen[96] 1984	13	200	24	0.76	9.2	-0.22	8.7	2.05			-2.2	1.34			

Midtbo et al.[207] 1988	10	240–480	384	−1.4			18.75*
Midtbo et al.[207] 1988	10	240–480	288	−4.6	−10.6	22.41*	
Midtbo et al.[207] 1988	25	240–480	192	−2.08	−0.72	25.64*	28.39*

TC = total cholesterol; TG = triglyceride; LDL = low-density lipoprotein; VLDL = very low density lipoprotein; HDL-C = high-density lipoprotein-cholesterol; APO = apoprotein; * = p < 0.05.

calculate the median value of mean percentage changes observed in individual studies is summarized in Table 14. This type of measurement only can be considered a gross approximation, because it does not attempt to take account of the relative quality or the relative sample size of each study, or the dose, duration, or drug administration.

It appears unlikely that any single mechanism will be found to explain the complex pattern of lipid changes that can occur with some of these agents, although all vasodilators are at least lipid neutral. No convincing evidence has yet been produced to support any of the various theories of production of these lipid changes. Understanding the mechanism by which these changes occur would make it easier to assess their importance. If it is accepted that any intervention changing plasma concentrations of lipoproteins also will alter the rate of development of atherosclerosis, then the changes must be of considerable significance.[2] Indeed, it appears that there is a greater than 2% increase in risk of cardiovascular events associated with every 1% increase in LDL-cholesterol or 1% decrease in HDL-cholesterol.[2,211]

With the new recommendations for dietary and other methods to control plasma lipid abnormalities,[211] many of the patients being seen in cardiac and hypertension clinics have plasma lipid levels that qualify them for consideration for such programs. The impact of methods for controlling plasma lipid abnormalities, however, clearly will be inhibited by some of the agents that are being used in the treatment of hypertension and other cardiovascular diseases.[10] Many considerations, including efficacy, cost, and relative frequency of side effects are in-

Table 14.
Calculated Approximations of the Extent of Drug Effect on Plasma Lipids (%)

	TC	TG	HDL	LDL
Thiazides	7	14	2	10
Propranolol	0	16	−11	−3
Atenolol	0	15	−7	−2
Pindolol	−1	7	−2	−3
α_1-blockers	−4	−8	5	−13
α_2-Stimulants	−7	—	—	—
Calcium channel blockers	0	0	0	0
ACE inhibitors	0	−5	5	0

TC = total cholesterol; TG = triglyceride; HDL = high-density lipoprotein; LDL = low-density lipoprotein.

Table 15.
Antihypertensive Drug Selection Considerations with Lipid Abnormalities

Lipid Abnormality	Avoid	Consider
Type II, IIa ↑LDL, ↑Cholesterol	Thiazide	Other drugs, especially α_1-blockers
Type IIb, ↑Cholesterol, ↓HDL, ↑Triglyceride, ↑LDL	β-blockers without ISA; thiazides	Other drugs, especially α_1-blockers
Type I, IV, V, ↑Triglyceride	β-blockers without ISA; thiazides	Other drugs
Type III, ↑Triglyceride, ↑Cholesterol	Thiazides	Other drugs

↑ = elevated; ↓ = low; HDL = high-density lipoprotein; LDL = low-density lipoprotein; ISA = intrinsic sympathomimetic activity.

volved in selecting a drug for any patient. Table 15 indicates the special additional considerations that are recommended for cardiac or hypertensive patients in whom common lipid abnormalities are detected.

References

1. Lardinois CK, Neuman SL: The effects of antihypertnsive agents on serum lipids and lipoproteins. Arch Intern Med 1988; 148: 1280-1288.
2. Houston MC: New insights and new approaches for the treatment of essential hypertension. Selection of therapy based on coronary heart disease risk factor analysis, hemodynamic profiles, quality of life, and subsets of hypertension. Am Heart J 1989; 117: 911-950.
3. Grimm RH: Treating hypertension and cardiovascular risk: are there trade-offs? Am Heart J 1990; 119: 729-732.
4. Krone W, Nagele H: Effects of antihypertensives on plasma lipids and lipoprotein metabolism. Am Heart J 1988; 116: 1729-1733.
5. Weidmann P, Ferrier C, Saxenhofer H, et al: Serum lipoproteins during treatment with antihypertensive drugs. Drugs 1988; 35 (Suppl 6): 118-134.
6. Dzau VJ: Treatment strategies: an evaluation of antihypertensive therapy. Am J Med 1989; 86 (Suppl lB): 113-115.
7. Johnson BF, Danylchuk MA: The relevance of plasma lipid changes with cardiovascular drug therapy. Med Clin N Amer 1989; 73: 449-473.
8. Working Group on Management of Patients with Hypertension and High Blood Cholesterol: National Education Programs Working Group Report on the Management of Patients with Hypertension and High Blood Cholesterol. Ann Intern Med 1991; 114: 224-237.

9. Veterans Administration Cooperative Study Group on Antihypertensive Agents: Effects of treatment on morbidity in hypertension. II. Results in patients with diastolic blood pressure averaging 90 through 114 mmHg. JAMA 1970; 213: 1143-1152.

10. 1988 Joint National Committee. The 1988 report of the Joint National Committee on detection, evaluation and treatment of high blood pressure. Arch Intern Med 1988; 148: 1023-1038.

11. Hypertension Detection and Follow-Up Program Cooperative Group: Five-year findings of The Hypertension Detection and Follow-Up Program. I. Reduction in mortality of persons with high blood pressure, including mild hypertension. JAMA 1979; 242: 2562-2574.

12. Medical Research Council Working Party: MRC trial of treatment of mild hypertension: principal results. Br Med J 1985; 291: 97-104.

13. Medical Research Council Working Party: Report of MRC Working Party on mild to moderate hypertension: adverse reactions to bendrofluazide and propranolol for the treatment of hypertension. Lancet 1981; 2: 539-542.

14. Murphy MB, Lewis PJ, Kohner EH, et al: Glucose intolerance in hypertensive patients treated with diuretics. A 14 year follow up. Lancet 1982; 2: 1293-1295.

15. Bloomgarden ZT, Ginsberg-Fellner F, Rayfield EJ, et al: Elevated hemoglobin A_{1c} and low-density lipoprotein cholesterol levels in thiazide-treated diabetic patients. Am J Med 1984; 77: 823-827.

16. Basabe J, Grant A, Johnson B, et al: Structural modification of therapeutic agents and their effect on insulin secretion. In Diabetes, Proceedings of the Seventh Congress of the International Diabetes Federation. Amsterdam, Excerpta Medica 1971; 476-484.

17. Spellacy WN, Cohn JE, Birk SA: Effects of diuril and dilantin on blood glucose and insulin levels in late pregnancy. Obstet Gynecol 1975; 45: 159-162.

18. Johnson BF, Munro-Faure AD, Slack J: Diuretic-induced hyper triglyceridemia. Lancet 1976; 1: 1019.

19. Johnson B, Bye C, Labrooy J, et al: Relation of antihypertensive treatment to plasma lipids and other risk factors in hypertensives. Clin Sci Mol Med 1974; 47: 9-10.

20. Ames RP, Hill P: Elevation of serum lipid levels during diuretic therapy of hypertension. Am J Med 1976; 61: 748-757.

21. Rosenthal T, Holtzman E, Segal P: The effect of chlorthalidone on serum lipids and lipoproteins. Atherosclerosis 1980; 36: 111-115.

22. van Brummelen P, Gevers Leuven JA, van Gent CM: Influence of hydrochlorothiazide on the plasma levels of triglycerides, total cholesterol and HDL cholesterol in patients with essential hypertension. Curr Med Res Opin 1979; 6: 24-29.

23. Gluck Z, Weidmann P, Mordasini R, et al: Increased serum low- density lipoprotein cholesterol in men treated short-term with the diuretic chlorthalidone. Metabolism 1980; 29: 240-425.

24. Goldman AI, Steele BW, Schnaper HW, et al: Serum lipoprotein levels during chlorthalidone therapy - a Veterans Administration-National

Heart, Lung and Blood Institute cooperative study on antihypertensive therapy: mild hypertension. JAMA 1980; 244: 1691-1695.

25. Crisp AJ, Kennedy PG, Hoffbrand BI, et al: Lipids and lipoprotein fractions after cyclopenthiazide and oxprenolol: a double-blind crossover study. Curr Med Res Opin 1980; 7: 101-103.

26. Mordasini R, Gluck Z, Weidmann P, et al: Zur pathogenese der diuretika-induzierten hyperlipoproteinamie. Klin Wochenschr 1980; 58: 359-363.

27. Joos C, Kewitz H, Reinhold-Kourniati D: Effects of diuretics on plasma lipoproteins in healthy men. Eur J Clin Pharmacol 1980; 17: 251-257.

28. Grimm RH, Leon AS, Hunninghake DB, et al: Effects of thiazide diuretics on plasma lipids and lipoproteins in mildly hypertensive patients. Ann Intern Med 1981; 94: 7-11.

29. Bauer JH, Brooks CS, Weinstein I, et al: Effects of diuretic and propranolol on plasma lipoprotein lipids. Clin Pharmacol Ther 1981; 30: 35-43.

30. Ames RP, Hill P: Antihypertensive therapy and the risk of coronary heart disease. J Cardiovasc Pharmacol 1982; 4 (Suppl 2): S206-S212.

31. Boehringer K, Weidmann P, Mordasini R, et al: Menopause-dependent plasma lipoprotein alterations in diuretic-treated women. Ann Intern Med 1982; 97: 206-209.

32. Grimm RH, Leon AS, Hunninghake DB, et al: Diuretics and plasma lipids: Effects of thiazides and spironolactone. In Noseda et al (eds): Lipoproteins and Coronary Atherosclerosis. Amsterdam, Elsevier, 1982; 371-376.

33. Meier A, Weidmann P, Mordasini R, et al: Reversal or prevention of diuretic-induced alterations in serum lipoproteins with β blockers. Atherosclerosis 1982; 41: 415-419.

34. Schiffl H, Weidmann P, Mordasini R, et al: Reversal of diuretic-induced increases in serum low-density lipoprotein cholesterol by the β-blocker pindolol. Metabolism 1982; 31: 411-415.

35. Valimaki M, Harno K, Nikkila EA: Serum lipoproteins and indices of glucose tolerance during diuretic therapy: a comparison between hydrochlorothiazide and piretanide. J Cardiovasc Pharmacol 1983; 5: 525-530.

36. Fagar A, Bergland G, Bondjers G, et al: Effects of antihypertensive therapy on serum lipoproteins, treatment with metoprolol, propranolol, and hydrochlorothiazide. Artery 1983; 11: 283-296.

37. Johnson BF, Romero L, Johnson J, et al: Comparative effects of propranolol and prazosin upon serum lipids in thiazide-treated hypertensive patients. Am J Med 1984; 76: 109-112.

38. Holtzman E, Rosenthal T, Goldbourt V, et al: Differential effects of metoprolol and chlorthalidone on serum lipoproteins. Isr J Med Sci 1984; 20: 1169-1176.

39. Johnson BF, Saunders R, Hickler R, et al: Effects of thiazide diuretics upon plasma lipoproteins. J Hypertens 1986; 4: 235-239.

40. Middeke M, Weisweiler P, Schwandt P, et al: Serum lipoproteins during antihypertensive therapy with β-blockers and diuretics: a controlled long-term comparative trial. Clin Cardiol 1987; 10: 94-98.

41. Trost BN, Weidmann P, Riesen W, et al: Comparative effects of doxazosin and hydrochlorothiazide on serum lipids and blood pressure in essential hypertension. Am J Cardiol 1987; 59: 99G-104G.

42. Hjortdahl P, von Krogh H, Daae L, et al: A 24 week multicenter double-blind study of doxazosin and hydrochlorothiazide in patients with mild to moderate essential hypertension. Acta Med Scand 1987; 221: 427-434.
43. Yoshino G, Iwai M, Kazumi T, et al: Comparison of the long-term effects of indapamide and trichlorothiazide on lipoprotein and apolipoprotein. Curr Ther Res 1987; 42: 607-612.
44. Holtzman E, Rosenthal T, Goldbourt U, et al: Do beta-blockers alter lipids and what are the consequences? J Cardiovasc Pharmacol 1987; 10 :S86-S92.
45. Lasser NL, Nash J, Lasser VI, et al: Effects of hypertensive therapy on blood pressure control, cognition and reactivity; a placebo-controlled comparison of prazosin, propranolol and hydrochlorothiazide. Am J Med 1989; 86 (Suppl 1B): 98-103.
46. Lehtonen A, Gordin A, Salo H: Comparison of sustained-release verapamil and hydrochlorothiazide in hypertension - effect on blood pressure and metabolic variables. Intl J Clin Pharm Ther Toxicol 1987; 25: 301-305.
47. Frithz G: Effect of pindolol on changes in serum lipids induced by hydrochlorothiazide. Eur J Clin Pharmacol 1989; 37: 221-223.
48. Pollare T, Lithell H, Berne C: A comparison of the effects of hydrochlorothiazide and captopril on glucose and lipid metabolism in patients with hypertension. N Engl J Med 1989; 321: 868-873.
49. Moser M: Lipid abnormalities and diuretics. AFP 1989; 40: 213-220.
50. Grimm RH, Neuton JD, McDonald M, et al: Beneficial effects from systematic dosage reduction of the diuretic, chlorthalidone: a randomized study within a clinical trial. Am Heart J 1985; 109: 858-864.
51. McKenney JM, Goodman RP, Wright JF Jr, et al: The effect of low-dose hydrochlorothiazide on blood pressure, serum potassium, and lipoproteins. Pharmacother 1986; 6: 179-184.
52. Frishman WH: Personal communication.
53. Schiffl H, Schollmeyer P: Metabolic consequences of long-term thiazide-based antihypertensive treatment of renal hypertension. Cardiology 1985; 72 (Suppl l): 54-56.
54. Lasser NL, Grandits G, Caggiula AW, et al: Effects of antihypertensive therapy on plasma lipids and lipoproteins in the Multiple Risk Factor Intervention Trial. Am J Med 1984; 76 (Suppl 2A): 52-66.
55. Stamler J: Population studies: In Levy R et al (eds): Nutrition, Lipids, and Coronary Heart Disease. New York, Raven Press 1979; 72.
56. Aranda P, Lopez de Novales E: Diuretics and the treatment of systemic hypertension. Am J Cardiol 1990; 65: 72H-76H.
57. Meyer-Sabellek W, Gotzen R, Heitz J, et al: Serum lipoprotein levels during long-term treatment with indapamide. Hypertension 1985; 7 (Suppl 2): 170-174.
58. Gerber A, Weidmann P, Bianchetti MG, et al: Serum lipoproteins during treatment with the antihypertensive agent indapamide. Hypertension 1985; 7 (Suppl II):II-164-II-169.
59. Leonetti G, Rappelli A, Salvetti A, et al: Long-term effects of indapamide: final results of a two year Italian multi-center study in systemic hypertension. Am J Cardiol 1990; 65: 67H-71H.

60. Hunninghake DB, Kibbard DM, Grimm RH, et al: Effects of spironolactone and hydrochlorothiazide, single and in combination, on plasma lipids and lipoproteins. (abstr) Circulation 1984; 70: II-118.

61. Schersten B, Thulin T, Kuylenstierna J, et al: Clinical and biochemical effects of spironolactone administered once daily in primary hypertension. Hypertension 1980; 2: 672-679.

62. Ames RP: Serum lipid and lipoprotein disturbances during antihypertensive therapy. Hosp Formul 1981; 16: 1476-1486.

63. Olefsky JM, Farquhar JW, Reaven GM: Reappraisal of the role of insulin in hypertriglyceridemia. Am J Med 1974; 57: 551-560.

64. Streja D, Mymin D: Effect of propranolol on HDL cholesterol concentrations. (letter) Br Med J 1978; 2: 1495.

65. Leren P, Foss PO, Helgeland A, et al: Effects of propranolol and prazosin on blood lipids. The Oslo Study. Lancet 1980; 2: 4-6.

66. Ruhling K, Schauer I, Thillmann K: Intraindividual variability of plasma cholesterol and triglycerides and the effect of propranolol treatment. Artery 1980; 8: 140-145.

67. Schauer I, Schauer U, Ruhling K: The effect of propranolol treatment on total cholesterol, HDL cholesterol, triglycerides. Postheparin lipolytic activity and lecithin: cholesterol acyl-transferase in hypertensive individuals. Artery 1980; 8: 146-150.

68. Day JL, Metcalfe J, Simpson N, et al: Adrenergic mechanisms in the control of plasma lipids in man. Am J Med 1984; 76:94-96.

69. Birnbaum J, DiBianco R, Becker KL, et al: Glucose and lipid metabolism during acebutolol and propranolol therapy of angina in nondiabetic patients. Clin Pharmacol Ther 1983; 333: 294-300.

70. Ponti GB, Carnovali M, Banderali G, et al: Effects of labetalol on the lipid metabolism in hypertensive patients. Curr Ther Res 1983; 33: 466-471.

71. Dujovne CA, DeCoursey S, Krehbiel P, et al: Serum lipids in normo- and hyperlipidemics after methyldopa and propranolol. Clin Pharmacol Ther 1984; 36: 157-162.

72. Leon AS, Agre J, McNally C, et al: Blood lipid effects of antihypertensive therapy: a double-blind comparison of the effects of methyldopa and propranolol. J Clin Pharmacol 1984; 24: 209-217.

73. Weber MA, Drayer JI, Kaufman CA: The combined α- and β- adrenergic blocker labetalol and propranolol in the treatment of high blood pressure: similarities and differences. J Clin Pharmacol 1984; 24: 103-112.

74. Durrington PN, Brownlee WC, Large CM: Short-term effects of β-adrenoceptor-blocking drugs with and without cardioselectivity and intrinsic sympathomimetic activity on lipoprotein metabolism in hypertriglyceridaemic patients and in normal men. Clin Sci 1985; 69: 713-719.

75. Flamenbaum W, Weber MA, McMahon FG, et al: Monotherapy with labetalol compared with propranolol. J Clin Hypertens 1985; 1: 56-69.

76. Harter HR, Meltzer VN, Tindira CA, et al: Comparison of the effects of prazosin versus propranolol on plasma lipoprotein lipids in patients receiving hemodialysis. Am J Med 1986; 80: 82-89.

77. Johnson BF, Romero L, Marwaha R: Hemodynamic and metabolic effects of the calcium channel blocking agent nitrendipine. Clin Pharmacol Ther 1986; 39: 389-394.

78. Velasco M, Hurt E, Silva H, et al: Effects of prazosin and propranolol on blood lipids and lipoproteins in hypertensive patients. Am J Med 1986; 80 (Suppl 2A): 109-113.

79. Harvengt C, Heller FR, Martiat PH, et al: Short-term effects of β-blockers atenolol, nadolol, pindolol, and propranolol on lipoprotein metabolism in normolipemic subjects. J Clin Pharmacol 1987; 27: 475-480.

80. Malini PL, Strocchi E, Cervi V, et al: The metabolic effects of enalapril. Clin Exp Hypetens 1987; 9: 675-679.

81. Northcote RJ, Packard CJ, Ballantyne D: The effect of sotalol on plasma lipoproteins and apolipoproteins. Clin Chimica Acta 1986; 158: 187-191.

82. Miller NE, Nanjee MN, Rajput-Williams J, et al: Double-blind trial of the long-term effects of acebutolol and propranolol on serum lipoproteins in patients with stable angina pectoris. Am Heart J 1987; 114: 1007-1010.

83. Lijnen P, Fagard R, Staessen J, et al: Serum cholesterol during ketanserin and propranolol administration in hypertensive patients. J Cardiovasc Pharmacol 1987; 10: 647-649.

84. Magarian EO, Dietz AJ, Freeman DS, et al: Effect of prazosin and beta-blockade monotherapy on serum lipids: A crossover, placebo-controlled study. J Clin Pharmacol 1987; 27: 756-761.

85. Fogari R, Zoppi A, Pasotti C, et al: Plasma lipids during antihypertensive therapy with different β-blockers. J Cardiovasc Pharmacol 1989; 14 (Suppl 7): S28-S32.

86. Leon AS, Hunninghake DB, Belcher J, et al: Comparative effects of prazosin and propranolol on blood lipid profiles in hypertensive, hypercholesterolemic patients: preliminary results. Am J Med 1989; 86 (1B): 36-40.

87. Alderman MH: Evaluation of efficacy of prazosin versus propranolol as initial antihypertensive therapy. Am J Med 1989; 86 (Suppl 1B): 45-49.

88. Sirtori CR, Johnson B, Vaccarino V, et al: Lipid effects of celiprolol, a new cardio-selective beta blocker versus propranolol. Clin Pharmacol Ther 1989; 45: 617-626.

89. Waal-Manning HJ: The effect of β-blockers on plasma lipids. Presented at Symposium on β-Blocker Therapy. Atlanta, Ga., January 13-14, 1981.

90. Northcote RJ, Ballantyne D: β-Adrenoceptor blockade and plasma lipoproteins. Comparison of the effects of propranolol and pindolol on plasma lipoproteins, including high-density lipoprotein subfractions. Clin Sci 1987; 72: 549-556.

91. Lehtonen A, Viikari J: Long-term effect of sotalol on plasma lipids. Clin Sci 1979; 57: 405S-407S.

92. Richard JL, Martin C, Jacotot : Teratolol does not affect biochemical markers of atherosclerosis in normo- and hyperlipidemic hypertensive patients. Am J Nephrol 1986; 6: 100-105.

93. Gundersen T, Kjekshust J, Stokke O, et al: Timolol maleate and HDL cholesterol after myocardial infarction. Eur Heart J 1985; 6: 840-844.

94. Leren P, Foss PO, Nordvik B, et al: The effect of enalapril and timolol on blood lipids. A randomized multicenter hypertension study in general practice in Norway. Acta Medica Scand 1988; 223: 321-326.

95. Giuntoli F, Scalabrino A, Galeone F, et al: Antihypertensive and metabolic effects of long-term treatment with acebutolol. Curr Ther Res 1984; 36: 188-194.

96. Lehtonen A: The effect of acebutolol on plasma lipids, blood glucose, and serum insulin levels. Intl J Clin Pharm Ther Toxicol 1984; 22: 269-272.

97. England JDF, Simons LA, Gibson JC, et al: The effect of metoprolol and atenolol on plasma high-density lipoprotein levels in man. Clin Exp Pharmacol Physiol 1980; 7: 329-333.

98. Rossner S, Weiner L: Atenolol and metoprolol: comparison of effects on blood pressure and serum lipoproteins, and side effects. Eur J Clin Pharmacol 1983; 24: 573-577.

99. Pasotti C, Zoppi A, Capra A, et al: Effect of β-blockers on plasma lipids. Intl J Clin Pharmacol Ther Toxicol 1986; 24: 448-452.

100. Lithell H, Weiner L, Selinus I, et al: Comparison of the effects of bisoprolol and atenolol on lipoprotein concentrations and blood pressure. J Cardiovasc Pharmacol 1986; 8 (Suppl 11): S128-S133.

101. Linden T, Camejo G, Wiklund O, et al: Effect of short-term beta blockade on serum lipid levels and on the interaction of LDL with human arterial proteoglycans. J Clin Pharmacol 1990; 30: S124-131.

102. Pasotti C, Capra A, Fiorella G, et al: Effects of pindolol and metoprolol on plasma lipids and lipoproteins. Br J Clin Pharmacol 1982; 13: 435S-439S.

103. Frishman WH, Michelson EL, Johnson BF, et al: Multiclinic comparison of labetalol to metoprolol in treatment of mild to moderate systemic hypertension. Am J Med 1983; 75 (Suppl): 54-67.

104. Materson BJ, Vlachakis ND, Glasser SP, et al: Influence of beta-2 agonism and beta-1 and beta-2 antagonism on adverse effects and plasma lipoproteins: results of a multicenter comparison of dilevalol and metoprolol. Am J Cardiol 1989; 63: 58I-63I.

105. Foss OP, Jensen K: The effect of captopril and metoprolol as monotherapy or combined with bendroflumethiazide on blood lipids. J Intern Med 1990; 227: 119-123.

106. Ferrara LA, Marotta T, Rubba P, et al: Effects of α-adrenergic and β-adrenergic receptor blockade on lipid metabolism. Am J Med 1986; 80: 104-108.

107. Eliasson K, Lins LE, Rossner S: Serum lipoprotein changes during atenolol treatment of essential hypertension. Eur J Clin Pharmacol 1981; 20: 335-338.

108. Lehtonen A, Marniemi J: Effect of atenolol on plasma HDL cholesterol subfractions. Atherosclerosis 1984; 51: 335-338.

109. Rouffy J, Jaillard J: Comparative effects of prazosin and atenolol on plasma lipids in hypertensive patients. Am J Med 1984; 76: 105-108.

110. Neusy AJ, Lowenstein J: Effects of prazosin, atenolol, and thiazide diuretic on plasma lipids in patients with essential hypertension. Am J Med 1986; 80: 94-99.

111. Rouffy J, Jaillard J: Effects of two antihypertensive agents on lipids, lipo-proteins, and apoproteins A and B. Comparison of prazosin and atenolol. Am J Med 1986; 80: 100-103.
112. Valimaki M, Maass L, Harno K, et al: Lipoprotein lipids and apoproteins during β-blocker administration: comparison of penbutolol and atenolol. Eur J Clin Pharmacol 1986; 30: 17-20.
113. Frick MH, Cox DA, Nimanen P, et al: Serum lipid changes in a 1 year, multicenter double-blind comparison of doxazosin and atenolol for mild to moderate essential hypertension. Am J Cardiol 1987; 59: 61G-67G.
114. Nash DT, Schonfeld G, Reeves RL, et al: A double-blind parallel trial to assess the efficacy of doxazosin, atenolol, and placebo in patients with mild to moderate systemic hypertension. Am J Cardiol 1987; 59: 87G-90G.
115. Ott P, Storm TL, Krusell LR, et al: Multicenter, double-blind comparison of doxazosin and atenolol in patients with mild to moderate hypertension. Am J Cardiol 1987; 59: 73G-77G.
116. Mazzola C, Guerrasio E: Doxazosin versus atenolol: a randomized compari-son of calculated coronary heart disease risk reduction. Am Heart J 1988; 116: 1797-1800.
117. Herpin D, Guillard O, Piriou A, et al: Effets compares tu pindolol t de l'atenolol sur la tension arterielle et le bilan lipidique en cas d'hypertension arterielle legere a moderee. Ann Med Interne 1988; 139: 484-487.
118. Takahashi H, Fukuyama M, Yoneda S, et al: Comparison of nisoldipine and atenolol in the treatment of essential hypertension. Arzn Forch/Drug Res 1989; 39: 379.
119. Superko HR, Wood PD, Krauss RM: Effect of alpha and selective beta-blockade for hypertension control on plasma lipoproteins, apoproteins, lipoprotein subclasses and postprandial lipemia. Am J Med 1989; 86 (Suppl 1B): 26-31.
120. Frithz G, Weiner L: Long-term effects of bisoprolol on blood pressure, serum lipids, and HDL-cholesterol in patients with essential hypertension. J Cardiovasc Pharmacol 1986; 8 (Suppl 11): S134-S138.
121. Frithz G, Weiner L: Effects of bisoprolol on blood pressure, serum lipids and HDL-cholesterol in essential hypertension. Am J Clin Pharmacol 1987; 32: 77-80.
122. Jurgensen HJ, Meinertz H, Faergeman O: Plasma lipids and lipoproteins in long-term α-adrenergic blockade. Acta Med Scand 1982; 211: 449-452.
123. van Brummelen P, Bolli P, Koolen MI, et al: Plasma lipid fractions during bopindolol treatment in hypertensive patients. J Cardiovasc Pharmacol 1986; 8 (Suppl 6): S42-S44.
124. Herrmann JM, Bischof F, Von Heymann F, et al: Effects of celiprolol on serum lipids in systemic hypertension. Am J Cardiol 1988; 61: 41C-44C.
125. Frishman WH, Schoenberger JA, Gorwit JI, et al: Multicenter comparison of dilevalol to placebo in patients with mild hypertension. Am J Hypertens 1988; 1: 295S-299S.
126. Simons LA, England JDF, Balasubramaniam, et al: Long-term treatment with slow release oxprenolol alone or in combination with other drugs: effects on blood pressure, lipoproteins, and exercise performance. Aust NZ J Med 1982; 12: 612-616.

127. Miettinen TA, Vanhanen H, Huttunen JK, et al: HDL cholesterol and β-adrenoceptor blocking agents in a 5 year multifactorial primary prevention trial. Br J Clin PHarmacol 1982; 13: 431S-434S.
128. Karmakoski J, Viikari J, Ronnemaa T: Effect of pindolol on serum lipoproteins in patients with coronary heart disease. Intl J Clin Pharmacol Ther Toxicol 1983; 21: 189-191.
129. Lehtonen A: The effects of trimazosin and pindolol on serum lipids, blood glucose, and serum insulin levels. Acta Med Scand 1985; 218: 213-216.
130. Carlson LA, Ribacke M, Terent A: A long-term study on the effect of pindolol on serum lipoproteins: a preliminary report. Br J Clin Pharmacol 1987; 24: 61S-62S.
131. Roman O, Pino ME, Valenzuela A: Effects of pindolol and clopamide on blood lipids in hypertensive patients. Cardiology 1987; 74: 219-225.
132. Ohman KP, Weiner L, von Schenck H, et al: Antihypertensive and metabolic effects of nifedipine and labetalol alone and in combination in primary hypertension. Eur J Clin Pharmacol 1985; 29: 149-154.
133. Farry JP, Fischl SJ, Tighe MJ: Effects of prazosin and labetalol on blood pressure control and blood lipid levels in patients with mild-moderate essential hypertension. Am J Med 1989; 86 (Suppl 1B): 41-44.
134. Frishman WH: Clinical significance of beta 1 selectivity and intrinsic sympathomimetic activity in a beta-adrenergic blocking drug. Am J Cardiol 1987; 59: 33F-37F.
135. Veterans Administration Cooperative Study Group: Comparison of propranolol and hydrochlorothiazide for the initial treatment of hypertension. II. Results of long-term therapy. JAMA 1982; 248: 2004-2011.
136. Barboriak JJ, Friedberg HD: Propranolol and hypertriglyceridemia. Atherosclerosis 1973; 17: 31-35.
137. Peden NR, Dow RJ, Isles TE, et al: Beta adrenoceptor blockade and responses of serum lipids to a meal and to exercise. Br Med J 1984; 1: 1788-1790.
138. Sakaguchi TN, Numura OK, Kanchisa T: Effect of chronic administration of propranolol on lipoprotein composition. Metabolism 1976; 25: 1071-1075.
139. Day JL, Metcalfe J, Simpson CN: Adrenergic mechanism in control of plasma lipid concentrations. Br Med J 1982; 284: 1145- 1148.
140. Cerasi E, Effendic E, Luft R: Role of adrenergic receptors in glucose-induced insulin secretion in man. Lancet 1969; 1: 301-302.
141. Furman BL, Tayo FM: Inhibitory effect of propranolol on insulin secretion. Br J Pharmacol 1973; 49: 145-147.
142. Eisner M, Dobrohorska H, Stachowski A: Effect of inderal on insulin secretion, glycemia and FFA concentration in normal subjects and diabetics. Pol Med Sci Hist Bull 1976; 15: 169-175.
143. Myers MG, Hope-Gill HF: Effect of d- and dl-propranolol on glucose-stimulated insulin release. Clin Pharmacol Ther 1979; 24: 303-308.
144. Goto Y: Effects of α- and β-blocker antihypertensive therapy on blood lipids: a multicenter trial. Am J Med 1984; 76: 72-78.

145. Fager G, Berglund G, Bondjers G: Effects of antihypertensive therapy on serum lipoproteins: treatment with metoprolol, propranolol and hydrochlorothiazide. Artery 1983; 11: 283-296.
146. Velasco M, Hurt E, Silva H: Effects of prazosin and propranolol on blood lipids and lipoproteins in hypertensive patients. Am J Med 1986; 80 (Suppl 2A): 109-113.
147. Lehtonen A: Long-term effect of pindolol on plasma lipids, apoproteins A, blood glucose, and serum insulin levels. Intl J Clin Ther Toxicol 1984; 22: 269-272.
148. Day JL, Simpson N, Metcalfe J: Metabolic consequences of atenolol and propranolol in treatment of essential hypertension. Br Med J 1979; 1: 77-80.
149. Kirkendall WM, Hammond JJ, Thomas JC, et al: Prazosin and clonidine for moderately severe hypertension. JAMA 1978; 240: 2553-2556.
150. Havard CW, Khokhar AM, Flax JS: Open assessment of the effect of prazosin on plasma lipids. J Cardiovasc Pharmacol 1982; 4 (Suppl 2): S238-S241.
151. Kokubu T, Itoh I, Kurita H, et al: Effect of prazosin on serum lipids. J Cardiovasc Pharmacol 1982; 4 (Suppl 2): S228-S232.
152. Kather H, Sauberlich P: Comparison of in vitro and in vivo effects of prazosin on lipid metabolism. Am J Med 1984; 76: 89-93.
153. Takabatake T, Ohta H, Maekawa M et al: Effects of long-term prazosin therapy on lipoprotein metabolism in hypertensive patients. Am J Med 1984; 76: 113-116.
154. Deger G: Effect of terazosin on serum lipids. Am J Med 1986; 80: 82-85.
155. Cambien F, Plouin PF: Prazosin does not alter levels of plasma lipids, glucose and insulin. J Cardiovasc Pharmacol 1985; 7: 516-519.
156. Torvik D, Madsbu HP: An open 1 year comparison of doxazosin and prazosin for mild to moderate essential hypertension. Am J Cardiol 1987; 59: 68G-72G.
157. Nakamura H: Effects of antihypertensive drugs on plasma lipids. Am J Cardiol 1987; 60: 24E-28E.
158. Pool JL: Plasma lipid-lowering effects of doxazosin, a new selective α1-adrenergic inhibitor for systemic hypertension. Am J Cardiol 1987; 59: 46G-50G.
159. Stamler R, Stamler J, Gosch FC, et al: Initial antihypertensive drug therapy: final report of random-ized controlled trial comparing α-blocker and diuretic. Hypertension 1988; 12: 574-581.
160. Rockhold FW, Goldberg MR, Thompson L, and the Pinacidil-Prazosin and Pinacidil-Placebo Research Groups: Beneficial effects of pinacidil on blood lipids: comparison with prazosin and placebo in patients with hypertension. J Lab Clin Med 1987; 114: 646-654.
161. Swislocki ALM, Hoffman BB, Sheu WHH, et al: Effect of prazosin treatment on carbohydrate and lipoprotein metabolism in patients with hypertension. Am J Med 1989; 86 (Suppl 1B): 14-18.
162. Lehtonen A, Himanen P, Saraste M, et al: Double-blind comparison of the effects of long-term treatment with doxazosin or atenolol on serum lipoproteins. Br J Clin Pharmacol 1986; 2 (Suppl 1): 77S-81S.

163. Frick MH, Halttunen P, Himanen P, et al: A long-term double-blind comparison of doxazosin and atenolol in patients with mild to moderate essential hypertension. Br J Clin Pharmacol 1986; 21 (Suppl 1): 55S-62S.

164. Torvik D, Madsbu HP: Multicenter 12 week double-blind comparison of doxazosin, prazosin and placebo in patients with mild to moderate essential hypertension. Br J Clin Pharmacol 1986; 21 (Suppl 1): 69S-75S.

165. Cubeddu LX, Pool JL, Bloomfield R, et al: Effect of doxazosin monotherapy on blood pressure and plasma lipids in patients with essential hypertension. Am J Hypertens 1988; 1: 158-167.

166. Giorgi G, Legramante JM, Fioravanti G, et al: A comparative study of doxazosin versus atenolol in mild to moderate hypertension. Am Heart J 1988; 116: 1801-1805.

167. Talseth T, Westlie L, Daae L, et al: Comparison of the effects of doxazosin and atenolol on blood pressure and blood lipids: a one year double-blind study in 228 hypertensive patients. Am Heart J 1988; 116: 1790-1795.

168. Nechwatal W, Berger J, Blumrich W, et al: A double-blind comparison of doxazosin and nitrendipine in patients with mild to moderate essential hypertension. Am Heart J 1988; 116: 1806-1813.

169. Taylor SH, Lee PS, Sharma SK: A comparison of doxazosin and enalapril in the treatment of mild and moderate essential hypertension. Am Heart J 1988; 116: 1820-1824.

170. Ames RP, Kiyasu JY: Alpha 1 adrenoreceptor blockade with doxazosin. Effects on blood pressure and lipoproteins. J Clin Pharmacol 1989; 29: 123-127.

171. Singleton W, Taylor CR: Effect of trimazosin on serum lipid profiles in hypertensive patients. Am Heart J 1983; 106: 1265-1268.

172. Taylor CR, Leader JP, Singleton W, et al: Profile of timazosin: an effective and safe antihypertensive agent. Am Heart J 1983; 106: 1269-1281.

173. Ferrier C, Baretta-Piccoli C, Weidmann P, et al: α1-adrenergic blockade and lipoprotein metabolism in essential hypertension. Clin Pharmacol Ther 1986; 40: 525-530.

174. Martinez TLR, Auriemo CRC, Machado AMO, et al: Effects of indoramin and metoprolol on plasma lipids and lipoproteins. J Cardiovasc Pharmacol 1986; 8 (Suppl 2): 76-79.

175. Luther RR, Glassman HN, Estep CB, et al: Terazosin, a new selective α1-blocking agent. Results of a long-term treatment on patients with essential hypertension. Am J Hypertens 1988; 1: 237S-240S.

176. Ferrara LA, Marotta T, Rubba PR, et al: Effects of alpha-adrenergic and beta-adrenergic receptor blockade on lipid metabolism. Am J Med 1986; 80 (Suppl 2A): 104-108.

177. Leren TP: Doxazosin increases low-density lipoprotein receptor activity. Acta Pharmacol Toxicol 1985; 56: 269-272.

178. Bricker LA, Kozlovskis PL, Levey GD: Adenosine 3,5-monophosphate and the regulation of rat hepatic sterol synthesis: A re-examination based on Sutherland criteria. Metabolism 1976; 23: 477-481.

179. Karlberg BE, Lins L-E, Rossner S: Clonidine in mild to moderate hypertension: effects on blood pressure and serum lipoproteins. J Hypertens 1985; 3 (Suppl 4): S69-S71.

180. Nilson-Ehle P, Ekberg M, Fridstrom P, et al: Lipoproteins and metabolic control in hypertensive Type II diabetics treated with clonidine. Acta Med Scand 1987; 229: 131-134.

181. Houston MC, Hays T, Nadeau J, et al: Effects of clonidine and atenolol monotherapy on serum lipids, lipoproteins and glucose in mild primary hypertension. (abstr) Clin Res 1987; 35: 348A.

182. Kaplan NM: Effects of guanabenz on plasma lipid levels in hypertensive patients. J Cardiovasc Pharmacol 1984; 6 (Suppl 5): S841-S846.

183. Weber MA, Drayer JIM, Deitch MW: Hypertension in patients with diabetes mellitus. Treatment with a centrally acting agent. J Cardiovasc Pharmacol 1984; 6 (Suppl 5): S823-S829.

184. McCarron DA: Step one antihypertensive therapy: a comparison of a centrally acting agent and a diuretic. J Cardiovasc Pharmacol 1984; 6 (Suppl 5): S853-S858.

185. Hauger-Klevene JH, Balossi EC, Scornavacchi JC: Effects of guanfacine on growth hormone, prolactin, renin, lipoproteins, and glucose in essential hypertension. Am J Cardiol 1986; 57: 27E-31E.

186. Hauger-Klevene JH: Hypolipaemic effect of guanfacine: two years' follow up. Drugs Exp Clin Res 1984; 10: 133-140.

187. Fillingim JM, Blackshear JL, Strauss A, et al: Guanfacine as monotherapy for systemic hypertension. Am J Cardiol 1986; 57: 50E-54E.

188. Velasco M, Silva H, Feldstein E, et al: Effects of prazosin and alphamethyldopa on blood lipids and lipoproteins in hypertensive patients. Eur J Clin Pharmacol 1985; 28: 513-516.

189. Weidmann P, Gerberg A, Mordasini R: Effects of antihypertensive therapy on serum lipoproteins. Hypertension 1983; 5 (Suppl III): 120-131.

190. Deming JB, Hodes ME, Baltazar A, et al: The changes in concentration of cholesterol in the serum of hypertensive patients during antihypertensive therapy. Am J Med 1958; 24: 882-892.

191. Gerber A, Weidmann P, Saner R, et al: Increased serum high-density lipoprotein cholesterol in hypertensive men treated with the potent vasodilator carprazidil. Metabolism 1984; 33: 342-346.

192. Hauger-Klevene JH, Reader C, Mayer E, et al: A comparative study of endralazine and captopril in essential hypertension: effect on renin levels, pulmonary function studies and lipid profiles. Intl J Clin Pharmacol Res 1986; 6: 275-281.

193. Johnson BF, Errichetti A, Urbach D, et al: The effect of once daily minoxidil on blood pressure and plasma lipids. J Clin Pharmacol 1986; 26: 534-538.

194. Ohman P, Aurell M, Asplund J, et al: A long-term follow up of patients with essential hypertension treated with captopril. Acta Med Scand 1984; 216: 53-56.

195. Weinberger MH: Influence of an angiotensin converting enzyme inhibitor on diuretic-induced metabolic effects in hypertension. Hypertension 1983; 5 (Suppl III): 132-138.

196. Saltvedt E, Andreassen P, Dahl K, et al: An improved serum lipid profile in hypertension during captopril treatment. (abstr) Postgrad Med J 1986; 62 (Suppl l): 78.

197. Ghirlanda G, Botta G, Bianchini G, et al: Influence of captopril on serum lipids in the long-term treatment of hypertension associated with hyperlipidemia. (abstr) Postgrad Med J 1986; 62 (Suppl 1): 79.

198. Perani G, Muggia C, Martignoni A, et al: Increase in plasma HDL cholesterol in hypertensive patients trated with enalapril. Clin Therap 1987; 9: 635-639.

199. Costa GB, Borghi C, Mussi A, et al: Use of captopril to reduce serum lipids in hypertensive patients with hyperlipidemia. Am J Hypertens 1988; 1: 221S-223S.

200. Sasaki J, Arakowa K: Effect of captopril on high density lipoprotein subfractions in patients with mild to moderate essential hypertension. Clin Therap 1989; 11: 129-134.

201. Sasaki J, Arakowa K: Effects of enalapril on serum lipoproteins in mild essential hypertension. Clin Therap 1989; 11: 38-42.

202. LaCourciere Y, Gagne C: Influence of zofenopril and low doses of hydrochlorothiazide on plasma lipoproteins in patients with mild to moderate essential hypertension. Am J Hypertens 1989; 2: 861-864.

203. Schoen R, Frishman WH, Shamoon H: Hormonal and metabolic effects of calcium-channel antagonists in man. Am J Med 1988; 84: 492-504.

204. Trost BN, Weidmann P: Effects of calcium antagonists on glucose homeostasis and serum lipids in nondiabetic and diabetic subjects. A review. J Hypertens 1987; 5 (Suppl 4): S81-S104.

205. Schulte K-L, Meyer-Sabellek WA, Haertenberger A, et al: Antihypertensive and metabolic effects of diltiazem and nifedipine. Hypertension 1986; 8: 859-865.

206. Perani G, Martignoni A, Muggia C, et al: Effects of nisoldipine treatment on plasma lipoproteins. Curr Ther Res 1987; 42: 601-606.

207. Midtbo K, Lauve O, Hals O: No metabolic side effects of long-term treatment with verapamil in hypertension. Angiology 1988; December: 1025.

208. Pool PE, Herron JM, Rosenblatt S, et al: Metabolic effects of antihypetensive therapy with a calcium antagonist. Am J Cardiol 1988; 62: 109G-112G.

209. Pollare T, Lithell H, Morlin C, et al: Metabolic effects of diltiazem and atenolol: results from a randomized double-blind study with parallel groups. J Hypertens 1989; 7: 551-559.

210. Osterloch I: The safety of amlodipine. Am Heart J 1989; 118: 1114-1119.

211. Expert Panel: Report of the National Cholesterol Education Program Expert Panel on Detection, Evaluation and Treatment of High Blood Cholesterol in Adults. Arch Intern Med 1988; 148: 36-69.

Chapter 12

Lipids, Vascular Disease, and Dementia With Advancing Age: Epidemiologic Considerations

William H. Frishman M.D., Peter Zimetbaum M.D.,
Wee Lock Ooi Dr. PH, Miriam Aronson Ed.D.

One of the most important issues in gerontologic planning and practice has been that of "compression of morbidity."[1] If, in fact, disability can be forestalled, the impact upon quality of life and cost of care would be substantial. This is especially important since persons over 80 are the fastest growing segment of our population. For these very old persons, the impact of ischemic heart disease has been relatively unaffected by the application of our increased knowledge regarding cardiovascular risk factors in general, and lipids in particular.

There is currently little dispute that elevations in serum lipids can influence the development of vascular disease in middle-aged persons. There are multiple studies of middle-aged male subjects showing that elevated cholesterol and lipid fractions correlate with the development of coronary or cerebrovascular events. More recently, intervention studies conducted by the Lipid Research Clinics[2] and Helsinki trials[3] have shown that drug therapy is efficacious in reducing vascular morbidity. However, no studies have shown conclusively a decrease in overall mortality with the lowering of serum cholesterol.

It is noteworthy that most lipid studies, both on risk evaluation and intervention, have concentrated on persons between the ages of 30 and 65 years. There have been very few studies evaluating the role of

From *Medical Management of Lipid Disorders: Focus on Prevention of Coronary Artery Disease,* edited by William H. Frishman, M.D. © 1992, Futura Publishing Inc., Mount Kisco, NY.

cholesterol as a risk factor for coronary heart disease (CHD) in the elderly (over age 65). Among these studies, the findings are varied and inconsistent, allowing no definitive conclusions to be drawn.

Although on a steady decline, ischemic heart disease (IHD) remains the leading cause of death in older persons.[4] Risk factors cited for ischemic heart disease include hypercholesterolemia, diabetes mellitus, hypertension, family/personal history, male gender, dietary indiscretion, increased truncal fat (increased waist:hip ratio), reduced HDL_2, and smoking. However, whether all or only some of these risk factors apply in the population over age 65 remains undetermined. It is not clear what the average cholesterol and lipid values are in the aged, whether these values remain stable over time, and whether they are associated with CHD. In addition, there is uncertainty as to whether the values assigned for therapeutic intervention by the National Cholesterol Education Program[5] are appropriate for this population. It is, therefore, time to attempt to answer questions about what is healthy versus what is pathological in people of more advanced age.

Lipids and Lipoproteins in the Elderly

Analysis of cholesterol and lipid values related to body weight shows that in later life, total cholesterol, triglycerides, LDL, and relative body weight decline in both sexes.[5] HDL does not change significantly in men but may fall in women after age 55.

The falling of lipid values is certainly due, in part, to selective mortality or premature demise of a proportion of the population with high lipid values. However, as noted by Hazzard,[6] this decline is probably authentic and related to a naturally declining body weight. Hershcopf et al,[7] in a longitudinal study, found that the drop in serum cholesterol levels was neither related solely to selective mortality nor to body weight, but to some other, as yet, undefined factor. The reduction in lipid values in the elderly could be related to changes in diet with advancing age.[8] Studies have shown that fat intake has dropped over time in the diet of the aged.[9] Men taking part in the Baltimore Longitudinal Aging Study reported eating fewer fatty acids and more polyunsaturated fatty acids.[10] While there was a drop in serum cholesterol in this study, it could not be attributed directly to a change in the type of fat eaten. Other than diet, cholesterol may also be influenced by alcohol intake, exercise, and body composition changes in the elderly (a decline in lean body mass and increase in fat tissue with increasing age.)[10]

Total Serum Cholesterol and LDL

Barrett-Connor et al studied 3187 subjects, aged 50-79 years, for 9 years and found that total serum cholesterol (LDL was not measured) remained a significant risk factor for CHD, unlike the finding of systolic hypertension that was not predictive of risk.[11]

The Framingham Study found that between ages 65-84 total serum cholesterol and LDL were significant risk factors for CHD in women but not definitively in men. In fact, total serum cholesterol at or above the 90th percentile was associated with almost twice the risk of IHD as those with total cholesterol less than 5.17 mm/L (200 mg/dl).[12]

The most recent analysis of the Framingham data has found an association between cholesterol and CHD in men as well as women. However, this association appeared to be stronger in middle-aged compared to elderly men.[13]

The Honolulu Heart Program conducted a 12-year longitudinal study of 1480 males of Japanese descent, aged 71 to 90. Baseline serum cholesterol level was correlated with the eventual development of cardiovascular disease. Univariate and multivariate analyses revealed that cholesterol remained an independent risk factor for CHD. In fact, comparison of middle-aged (< 60 years) with older males showed no significant difference in the predictive value of serum cholesterol for CHD in these groups.[14]

The Kaiser Permanente Coronary Heart Disease in the Elderly Study is a study of mortality from CHD in a cohort of 7445 white adult members of the Kaiser Permanente Medical Care Program between the ages of 60 and 79 years.[15] Over a mean follow-up of 10.1 years, the investigators examined whether an association existed between total blood cholesterol levels and mortality from CHD in white male members of the cohort (n=2746).[15] The relative risk for mortality from coronary artery disease in men in the highest quartile was 1.5 compared with those in the three lowest quartiles combined. The relative risk did not change greatly with age, ranging from 1.4 in men 60-64 years of age to 1.7 in mean 75-79 years of age. However, because mortality from CHD increased with age, the excess risk for such mortality attributable to elevated serum cholesterol increased fivefold over 20 years (2.2 deaths per 1000 person-years to 11.3 deaths per 1000 person-years).

The Glostrup population studies investigated cholesterol in subjects aged 70, and then 10 years later at age 80.[16] Total mortality in 80 year olds was not associated with cholesterol values at age 70. Yet, further analysis dividing death into CHD and non-CHD revealed a J-shaped curve for both sexes, showing highest quartile cholesterol values associated with cardiovascular disease and lowest quartile values with cancer mortality.

The opinion that cholesterol and LDL are no longer risk factors for CHD in old age is supported by the 7 Countries Study that showed a decrease in the association between cholesterol and CHD with advancing age in subjects aged 50-69 years.[17]

The Stockholm Prospective Study, a 9-year follow-up study of 3168 men of all ages, found that there was a linear association between total cholesterol and CHD in those under but not over 60 years of age.[18]

In a report from a recent workshop sponsored by the National Heart, Lung and Blood Institute, data were pooled from 23 different population studies to assess whether cholesterol was a risk factor for CHD in male and female subjects under and over 65 years of age.[19] CHD mortality rates were calculated for each study using the NCEP definition[5] of high-risk cholesterol values 6.21 mm/L (> 240 mg/dl) and low risk values 5.17 mm/L (< 200 mg/dl). Subjects were stratified by age (≥ 65 years and < 65 years) and gender. Unadjusted relative risks (risk ratios) were calculated for number of CHD deaths in each age-gender stratum and 95% confidence limits constructed for these relative risks. Rates of fatal CHD were also used to calculate unadjusted absolute or attributable risk by subtracting CHD rates in the two cholesterol groups for each stratum. Data in each stratum were pooled by summing the number of events for all studies and by dividing by the total number of persons at risk in all studies. This approach does not constitute a formal meta-analysis because differences in length of subject follow-up, sampling methods, and population characteristics were not accounted for.

In men under age 65, the crude relative risk ratio for cholesterol 6.21 mm/L (> 240 mg/dl) was greater than 1.0 for 22 out of 23 studies and averaged 2.27. In contrast, in men over the age of 65, the risk ratio was 1.60, still reflecting a positive association. In comparing attributable or absolute risk, a larger number of CHD deaths were seen in older men compared to younger men. There appeared to be no racial differences.

It was concluded from this analysis that cholesterol screening in middle-aged men could identify subjects at increased risk of developing CHD, and that screening of older men could identify subjects at somewhat lower risk (risk ratio). However, a larger number of those identified in the older age group would develop the disease.

In the same workshop[19] the results of 13 studies were pooled to assess cholesterol as a possible risk factor in middle-aged and older women. The average relative risk was 3.06 in younger women. There were no gender differences in relative risk ratios in those studies where men and women were assessed together. In older women, the average relative risk ratio for all studies combined was 1.53 and appeared to be less impressive than that seen in older men. However, the attributable risk differences were nearly twice that seen in middle-aged women. Based on this analysis, it was concluded that the relationship between total cholesterol and CHD risk was less important in women than in men of all ages.

HDL

Gordon et al[20] reanalyzed data from the British Regional Heart Study, Framingham, Lipid Research Clinics Prevalence Mortality Follow Up and Primary Preventive Trials, and Multiple Risk Factor Intervention Trial (MRFIT), looking for a correlation between HDL and cardiovascular disease. They found that for these five major studies, HDL had a significant inverse association with CHD. In fact, in Framingham's subjects aged 50-79, men in the bottom 75% of HDL values had 70% more myocardial infarctions than those in the top 25%.[21] This association was stronger in women, where those in the top 25% of HDL levels (> 1.68 mm/L [> 65 mg/dl]) had one sixth the number of myocardial infarctions as those in the lowest 25% (1.19 mm/L [> 46 mg/dl]).[21] It was also found that subjects with low HDL, even in the presence of low total cholesterol, had an increased incidence of myocardial infarctions.[21]

The Helsinki Heart Study[3] treated a hypercholesterolemic middle-aged male cohort with gemfibrozil. They found the greatest reduction in cardiovascular risk in those subjects with pretreatment hypertriglyceridemia and low HDL, although overall mortality risk did not change. Elevated triglycerides were not found to be an independent risk factor, suggesting that correction of low HDL values conferred the greatest cardioprotective effect.

Nonetheless, there is currently little data regarding the risk or correction of isolated low HDL levels. Framingham has provided some evidence that low HDL is correlated with the risk of myocardial infarction in the elderly.[22] The Bronx Longitudinal Aging Study, a prospective population study in the old old (mean age 79) has shown that low HDL levels are independently associated with development of myocardial infarction, cardiovascular disease, and death in men but not in women.[23] It has been suggested that HDL_2 might be the lipoprotein most associated with increased risk of IHD in the elderly.[24,25] However, until more studies corroborate these findings, it is premature to draw conclusions.

Triglycerides

As opposed to LDL, total cholesterol, and HDL, the issue of triglycerides as a risk factor for cardiovascular disease in the middle-aged population, let alone the elderly, is as yet unresolved.

A current epidemiologic review involving triglycerides found that case control studies show a univariate association between elevated triglycerides and IHD.[26] However, this association is not maintained in most of the large longitudinal studies or during multivariate analyses involving other lipid fractions. Most likely triglycerides interact with other lipid fractions (i.e., HDL) in an inverse fashion to increase the risk of CHD.[27]

Framingham, a study involving older cohorts, showed that triglycerides are an independent risk factor in both sexes,[28] the significance being greater in women than men.[29] However, the correlation is higher in males when their HDL levels are < 1.03 mm/L (< 40 mg/dl). In conclusion, it was suggested that individuals with very high triglyceride levels (top 10%) in the presence of a total cholesterol/HDL ratio > 3.5 should be considered at risk for IHD.[28]

The Glostrup population study found that after 10 years of follow-up, at which time all subjects were 80 years old, triglyceride values in the top 25th percentile were an independent risk factor for cardiovascular disease in men and cerebrovascular disease in women.[16] The authors point out, however, that the predictive value of elevated triglycerides might reflect a depressed HDL level.

The Bronx Longitudinal Aging Study did not find an independent association between high triglycerides and the development of myocardial infarction, cardiovascular disease, and death in either men or women.[23]

In summary, the role of triglycerides, if any, in the development of CHD has not been elucidated. It is suspected that in some cases there is an inverse relation between triglycerides and HDL, however, the significance of this observation in the elderly population is currently unknown.

HDL/LDL

The concept that a low LDL and high HDL is somehow protective, and the reverse detrimental, suggests that the ratio of HDL to LDL or to total cholesterol would be a good index of one's lipoprotein-related risk for CHD. Results from the type II Coronary Intervention Study support this idea, having found that changes in the HDL-C/TC or LDL-C ratio were the best predictors of CHD.[30] The endpoint used to determine CHD was angiographic evidence of CHD progression with or without evidence of regression. The subjects with highest HDL-C/TC ratio had progression rates one third to one half less than those with the lowest rates. The significance of these results, indicating a relationship between HDL-C/LDL-C ratio and CHD, was maintained with subsequent logistic regression analysis. The usefulness of this ratio has also been supported by numerous reports from Framingham.[31]

Information regarding differences in the HDL-C/LDL-C ratio for the North American population relating to age, sex, and race have been provided by the Lipid Research Clinics Program Prevalence Study.[32] Their data showed that for females not taking gonadal hormones, the HDL-C/TC or LDL-C ratio declined from young adolescence to 55-59 years, at which point values increased slightly with the oldest reported age group being 70+ years. The same trend was observed in males; however, the shift from decreasing to slightly increasing values occurred at age 50-54 years. It is noteworthy that this ratio is most helpful when used to evaluate lipid values within but not at the extremes of the spectrum. This stipulation is added because we have not yet determined which lipoprotein fraction is of absolute greatest importance, e.g., does the protective value of high HDL outweigh the risk of a high LDL, and does a low LDL eliminate the risk associated with a low HDL? This question becomes further complicated by the notion that the relative importance of the individual lipid fraction might change with age.

Other Risk Factors for CHD in the Elderly, and Their Association with Hyperlipidemia

Data from 26 years of follow-up in the Framingham Study indicate that CHD morbidity for men is far in excess of that for women until old age.[33] There is a 40-fold increase in the incidence of CHD in the oldest female age group (75-84 years) as compared to the youngest (35-44 years). In men, the difference in incidence is 6-fold between the oldest and youngest age groups. In early middle age (35-44 years), men have six times as much CHD morbidity as women, but by age 75, the gap is essentially closed. Thus, it is true that up to approximately the middle seventh decade of life, women enjoy some protection from CHD compared to men. However, by the late seventh decade, the risk appears to be equal.[33] As a result of these findings, the question arises as to whether lipoproteins no longer affected by estrogen in the postmenopausal female, begin to exert an effect as a risk factor in this older age group.

The Framingham Study performed the most extensive characterization of variables affecting the occurrence of and mortality from CHD in the elderly (≥ 65 years).[34] Multivariate analysis found that male sex conferred 1.7 times the risk as female gender. Systolic blood pressure >170 mmHg correlated with a 2.8 increase in risk for males and a 1.8 increase in risk for females. Elevated diastolic blood pressure was significant only in men. Left ventricular hypertrophy by ECG doubled the risk, as did a blood glucose level of >175 mg/dl compared to <90 mg/dl. As noted earlier, total serum cholesterol was also associated with increased risk, as was a Metropolitan Life relative weight of 130% or greater. Cigarette smoking of at least 20 cigarettes per day caused a slight increase in risk. In general, the significance of these risk factors was similar for males and females, however, casual blood glucose levels between 125–174 mg/dl had a 1.8 compared to a 0.9 increase in risk for females compared to males.

Hyperlipidemia and Other Vascular Events

Other cardiovascular endpoints that may be related to lipid abnormalities include stroke and dementia. In Western populations, thrombotic strokes are more prevalent than hemorrhagic strokes, whereas in

Asian populations hemorrhagic strokes are quite common. The Framingham study found that in subjects > 65 years, total cholesterol and LDL varied inversely with the incidence of stroke, and in particular, thrombotic infarction.[35] This relationship is most significant in the 75- to 84-year-old cohort, and pertains predominantly to women. There was no association between triglycerides or HDL and the incidence of cerebrovascular disease. The Glostrup Study, as mentioned earlier, found that females had elevated triglycerides associated with cerebrovascular disease of unspecified type.[16]

Data from the MRFIT[36] as well as the Honolulu Heart Program [37] show an inverse association between lowest quintile serum cholesterol levels (for their respective cohorts) and intracerebral hemorrhage. In MRFIT but not the Honolulu Heart Program, the association between cholesterol and stroke was greater among hypertensive men.

Adams et al demonstrated low HDL concentrations in patients having suffered a cortical but not lacunar stroke.[38] Kostner et al,[39] using multivariate analysis to stratify cardiovascular disease risk factors, found that serum apoprotein A-I, apoprotein A-II, and HDL were independent risk factors for ischemic stroke that gained strength when associated with elevated blood pressure and body weight index. Elevated triglycerides also proved significant when combined with hypertension and body weight index.

The principal types of dementia affecting the elderly are Alzheimer's disease and multi-infarct dementia. Muckle and Roy[40] suggested that the presence of a low HDL was a useful factor to help discriminate multi-infarct dementia from Alzheimer's disease. Their findings were supported by Erkinjuntti et al[41] who found that in women, HDL values were lower in association with multi-infarct dementia than with Alzheimer's disease. The patients in this study with dementia were over 65 years of age. However, for younger male patients with dementia and brain infarcts, an association between elevated triglycerides and stroke was demonstrated.[41]

The Bronx Longitudinal Aging Study did not find any association between serum lipids and lipoproteins and the development of all-cause dementia and stroke in subjects over the age of 80 years.[23]

There is obviously little consensus regarding the importance and/ or mechanism of lipids in the pathophysiology of stroke or dementia. Many studies of middle-aged cohorts have found low HDL values in subjects suffering cerebrovascular accidents. However, studies of older cohorts, such as Glostrup,[16] Framingham,[35] and the Bronx Aging Study[23] do not identify HDL as a risk factor although the significance of elevated triglycerides in the Glostrup Study may be associated with a low HDL. The Framingham data, using the more specific atherosclerosis-related endpoint of thrombotic brain infarction, found an inverse relationship between total cholesterol and cerebrovascular disease, particularly in women. This finding is in direct contradistinction to cholesterol's association in Framingham's elderly women regarding CHD mortality. Low cholesterol levels are also associated with hemorrhagic stroke.

Therefore, because these studies have yielded results that were unclear and conflicting, no conclusions or clinical decisions can be made regarding the relationship of lipids to the development of cerebrovascular disease in the elderly. Further study is required.

Implications for Therapy and Future Directions

The final and most basic question is, why bother investigating lipids in the elderly? Many clinicians feel that even if elevated, the effort involved for the patient to lower these values may not be worth the gain. Smith et al,[42] in their argument to treat hyperlipidemia in the elderly, note that many other factors aside from elevated cholesterol develop as one ages and contribute to cardiovascular morbidity. Thus, the relative importance or risk from hypercholesterolemia seems to be diluted with age as the pool of risk factors increases. However, they point out that when comparing elderly people at either end of the spectrum of cholesterol values, the absolute risk of CHD for those with high cholesterol is significantly greater than for those with low values. Thus, while many other factors contribute to IHD morbidity as one grows older, the risk imparted by an elevated cholesterol may be no less lethal than in the middle-aged population. Another way of phrasing this argument is that in the elderly, although the relative risk of lipids may decrease, the attributable risk or the benefit expected from improving lipid profiles may be significant.[14,34] The importance of attributable risk analysis may be provided from follow-up of subjects in the MRFIT.[43] This analysis found that with aging, the attributable risk of cholesterol increased, while the relative risk (risk ratio) decreased. It is important to note that the oldest subjects in this study were 60, and although extrapolations to older ages have been performed,[19,44] data are limited in the population over 65 years of age. The Kaiser Permanente Study did evaluate an elderly male population, demonstrating an increased attributable risk for cholesterol with increasing age, while no change in relative risk was demonstrated.[15] Attributable risk analysis is lacking for the other lipid subfractions, most notably HDL.

The Bronx Aging Study, a 10-year nonintervention study of an ambulatory, nondemented cohort, has been testing the hypotheses that lipids remain a risk factor for cardiovascular disease and become a risk factor for dementia in the very elderly (mean age 79 at entry).[23,45] Baseline lipid and lipoprotein values from this study are shown in Tables 1–4.[46] The results of this study suggest that HDL-C is independently associated with myocardial infarction, cardiovascular disease, and death in men; LDL-C is independently associated with the occurrence of myocardial infarction in women.[23] No association between lipids and the development of dementia has been seen.[23]

Beyond prevalence and phenomenological data, clinical trials are needed to determine whether dietary and/or drug therapy are efficacious in reducing vascular mortality or the development of dementia in the elderly before treatment can be recommended as the standard of care.[47,48] In essence, it must be determined whether lowering of cholesterol would lead to compression of morbidity without sacrifice in the quality of life.[49] To address this issue, the National Heart Blood and Lung Institute has initiated a pilot study that proposes the use of HMG CoA reductase inhibitors for treating hypercholesterolemia in the elderly (age 65-75 years). The study is a double-blind, placebo-controlled multicenter trial primarily looking at the effect of lowering LDL-cholesterol in the elderly. If this project can successfully be carried out, some of the controversies regarding treatment of hyperlipidemia in the elderly may be resolved.

The final issue is whether or not screening for abnormal levels is indicated in the older population. Garber et al recommend against this practice because of the inconsistent and scarce data currently available.[49] The clinician must be willing to initiate dietary or pharmacological therapy in the elderly patients with abnormal lipid profiles before screening can be recommended. Until intervention data are available, it will be left to the physician to decide if the individual patient, no matter what his/her age, can tolerate diet restriction and medication without compromise to other health parameters.

Table 1.
Cholesterol Baseline (Means ± Standard Deviations) and Percentiles for the Bronx Aging Study Cohort with Respect to Gender and Age

	Mean ± SD (mg/dl)	5%	10%	25%	50%	75%	90%	95%
Total (n = 443)	224 ± 45	155	168	194	222	253	281	301
Male (n = 162)	207 ± 40	151	160	179	204	228	255	275
Female (n = 281)	234 ± 44	157	183	204	235	263	292	314
75–80 Yrs (n = 292)	224 ± 45	151	169	195	224	252	280	301
81–85 Yrs (n = 151)	224 ± 45	157	167	192	218	255	284	301

Conversion factor for cholesterol is 0.02586 mm/L for 1 mg/dl. (From ref. 43, with permission.)

Table 2.
HDL-Cholesterol Baseline (Means ± Standard Deviations) and Percentile for the Bronx Aging Study Cohort with Respect to Gender and Age

	Mean ± SD (mg/dl)	5%	10%	25%	50%	75%	90%	95%
Total (n = 438)	43 ± 14	24	28	32	42	52	63	70
Male (n = 162)	38 ± 12	20	24	30	37	45	55	58
Female (n = 276)	46 ± 14	28	30	36	46	55	66	72
75–80 Yrs (n = 290)	43 ± 14	24	28	32	42	53	64	20
81–85 Yrs (n = 148)	43 ± 14	24	28	32	43	52	61	68

Conversion factor for cholesterol is 0.02586 mm/L for 1 mg/dl. (From ref. 43, with permission.)

Table 3.
LDL-Cholesterol Baseline (Means ± Standard Deviations) and Percentile for the Bronx Aging Study Cohort with Respect to Gender and Age

	Mean ± SD (mg/dl)	5%	10%	25%	50%	75%	90%	95%
Total (n = 437)	151 ± 39	90	102	126	151	177	202	223
Male (n = 161)	141 ± 37	87	98	115	139	159	187	205
Female (n = 276)	158 ± 59	91	105	133	157	184	206	226
75–80 Yrs (n = 289)	151 ± 40	87	101	122	151	176	201	223
81–85 Yrs (n = 148)	152 ± 38	94	103	127	150	178	205	214

Conversion factor for cholesterol is 0.02586 mm/L for 1 mg/dl. (From ref. 43, with permission.)

Table 4.
Triglyceride Baseline (Means ± Standard Deviations) and Percentile for the Bronx Aging Study Cohort with Respect to Gender and Age

	Mean ± SD (mg/dl)	5%	10%	25%	50%	75%	90%	95%
Total (n = 443)	136 ± 75	60	69	87	114	165	228	272
Male (n = 162)	138 ± 69	60	66	89	120	172	230	257
Female (n = 281)	135 ± 77	60	70	85	111	161	227	287
75–80 Yrs (n = 292)	139 ± 80	58	67	87	114	169	237	279
81–85 Yrs (n = 151)	129 ± 62	61	75	86	115	164	201	230

Conversion factor for triglycerides is 0.01129 mm/L for 1 mg/dl. (From ref. 43, with permission.)

References

1. Fries JF: Aging, natural death and the compression of morbidity. N Engl J Med 1980; 303: 130-135.
2. The Lipid Research Clinics Coronary Primary Prevention Trial Results. 1. Reduction in incidence of coronary heart disease. 2. The relationship of reduction in incidence of coronary heart disease to cholesterol lowering. JAMA 1984; 251: 351-364, 365-374.
3. Heikki Frick M, Eld O, Haapa K, et al: Helsinki Heart Study: Primary Prevential Trial with gemfibrizol in middle-aged men with dyslipidemia. N Engl J Med 1987; 317: 1237-1245.
4. Wenger NK, Furberg CD, Pitt E: Coronary Heart Disease in the Elderly. New York, Elsevier, 1986; 11-412.
5. Report of the National Cholesterol Education Program Expert Panel on Detection, Evaluation and Treatment of High Blood Cholesterol in Adults. Arch Intern Med 1988; 148: 36-69.
6. Hazzard W: Aging and atherosclerosis: teasing out the contributions of time, secondary aging and primary aging. Clinics Ger Med February 1985; 1: 251-285.
7. Hershcopf RJ, Elah D, Andres R, et al: Longitudinal changes in serum cholesterol in man: an epidemiologic search for an etiology. J Chron Dis 1982; 35: 101-114.
8. Myrianthopoulos M: Dietary treatment of hyperlipidemia in the elderly. Clinics in Ger Med 1987; 3: 343-353.
9. Elahi VK, Elahi D, Andres R, et al: A longitudinal study of nutritional intake in men. J Gerentol 1983; 38: 162-180.
10. Shock NW, Greulich RC, Andres R, et al: Normal human aging: The Baltimore Longitudinal Aging Study. NIH Publications 1984; 84-2450, 95-167, 208-209.
11. Barrett-Connor E, Saurez L, Khaw K-T, et al: Ischemic heart disease risk factors after age 50. J Chron Dis 1984; 37: 903-908.
12. Castelli WP, Garrison RJ, Wilson PWF, et al: Incidence of coronary heart disease and lipoprotein cholesterol levels, The Framingham Study. JAMA 1986; 256: 2835-2838.
13. Castelli WP, Wilson WF, Levy D, et al: Cardiovascular risk factors in the elderly. Am J Cardiol 1989; 63: 12H-19H.
14. Benfante R, Reed D: Is elevated serum cholesterol level a risk factor for coronary heart disease in the elderly? JAMA 1990; 263: 393-396.
15. Rubin SM, Sidney S, Black DM, et al: High blood cholesterol in elderly men and the excess risk for coronary heart disease. Ann Intern Med 1990; 113: 916-920.
16. Agner E, Hansen PF: Fasting serum cholesterol and triglycerides in a ten year prospective study in old age. Acta Med Scand 1983; 214: 33-41.
17. Mariott S, Capolaccia R, Farchi G, et al: Age, period, cohort and geographical area effects on the relationship between risk factors and coronary heart disease mortality. 15 year follow up of the European cohorts of the Seven Countries Study. J Chron Dis 1986; 39: 229-242.

18. Carlson LA, Bottiger LE: Ischaemic heart disease in relation to fasting values of plasma triglycerides and cholesterol: The Stockholm Prospective Study. Lancet 1972; 1: 865-868.

19. Manolio TA, Pearson TA, Wenger NK, et al: Cholesterol and heart disease in older persons and women: overview of an NHLBI workshop. In Harlan WR (ed): Proceedings of the National Heart, Lung, Blood Institute of National Institutes of Health, Cholesterol and Heart Disease in Older People and in Women. Ann Epidem 1992; 2: 1-176.

20. Gordon DJ, Probstfield J, Garrison RJ, et al: High density lipoprotein cholesterol and cardiovascular disease. Four prospective American studies. Circulation 1989; 79: 8-15.

21. Abbott RD, Wilson PWF, Kannel WB, et al: High density lipoprotein cholesterol, total cholesterol screening, and myocardial infarction. Arteriosclerosis 1988; 8: 207-211.

22. Gordon DJ, Rifkind BM: High density lipoprotein - The clinical implications of recent studies. N Engl J Med 1989; 321: 1311-1316.

23. Zimetbaum P, Frishman WH, Ooi WL et al: Plasma lipids and lipoproteins and the incidence of cardiovascular diseases in the old old: The Bronx Longitudinal Aging Study. Arteriosclerosis & Thrombosis 1992; in press.

24. Musliner TA, Krauss RM: Lipoprotein subspecies and risk of coronary disease. Clin Chem 1988; 34: B78-B83.

25. Ostlund RE, Staten M, Kohrt WM, e` al: The ratio of waste:hip circumference, plasma insulin level, and glucose intolerance as independent predictors of the HDL_2 cholesterol level in older adults. N Engl J Med 1990; 322: 229-234.

26. Austin MA: Plasma triglyceride as a risk factor for coronary heart disease. Am J Epidemiol 1989; 129: 249-259.

27. Grundy SM, Vega GI: Fibric acids: Effects on lipids and lipoprotein metabolism. Am J Med 1987; 83: 9-20.

28. Castelli WP: The triglyceride issue: A view from Framingham. Am Heart J 1986; 112: 432-437.

29. Castelli WP: Cholesterol and lipids in the risk of coronary artery disease - The Framingham Heart Study. Can J Cardiol 1988; 4 (Suppl A): 5A-10A.

30. Levy RI, Brensike JF, Epstein SE, et al: The influence of changes in lipid values induced by cholestyramine and diet on progression of coronary artery disease: results of the NHLBI Type II Coronary Intervention Study. Circulation 1984; 69: 325-337.

31. Kannel WB: High density lipoproteins: epidemologic profile and risks of coronary artery disease. Am J Cardiol 1983; 52: 9B-12B.

32. Green MS, Heiss G, Rifkind BM, et al: The ratio of plasma high density lipoprotein cholesterol to total and low density lipoprotein cholesterol: age-related changes and race and sex differences in selected North American populations. The Lipid Research Clinics Program Prevalence Study. Circulation 1985; 72: 93-104.

33. Lerner DJ, Kannel WB: Patterns of coronary heart disease morbidity and mortality in the sexes: A 26 year follow up of the Framingham population. Am Heart J 1986; 3: 383-390.

34. Harris T, Cook EF, Kannel WB, et al: Proportional hazards analysis of risk factors for coronary heart disease in individuals aged 65 or older. The Framingham Heart Study. J Am Geriatr Soc 1988; 36: 1023-1028.
35. Wolf PA, Kannel WB, Vecter J: Current status of risk factors for stroke. Neurol Clinics 1983; 1: 317-343.
36. Iso H, Jacobs DR Jr., Wentworth D, et al: Serum cholesterol levels and six year mortality from stroke in 350,977 men screened for the Multiple Risk Factor Intervention Trial. N Engl J Med 1989; 320: 904-910.
37. Yano K, Reed DM, MacLean CJ: Serum cholesterol and hemorrhagic stroke in the Honolulu Heart Program. Stroke 1989; 20: 1460-1465.
38. Adams RJ, Carrol RM, Nichols FT, et al: Plasma lipoproteins in cortical versus lacunar infarction. Stroke 1989; 20: 448-452.
39. Kostner GM, Marth E, Pfeiffer KP, et al: Apolipoproteins A-I, A-II and HDL phospholipids but not Apo-B are risk indicators for occlusive cerebro-vascular disease. Europ Neurol 1986; 25: 346-354.
40. Muckle TJ, Roy JR: High density lipoprotein cholesterol in differential diagnosis of senile dementia. Lancet 1985; i: 1191-1192.
41. Erkinjuntti T, Sulkava R, Tilvis R: HDL cholesterol in dementia. The Lancet 1985; ii: 43.
42. Smith DA, Karmally W, Brown WV: Treating hyperlipidemia. Part 1: whether and when in the elderly. Geriatrics 1987; 42: 33-44.
43. Malenka DJ, Baron JA: Cholesterol and coronary heart disease. The attributable risk reduction of diet and drugs. Arch Intern Med 1989; 149: 1981-1985.
44. Gordon DJ, Rifkind BM: Treating high blood cholesterol in the older patient. Am J Cardiol 1989; 63: 48H-52H.
45. Aronson MK, Ooi WL, Morganstern H, et al: Women, myocardial infarction and dementia in the very old. Neurology 1990; 40: 1102-1106.
46. Frishman WH, Ooi WL, Derman M, et al: Serum lipids and lipoproteins in advanced age: Intra-individual changes. Ann Epidemiol 1992; 2: 43-50.
47. Denke MA, Grundy SM: Hypercholesterolemia in elderly persons: resolving the treatment dilemma. Ann Intern Med 1990; 112: 780-792.
48. Kafunek SD, Kwiterovich PO: Treatment of hypercholesterolemia in the elderly. Ann Intern Med 1990; 112: 723-725.
49. Garber AM, Sox HC Jr., Littenberg B: Screening asymptomatic adults for cardiac risk factors: the serum cholesterol level. Ann Intern Med 1989; 110: 622-639.

Index

Acebutolol, 266

N-Acetylcysteine, 16

Acyl coenzyme A transferase (ACAT) inhibitors, 241

Adolescents
dietary therapy in, 32, 78-79, 79
lipid-lowering therapy in, 28-30
lipoproteins (LDL) classification system for, 31

Adrenergic blocking agents
alpha₁-, 271-272, 273-276
alpha-beta-, 270
beta-, 261, 262-264, 265, 266-269

Adrenergic neuron blockers, 278, 280

Age and exercise effects, 96-97

Aging and lipid profile, 302-308, see also Elderly persons

Alcohol consumption, 10, 11, 62-63

Alpha₁-adrenergic blocking agents, 271-272, 273-276, 286

Alpha₂ agonists, 286

Alpha-beta-adrenergic agents, 270

Alprenolol, 268

Alzheimer's disease, 309-310

American Diabetes Association dietary recommendations, 75-77

American Dietetic Association, 80-81

American Heart Association step-one diet, 58, 75-77, 221-222

Amlodipine, 284

Angiotensin-converting enzyme (ACE) inhibitors, 280-281, 282, 286

Antibiotics, 227-230
in combination therapy, 163-164, 191-192

Antihypertensive drugs. See Cardiovascular drugs and individual types

Apolipoproteins, laboratory measurement, 19

Apoprotein B-100, 14-15, 112-114

Aspirin, 186

Atenolol, 266-267, 286

Atherogenesis, theories of, 205-206

Atherosclerosis, 131-132
bile-acid sequestrant therapy and, 108-109
diet and etiology, 45-50
estrogen and, 233-234
regression studies, 53-56, 115-116, 209
see also Coronary artery disease; Coronary heart disease

Baltimore Longitudinal Aging Study, 302-303

B-complex vitamins. See Nicotinic acid

Beta-adrenergic blocking agents, 210, 261, 262-264, 265, 266-269, 271

Bezafibrate. See Fibric acid derivatives (FAD)

Bile-acid sequestrants, 210
  adverse effects, 117-118
  chemistry, 103-104
  clinical experiences, 106-116
  clinical use, 116-117
  in combination therapy, 137-
    139, 138, 162-163, 166, 188-
    189, 193, 197, 211, 212
  pharmacokinetics, 105-106
  pharmacology, 104-105
  vs. pravastatin, 172
Bisoprolol, 267
Blood abnormalities and FAD
    drugs, 144-145
Bopindolol, 268
Broad beta disease (dysbetalipo-
    proteinemia), 13, 160
Bronx Longitudinal Aging Study,
    306, 309, 312-315
Bypass procedures
  ileal, 56, 105-106, 118
  coronary artery, 33-34

Calcium channel blockers, 281,
    283, 284-285, 286
Cancer risk and estrogen therapy,
    236-237, 238-239
Captopril, 281, 282
Cardiac transplantation, 34-35,
    167
Cardiovascular drugs
  adrenergic neuron blockers, 278,
    280
  alpha$_1$-adrenergic blockers,
    271-272, 273-277
  alpha-beta-adrenergic blockers,
    270
  angiotensin-converting enzyme
    (ACE) inhibitors, 280-281

beta-adrenergic blockers, 261,
    262-264, 265
  calcium channel blockers, 281,
    283, 284-285
  centrally acting drugs (alpha$_2$-
    agonists), 278, 279
  combination regimens, 283
  direct vasodilators, 280
  diuretics, 254-261
Cataracts as side effect, 168
Celiprolol, 268
Centrally acting vasodilators, 278,
    279
Children
  dietary therapy in, 32, 78-79, 79
  lipid-lowering drugs in, 28-30,
    110-111, 213
  low-density lipoproteins (LDL)
    classification system for, 31
Chlorthalidone, 256-257, 280
Cholelithiasis/cholecystitis as side
    effect, 144-145, 170, 214
Cholesterol
  aging and serum levels, 303-305
  in atherogenesis, 205-206
  dietary and serum levels, 50-52
  dietary manipulation and serum
    levels, 51-52
  FAD drugs and secretion, 130
  HDL. See High-density lipopro-
    teins (HDL)
  laboratory methods and accu-
    racy, 18-19
  LDL. See Low-density lipopro-
    teins (LDL)
  reverse transport principle, 208
  synthetic pathway, 157
Cholesterol ester transfer protein
    (CETP), 8-9, 242

Cholesterol-Lowering Atherosclerosis Study, 54, 114-116, 188-189
Cholestyramine, 103-118, *see also* Bile-acid sequestrants
Chylomicronemia, 14, 25-26
Chylomicrons, 6-7
Cirrhosis, 10
Clofibrate. *See* Fibric acid derivatives (FAD)
Clonidine, 278, 279
Coagulopathic side effects, 169
Colestipol, 103-118
    in combination therapy, 162-163, 166
Compression of morbidity, 301
Consumer issues and diet therapy, 65
Cooperative Lipoprotein Phenotyping Study, 49
Coronary angioplasty, 34
Coronary artery bypass grafts, 33-34
Coronary artery disease
    age and, 28-30
    cholesterol ester transfer protein (CETP) and, 8-9
    in diabetes mellitus, 27
    estrogen and, 233-234
    gender and, 28
    hyperlipidemia as risk factor, 16-17
    lipoprotein(a) and, 15-16
    low-density lipoproteins (LDL) and risk, 20, 22-24
    non-LDL risk factors, 25
    risk assessment, 17-18, *see also* Risk and risk management
    systemic hypertension and, 30-32

see also Atherosclerosis; Coronary heart disease
Coronary Drug Project, 16-17, 187-189, 198-199
Coronary heart disease
    dietary risk factors, 46-50
    in elderly persons, 302-308
    nicotinic acid in, 187-190
    in women, 77-78
Cyclopenthiazide, 256-257

Dementia and aging, 308-310
Diabetes mellitus, 9-11, 27
    ACE inhibitors in, 281-283
    dietary therapy, 63-64, 73-74, 75
    and dietary fiber, 62
    FAD drug therapy in, 139-141
    fish oil supplementation in, 60
    lovastatin in, 164
    nicotinic acid in, 193-194, 196
    probucol in, 212
    thiazide diuretics and exacerbation, 254-255
Dietary fiber, 61-62
    components, 218
    psyllium supplementation, 217-223
    types, 217-218
Dietary therapy, 116, 154, 166, 192
    alcohol consumption, 62-63
    in children and adolescents, 30, 32
    cholesterol-lowering trials, 57-58
    cholesterol reduction and diet, 51-52
    consumer issues, 65

diabetes and glucose tolerance, 63-64
diet as risk factor, 45-51
fiber and lipid reduction, 61-62, 219-222
fish oils and coronary heart disease, 59-61
lipid profile assessment, 72-77
morbidity and cholesterol reduction, 52-53
NCEP step-one program, 66-81
patient assessment and education, 66-81
psyllium supplementation and, 219-222
regression of coronary heart disease, 53-56
trends in U.S. diet, 64-65
Dietitian referral, 80-81
Dilevalol, 268
Diltiazem, 284
Diuretics, 210, 254-255
chlorthalidone, 256t-257
mechanisms of hyperlipidemic effect, 259, 261
nonthiazides, 260
thiazides, 255, 256-257, 258
Doxazosin, 272, 275-276
Drug interactions, 167-168, 223-224
Drug therapy. See Pharmacological approaches
Dysbetalipoproteinemia (broad beta disease), 13, 160

Elderly patients, 30
dietary therapy in, 78
epidemiologic studies of vascular disease, 301-308
exercise effects, 96
stroke and dementia, 308-310
Enalapril, 282
Epidemiologic studies
diet and CHD risk, 46-50
elderly individuals and cardiovascular disease, 301-308
Epstatin. See Pravastatin
Estrogen therapy, 232-234
in males, 238
mechanism of action, 234-236
potential uses and risks, 236-238
recommendations, 238-239
Exercise, 131
general effects, 89-91, 92t-93t
and HDL, 91, 94-96
and LDL, 91
and triglycerides, 96-97
Expanded Clinical Evaluation of Lovastatin (EXCEL) study, 161
Expert Panel on Blood Cholesterol Levels in Children and Adolescents, 78-79
Familial Atherosclerosis Treatment Study (FATS), 190

Fat intake assessment form, 67
Fatty acid composition and serum cholesterol, 57-58
FDA. See U.S. Food and Drug Administration Fenofibrate, See Fibric acid derivatives (FAD)
Fiber. See Dietary fiber
Fibric acid derivatives (FAD), 125-126
adverse effects, 144-145
clinical experience, 132-142
clinical use, 142-143

in combination therapy, 137-
    139, 138t, 163, 167-168, 212
in diabetes mellitus, 164
mechanism of action, 127-132
pharmacokinetics, 126-127
vs. pravastatin, 172
Fish oil therapy, 34, 59-61
Framingham Study, 47, 232, 305,
    306, 308
Frederickson phenotypes, 11
Furosemide, 260

Gallbladder disease as side effect,
    144-145, 170, 214
Gemfibrozil, 25, 125-145, 159,
    164, 167, 172, 305, see also Fi-
    bric acid derivatives (FAD)
Gender differences, 8, 77-78, 96,
    305, 308
Genetic causes of hyperlipopro-
    teinemia, 11-15, 12t
Glostrup population studies, 304,
    306
Glucose intolerance. See Diabetes
    mellitus
Guanabenz, 279

HDL
    alcohol consumption and, 63
    cholestyramine therapy and,
        111-112
    and dietary fiber, 61-62
    dietary therapy and, 50, 73-74
    in elderly persons, 305-306, 307
    estrogen and, 233-235
    exercise effects, 91, 94-96
    in hypertriglyceridemia, 129-130
    metabolism, 8
    nicotinic acid and, 184-186
    and omega-3 fatty acids, 59

protective effect, 8
reduced levels, 17-18, 26-27
simvastatin and, 170
thiazide diuretics and, 255
HDL-C and nicotinic acid, 184
HDL-infusion technique, 241-242
HDL:LDL ratio in elderly persons,
    307
Heart transplantation, 34-35, 167
Helsinki Heart Study, 16-17,
    52-53, 126-145, 114-116, 305
Hepatitis, 10
High density lipoprotein. See HDL
High-risk status criteria, 25
HMG-CoA reductase, 130
HMG-CoA reductase inhibitors,
    153-154, 172-173
    in combination therapy, 137-
        138, 138t, 197-198
    lovastatin, 154-169, see also Lo-
        vastatin
    pravastatin, 171-172
    simvastatin, 169-171
    structural formulas, 155
Honolulu Heart Program, 48-50,
    303, 309
Hormonal therapy
    estrogens and progestogens,
        232-239
    thyroxine, 230-231
Hydralazine, 280
Hydrochlorothiazide. See Thiazide
    diuretics
7-alpha-Hydroxylase inhibitors,
    242
Hypercholesterolemia, 9
    in children and adolescents,
        28-30
    in elderly individuals, 30
    dietary recommendations, 76t

FAD drugs in, 134-137
familial, 14, 56, 76, 191-192
heterozygous familial, 107-111,
    158-159, 192-193, 210
homozygous, 76t, 159, 193
hypertension and, 30
and metabolic training effect, 46
patient selection for treatment,
    20-25
polygenic, 241
see also Bile-acid sequestrants;
    Hyperlipidemia; Hyperlipo-
    proteinemia
Hyperchylomicronemia, dietary
    recommendations, 77
Hyperlipidemia
    familial combined, 159-160
    familial dysbetalipoproteinemia,
        160
    polygenic, 160-162
    as risk factor, 16-17
    thiazide-induced, 254-258
    treatment rationales, 16-17
    see also Hypercholesterolemia;
        Hyperlipoproteinemia
Hyperlipoproteinemia
    acquired causes, 9-11
    classification, 11-13, 12
    familial and lipoprotein(a),
        15-16
    genetic causes, 11-15, 12
    phenotypic, 191-192
    simvastatin in, 170
Hypersensitivity, 169
Hypertension
    hyperchoslesterolemia and, 30
    lipid effects of antihypertensive
        drugs, 254-283
Hypertriglyceridemia
    borderline, 26

in diabetes mellitus, 140-141
exercise and, 96-07
familial, 13, 26, 76, 191-192
fibric acid derivatives (FAD) in,
    128-136
lovastatin in, 165-166
patient selection for treatment,
    26-27
in renal disease, 141-142
Hypothyroidism, 10, 230-231

IDL, 47, 109-110, 192
Immunosuppressive therapy,
    167-168
Indapamide, 260
Indoramin, 277
Insulin synthesis and secretion, 90,
    259, 261, 271, see also Diabetes
    mellitus
Intermediate-density lipoproteins.
    See IDL

Japanese diet study, 47-48, 303, see
    also Honolulu Heart Study

Kaiser Permanente Coronary
    Heart Disease in the Elderly
    Study, 303

Labetalol, 265
Laboratory evaluations, techniques
    and accuracy, 18-19
LDL
    in atherogenesis, 205-206
    bile-acid sequestrant therapy
        and, 107-109, 113-114
    classification system for chil-
        dren and adolescents, 31
    dietary fiber and, 61-62

dietary therapy and, 55-56,
  73t-74t
in elderly persons, 307
exercise effects, 91
laboratory measurement, 19
lovastatin and, 158
metabolism, 8-9
nicotinic acid and, 182, 184
omega-3 fatty acids and, 59
oxidation of, 206
as parameter for intervention,
  20, 22-24
as risk predictor, 17-18
simvastatin and, 170
thiazide diuretics and increase,
  255, 258
LDL-apheresis, 239-240
Lecithin cholesterol acyl transferase (LCAT), 8-9
Leiden Intervention Trial, 54
Lifestyle Heart Trial, 54-55
Lipid profile and aging, 302-308
Lipid profile assessment, 72-77
Lipid Research Clinics Coronary
  Prevention Trial, 16-17, 52,
  64-65, 107-109, 233
Lipid Research Clinics Prevalence
  Study, 305, 307
Lipoprotein(a), 15-16, 165
Lipoprotein lipase, 242
Lipoprotein metabolism, 4
  endogenous pathway, 7-9
  exogenous pathway, 6-7
Lipoproteins
  classes and composition, 4, 5,
    112-114
  effects of menopause, 232
  see also HDL, IDL, LDL, VLDL
  Los Angeles VA study, 53
Lovastatin

adverse effects, 161, 166-169
chemistry, 154, 155
clinical experiences, 157-166
clinical use, 166
in combination therapy, 162-
  164, 197-198, 212
pharmacokinetics, 157
pharmacology, 154
post coronary angioplasty, 34
Low density lipoprotein. See LDL

Medical Research Council Trial,
  254-255
Mediterranean advantage concept,
  47
Men, estrogen therapy in, 238, see
  also Gender differences
Menopause, 232-239
Mepindolol, 268
Metabolic training, 46
Methyldopa, 278
Metoprolol, 267, 271
Mevinolin. See Lovastatin
Minoxidil, 280
Monounsaturated fats, 57-58
Multi-infarct dementia, 309-310
Multiple Risk Factor Intervention
  Trial (MRFIT), 153, 305, 309
Myocardial infarction, 108,
  187-189
  cholesterol-lowering therapy
    and, 33
  in elderly persons, 310-312
  exercise in postinfarction period,
    92-93
  postinfarction lipid-lowering
    therapy, 33, 171
Myopathy as side effect of lovas-
  tatin therapy, 167

Nadolol, 264, 280
National Cholesterol Education
    Program, 153, 187
    recommendations, 19-35, 79
    step-one diet, 57-81
    step-two diet, 70
National Diet-Heart Study, 52
National Exercise and Heart Dis-
    ease Project, 95
National Heart, Lung, and Blood
    Institute, 108-109, 304
National Institutes of Health,
    64-65, 153
Neomycin, 227-230
    in combination therapy, 163-
    164, 191-192
Nephrotic syndrome, 10, 141-142,
    165, 194, 212-213
Nicotinic acid, 16, 25, 181-182
    adverse effects, 186, 196,
    198-199
    clinical experience, 187-195
    clinical use, 195-199
    in combination therapy, 163,
    197-198
    myocardial infarction mortality
    and, 187-189
    pharmacology, 182-187
    pharmocokinetics, 182
    slow-release forms, 196-197
    vs. nicotinamide, 183, 186
Nifedipine, 284
Ni-Hon-San Study, 48, 49-50
Nisoldipine, 284
Nitrendipine, 284
Nonpharmacological approaches
    dietary therapy, 45-81
    exercise, 89-97
Norwegian diet study, 47
Nurses' Health Study, 232-233

Nutritional counseling, 66-71
Nutritional knowledge assessment
    form, 67

Obesity, 10, 64, 75, see also Diabe-
    tes mellitus
Omega-3 polyunsaturated fatty
    acids, 59-61

Oral contraceptives, 10
Oslo Study, 53
Oxprenolol, 268t

Pancreatitis and side effect, 142
Patient education
    assessment for adherence,
    70-71, 71
    individualization, 71-72
    nutritional counseling, 66-70
Penbutolol, 268
Pharmacological approaches
    antibiotics, 227-230
    bile acid sequestrants, 103-119
    in children, 30
    gemfibrozil and other FAD
    drugs, 125-145
    HMG-CoA reductase inhibitors,
    153-173
    hormonal therapy, 230-239
    lipid-lowering drugs, 27-34
    nicotinic acid, 16, 25, 181-199
    probucol, 205-214
    psyllium, 217-223
    see also Drug interactions and in-
    dividual drugs and drug classes
Pinacidil, 279, 280
Pindolol, 265, 268-269, 286
Piretanide, 260
Plant sterols, 240-241
Plasmapheresis, 239-240

Platelet aggregation, 53, 130-131
Polyunsaturated fatty acids, 57-58
   omega-3, 59-61
Pooling Project. *See* Cooperative
   Lipoprotein Phenotyping
   Study
Postmenopausal Estrogen/Proges-
   tin Interventions (PEPI) trial,
   239
Pravastatin, 171-172
Prazosin, 272, 273-274
Probucol
   adverse effects, 213-214
   chemistry, 206-207
   clinical experiences, 209-213
   clinical use, 213
   in combination therapy, 163,
      211-212
   mechanisms of action, 207-209
   pharmacokinetics, 207
   vs. simvastatin, 169-170
Probucol Quantitative Regression
   Swedish Trial (PQRST), 209
Progestogen therapy, 232-239
Propanolol, 261, 262-263, 286
Prostaglandins and nicotinic acid,
   186-187
Psyllium, 218-219
   adverse reactions, 222-223
   clinical experiences, 219-222
   clinical recommendations, 223
   mechanism of action, 222
Puerto Rico Heart Health Program, 48

QT interval depression and pro-
   bucin, 213-214

Regression trials, 209

Renal failure, 10, 141-142, *see also*
   Nephrotic syndrome
Reserpine, 280
Risk and risk management, 3-4
   assessment of risk, 17-18
   in elderly persons, 300-308
   estrogen therapy and, 235t
   hyperlipoproteinemia, 9-15
   hypertriglyceridemia, 25-26
   laboratory methods, 18-19
   lipoprotein(a), 15-16
   lipoprotein structure and func-
      tion, 4-9
   low HDL levels, 26-27
   patient selection, 20-25
   screening, 19-20
   special problems, 27-35
   treatment rationales, 16-17

Screening, 19-20
   in elderly persons, 311
Serum total cholesterol
   in aging individuals, 303-305
   diet and, 50-53, 73-74
   measurement, 18-19
7-alpha-hydroxylase inhibitors,
   242
Seven Countries Study, 46-47
Simvastatin, 169-171
beta-Sitosterol, 240-241
Sotalol, 264
Stearic acid, 58
Stockholm Prospective Study, 304
Stroke, 308-310
Synvolin. *See* Simvastatin

Teratolol, 264
Terazosin, 277
Thiazide diuretics, 254-255, 256-
   257, 258, 261, 286

in combination therapy, 283
Thyroxine therapy, 230-231
Timolol, 264t
Total serum cholesterol. *See* Serum
    total cholesterol
Trans fatty acids, 57-58
Triglycerides
    in elderly persons, 306-307
    estrogen and, 235
    exercise effects, 96-97
    laboratory studies, 19
    lovastatin and, 165-166
    nutritional intervention effects,
    73-74
    see also Hypertriglyceridemia
Trimazosin, 277

U.S. Food and Drug Administra-
    tion, 65, 154

VA Los Angeles study, 53
Vasodilating drugs. *See* Cardiovas-
    cular drugs
Verapamil, 284-285
Very low density lipoprotein. *See*
    VLDL
Veterans Administration-NHLBI
    Cooperative Study, 259
Visual side effects, 168
Vitamin supplementation, 105, 119
VLDL

bile-acid sequestrants and, 111,
    117-117
exercise effects, 90
fibric acid derivatives (FAD),
    126-128
in hypercholesterolemia, 9
lovastatin and, 159-160
nicotinic acid and, 182-184
nutritional intervention effects,
    73-74
omega-3 fatty acids and, 59
synthesis and secretion, 7-8
thiazide diuretics and, 255
VLDL-Tg, 182-184, 195
VLDL-infusion technique, 241-242

Western Electric Study, 48-49
Women
    cholesterol and risk, 305
    dietary modification in, 77-78
    postmenopausal, 232-239, 258
    see also Gender differences
World Health Organization FAD
    drug trial, 144
World War I and II CHD regres-
    sion studies, 54

Xanthomas, 208, 213

Zofenopril, 282
Zutphen study, 48